Sid Kimel

Depression

DEPRESSION

Causes and Treatment

AARON T. BECK, M. D.

*Professor of Psychiatry,
University of Pennsylvania School of Medicine;
Chief of Section, Department of Psychiatry,
Philadelphia General Hospital, Philadelphia*

University of Pennsylvania Press

Philadelphia

TO PHYLLIS

First *University of Pennsylvania Press* edition, 1970

Second Printing, 1974
Third Printing, 1975

First published in 1967 under the title
Depression: Clinical, Experimental, and Theoretical Aspects

Library of Congress Catalog Card Number: 67-23826

ISBN: (clothbound edition) 0-8122-7652-3
ISBN: (paperbound edition) 0-8122-1032-8

Contents

v

9. Biological Studies of Depression   *125*

    MANIC-DEPRESSIVE DISORDER AND CONSTITUTION   *126*

    HEREDITY IN MANIC-DEPRESSIVE DISORDER   *128*

    Identical Twin Studies   *128*
    Identical Twins Reared Separately   *130*
    Pedigree Studies   *131*
    Summary   *132*

    BIOCHEMICAL STUDIES OF DEPRESSION   *132*

    Early Studies (1903-1939)   *132*
       Blood glucose.   Glucose tolerance.   Acidity and alkaline reserve.
       Serum calcium and phosphorous.   Nitrogenous substances.   Lipoidal
       substances.   Chlorides.   Critique of studies
    Recent Studies (1940-1966)   *134*
       Differences between manic and depressive phases.
       Studies of continued cycles.   Studies during depressive episodes.
       Responses of normal subjects to stress.   Summary

    ENDOCRINE STUDIES   *139*

    Steroid Metabolism   *139*
    Thyroid Function   *141*

    AUTONOMIC FUNCTION   *142*

    Blood Pressure Responses to Mecholyl   *142*
    Salivation Studies   *143*

    NEUROPHYSIOLOGICAL STUDIES   *145*

    Sedation Threshold   *145*
    EMG Studies   *146*
    EEG Sleep Studies of Depressed Patients   *147*
    EEG Arousal Response   *151*

    CONCLUSIONS   *152*

10. Psychological and Psychodynamic Studies   *154*

    PSYCHOMOTOR PERFORMANCE   *154*

    CONCEPTUAL PERFORMANCE   *155*

    PERCEPTUAL THRESHOLD   *156*

    DISTORTION OF TIME JUDGMENT   *156*

    DISTORTION OF SPATIAL JUDGMENT   *157*

    FACTOR ANALYTIC STUDIES   *158*

    EXPERIMENTAL STUDIES   *160*

    FAMILY BACKGROUND AND PERSONALITY   *161*

    SELF-CONCEPT   *164*

    SUMMARY   *164*

Contents

Preface

Depression ranks as one of the major health problems of today. Millions of patients suffering from some form of this disorder crowd the psychiatric and general hospitals, the outpatient clinics, and the offices of private practitioners. Depression may appear as a primary disorder or it may accompany a wide variety of other psychiatric or medical disorders. Not only is depression a prominent cause of human misery but its by-product, suicide, is a leading cause of death in certain age groups.

In an attempt to check the suffering inflicted by this disorder, numerous studies have been conducted to determine its cause and cure. In the past ten years, there has been a landslide of reports, particularly in the area of the drug treatment of depression. When the thousands of clinical and controlled studies have been sifted, the question naturally arises: What has definitely been established regarding the nature, the causes, and the treatment of depression?

In attempting to demarcate the body of knowledge regarding depression, to separate what is known from what is alleged or simply taken for granted, I surveyed the broad spectrum of the studies ranging from the molecular level to the interpersonal relations. I extracted from the mass of the literature a group of representative studies of the clinical, biological, psychological, theoretical and therapeutic aspects of depression.

In the clinical section (Part I) I have summarized those studies that combined thoroughness with statistical presentation of the data. Part II critically reviews the biological and psychological studies of depression. I paid particular attention to the sampling techniques, research design, and treatment of the data. Because of space limitations, many reports that were of a preliminary nature or that were duplicated by other reports were omitted. In the review of the literature concerning the theories of depression (Part IV), I included only a representative sample and made no attempt to provide the comprehensive coverage that is already available in other monographs.

Part V includes a critical review of current knowledge regarding the treatment of depression by drug therapy and electroconvulsive therapy. Because of the numerous articles on the drug treatment, I have not dealt with specific articles but have here summarized the reviews of the controlled studies of depression.

In addition to reviewing the literature I have presented some of the findings of a five-year research project conducted at the University of Pennsylvania and supported in part by a grant from the National Institute of Mental Health. In the course of this investigation, more than one thousand patients were studied and considerable data were accumulated regarding the clinical and psychological aspects of depression. Additional data were collected in the course of the psychotherapy of depressed patients. The findings of the studies have for the most part been already reported in various journal articles. The entire research investigation is summarized for the first time in a unified form in Part III. Other findings from the investigation are included in Parts I and II.

Our systematic investigation of depression provided the basis for my theoretical formulations in Chapters 17 and 18. In outlining the techniques for the psychotherapy of depression in Part V, I drew on these conceptualizations and my practical experience in treating depressed patients.

It is my pleasure to acknowledge the contributions of my colleagues who participated in the depression research project described in Part III: John K. Erbaugh, Seymour Feshbach, Marvin Hurvich, William Kanar, Armin Loeb, Myer Mendelson, John E. Mock, Brij Sethi, Robert Tuthill, and Clyde Ward.

Warm thanks are also extended to Ruth Lazarus and Richard Segal for their assistance in the search for titles and compilation of the bibliography. I am also grateful to Polly Fischer, Estelle Gross, and Judy Kinman for their assistance in the preparation of the manuscript.

I am deeply appreciative to Albert J. Stunkard for his encouragement and his helpful comments and suggestions. I am also indebted to Leon J. Saul and Marvin Stein, whose support and interest stimulated my venture into the systematic study of depression.

Finally, I am thankful to Estelle Marcus for her careful typing of the successive drafts of this book.

The author wishes to express his gratitude for permission to reproduce material that originally appeared in the following publications: *Acta Psychiatrica Scandinavica, American Journal of Psychiatry, Archives of General Psychiatry, Comprehensive Psychiatry, Journal of the American Medical Association,* and *Psychosomatic Medicine.*

AARON T. BECK, M.D.

Philadelphia, Pennsylvania

Part I.
CLINICAL ASPECTS
OF DEPRESSION

Chapter. 1
The Definition of Depression

PARADOXES OF DEPRESSION

Depression may someday be understood in terms of its paradoxes. There is, for instance, an astonishing contrast between the depressed person's image of himself and the objective facts. A wealthy man moans that he doesn't have the financial resources to feed his children. A widely acclaimed beauty begs for plastic surgery in the belief that she is ugly. An eminent physicist berates himself "for being stupid."

Despite the torment experienced as the result of these self-debasing ideas, the patients are not readily swayed by objective evidence or by logical demonstration of the irrationality of these ideas. Moreover, they often perform acts that seem to enhance their suffering. The wealthy man puts on rags and publicly humiliates himself by begging for money to support himself and his family. A clergyman with an unimpeachable reputation tries to hang himself because "I'm the world's worst sinner." A scientist whose work has been confirmed by numerous independent investigators, publicly "confesses" that his discoveries were a hoax.

Attitudes and behaviors such as these are particularly puzzling—on the surface, at least—because they seem to contradict some of the most strongly established axioms of human nature. According to the "pleasure principle," the patient should be seeking to maximize his satisfactions and minimize his pain. According to the time-honored concept of the instinct of self-preservation, he should be attempting to prolong his life rather than to terminate it.

Although depression (or melancholia) has been recognized as a clinical syndrome for over 2,000 years, as yet no completely satisfactory explanation of its puzzling and paradoxical features has been found. There are still major unresolved issues regarding its nature, its classification, and its etiology. Among these are the following:

1. Is depression an exaggeration of a mood experienced by the normal, or is it qualitatively as well as quantitatively different from a normal mood?

3

2. Is depression a well defined clinical entity with a specific etiology and a predictable onset, course, and outcome, or is it a "wastebasket" category of diverse disorders?

3. Is depression a type of reaction (Meyerian concept), or is it a disease (Kraepelinian concept)?

4. Is depression caused primarily by psychological stress and conflict, or is it related primarily to a biological derangement?

There are no universally accepted answers to these questions. In fact, there is sharp disagreement among clinicians and investigators who have written about depression. There is considerable controversy regarding the classification of depression and a few writers see no justification for using this nosological category at all. The nature and etiology of depression are subject to even more sharply divided opinion. Some authorities contend that depression is primarily a psychogenic disorder; others maintain just as firmly that it is caused by organic factors. A third group supports the concept of two different types of depression: a psychogenic type and an organic type.

The importance of depression is recognized by everyone in the field of mental health. According to Kline (1964), more human suffering has resulted from depression than from any other single disease affecting mankind. Depression is second only to schizophrenia in first and second admissions to mental hospitals in the United States, and it has been estimated that the prevalence of depression outside hospitals is five times greater than that of schizophrenia (Dunlop, 1965). A systematic survey of the prevalence of depression in a sharply defined geographical area indicated that 3.9 per cent of the population more than 20 years of age was suffering from depression at a specified time (Sørenson and Strömgren, 1961).

DESCRIPTIVE CONCEPTS OF DEPRESSION

The condition that today we label depression has been described by a number of ancient writers under the classification of "melancholia." The first clinical description of melancholia was made by Hippocrates in the fourth century B. C. He also referred to swings similar to mania and depression (Jelliffe, 1931).

Aretaeus, a physician living in the second century, A.D., described the melancholic patient as "sad, dismayed, sleepless. . . They become thin by their agitation and loss of refreshing sleep. . . At a more advanced stage, they complain of a thousand futilities and desire death." It is noteworthy that Aretaeus specifically delineated the manic-depressive cycle. Some authorities believe that he anticipated the Kraepelinian synthesis of manic-depressive psychosis, but Jelliffe discounts this hypothesis.

Plutarch, in the second century A.D., presented a particularly vivid and detailed account of melancholia:

He looks on himself as a man whom the Gods hate and pursue with their anger. A far worse lot is before him; he dares not employ any means of averting or of remedying the evil, lest he be found fighting against the gods. The physician, the consoling friend, are driven away. 'Leave me,' says the wretched man, 'me, the impious, the accursed, hated of the gods, to suffer my punishment.' He sits out of doors, wrapped in sackcloth or in filthy rags. Ever and anon he rolls himself, naked, in the dirt confessing about this and that sin. He has eaten or drunk something wrong. He has gone some way or other which the Divine Being did not approve of. The festivals in honor of the gods give no pleasure to him but fill him rather with fear or a fright.*

Pinel at the beginning of the nineteenth century described melancholia as follows:

The symptoms generally comprehended by the term melancholia are taciturnity, a thoughtful pensive air, gloomy suspicions, and a love of solitude. Those traits, indeed, appear to distinguish the characters of some men otherwise in good health, and frequently in prosperous circumstances. Nothing, however, can be more hideous than the figure of a melancholic brooding over his imaginary misfortunes. If moreover possessed of power, and endowed with a perverse disposition and a sanguinary heart, the image is rendered still more repulsive.

These accounts bear a striking similarity to modern textbook descriptions of depression; they are also similar to contemporary autobiographical accounts such as that by Clifford W. Beers (1928). The cardinal signs and symptoms used today in diagnosing depression are found in the ancient descriptions: disturbed mood (sad, dismayed, futile); self-castigations ("the accursed, hatred of the gods"); self-debasing behavior ("wrapped in sackcloth or dirty rags. . . he rolls himself, naked, in the dirt"); wish to die; physical and vegetative symptoms (agitation, loss of appetite and weight, sleeplessness); and delusions of having committed unpardonable sins.

The foregoing descriptions of depression include the typical characteristics of this condition. There are few psychiatric syndromes whose clinical descriptions are so constant through successive eras of history.† It is noteworthy that the historical descriptions of depression indicate that its manifestations are observable in all aspects of behavior, including the traditional psychological divisions of affection, cognition, and conation.

Because the disturbed feelings are generally a striking feature of de-

* Quoted by Zilboorg (1941).
† For a complete presentation of the descriptions of depression through the ages, see Robert Burton, (1621).

pression, it has become customary in recent years to regard this condition as a "primary mood disorder" or as an "affective disorder." The central importance ascribed to the feeling component of depression is exemplified by the practice of utilizing affective adjective check lists to define and measure depression. The representation of depression as an affective disorder is as misleading as it would be to designate scarlet fever as a "disorder of the skin" or as a "primary febrile disorder." There are many components to depression other than mood deviation. In a significant proportion of the cases, no mood abnormality at all is elicited from the patient. In our present state of knowledge, we do not know which component of the clinical picture of depression is primary, or whether they are all simply external manifestations of some unknown pathological process.

Depression may now be defined in terms of the following attributes:

1. A specific alteration in mood: sadness, loneliness, apathy.

2. A negative self-concept associated with self-reproaches and self-blame.

3. Regressive and self-punitive wishes: desires to escape, hide, or die.

4. Vegetative changes: anorexia, insomnia, loss of libido.

5. Change in activity level: retardation or agitation.

SEMANTICS OF DEPRESSION

One of the difficulties in conceptualizing depression is essentially semantic, viz., that the term has been variously applied to designate: a particular type of feeling or symptom; a symptom-complex (or syndrome); and a well-defined disease entity.

Not infrequently, normal people say they are depressed when they observe any lowering of their mood below their baseline level. A person experiencing a transient sadness or loneliness may state that he is depressed. Whether this *normal* mood is synonymous with, or even related to, the feeling experienced in the abnormal condition of depression is open to question. In any event, when a person complains of feeling inordinately dejected, hopeless, or unhappy, the term *depressed* is often used to label this subjective state.

The term depression is often used to designate a complex pattern of deviations in feelings, cognition, and behavior (described in the previous section) that is not represented as a discrete psychiatric disorder. In such instances it is regarded as a syndrome, or symptom-complex. The cluster of signs and symptoms is sometimes conceptualized as a psychopathological dimension ranging in intensity (or in degree of abnormality) from mild to severe. The syndrome of depression may at times appear as a concomitant of a definite psychiatric disorder such as schizophrenic reaction; in such a case, the diagnosis would be "schizophrenic reaction with depression." At times, the syndrome may be secondary to, or a manifestation of, organic disease of the brain such as general paresis or cerebral artereosclerosis.

Finally, the term depression has been used to designate a discrete nosological entity. The term is generally qualified by some adjective to indicate a particular type or form, as for example: reactive depression, agitated depression, or psychotic-depressive reaction. When conceptualized as a specific clinical entity, depression is assumed to have certain consistent attributes in addition to the characteristic signs and symptoms; these attributes include a specifiable type of onset, course, duration, and outcome.

In medicine, a clinical entity or disease is assumed to be responsive to specific forms of treatment (not necessarily discovered as yet), and to have a specific etiology. There is a considerable body of evidence indicating that the clinical entity depression responds to certain drugs and/or electroconvulsive therapy (ECT), but there is no consensus as yet regarding its etiology.

DEPRESSION AND NORMAL MOODS

There is little agreement among authorities regarding the relationship of depression to the changes in mood experienced by normal individuals. The term, *mood,* is generally applied to a spectrum of feelings extending from elation and happiness at one extreme, to sadness and unhappiness at the other. The particular feelings encompassed by this term, consequently, are directly related to either happiness or sadness. Subjective states, such as anxiety or anger, that do not fit into the happiness-sadness categories are not generally included. Some authors (Hinsie and Campbell, 1960) believe that all individuals have mood-swings and that normal individuals may have "blue" hours or "blue" days. This belief has been supported by systematic studies of oscillations in mood in normal subjects (Wessman and Ricks, 1966).

The episodes of low mood or of feeling blue experienced by normal individuals are similar in a number of ways to the clinical states of depression. First, there is a similarity between the descriptions of the subjective experience of normal low mood and of depression. The words used to describe normal low mood tend to be the same used by depressives to describe their feelings—blue, sad, unhappy, empty, low, lonely. It is possible, however, that this resemblance may be due to the depressed patient's drawing on his familiar vocabulary to describe a pathological state for which he has no available words. Some patients, in fact, state that their feelings during their depressions are quite distinct from any feelings they have ever experienced when not in a clinical depression.

Second, the behavior of the depressed patient resembles that of a person who is sad or unhappy, particularly in the mournful facial expression and the lowering of the voice. Third, some of the vegetative and physical manifestations characteristic of depression are occasionally seen in individuals who are feeling sad but who would not be considered clinically depressed. A person who has failed an examination, lost a job, or been jilted, may not only feel discouraged and forlorn, but may experience anorexia, insomnia, and fatigability. Finally, many individuals experience blue states that seem to oscillate in a consistent or rhythmic fashion, independently of external stimuli, suggestive of the rhythmic variations in the intensity of depression (Wessman and Ricks, 1966).

The resemblance between depression and the low mood of normals has led to the concept that the pathological is simply an exaggeration of the normal. On the surface, this view seems plausible. As will be discussed in Chapter 2, each symptom of depression may be graded in intensity along a dimension, and the more mild intensities are certainly similar to the phenomena observed in normal individuals who are feeling blue.

In rebuttal to this *continuity hypothesis,* it could be contended that many pathological states that seem to be on a continuum with the normal state are different in their essential character from the normal state. To illustrate this, an analogy may be made between the deviations of mood and deviations of internal body temperature. While pronounced changes in body temperature are on the same continuum as are normal temperatures, the underlying factors producing the large deviations are not an extension of the normal state of health: A person may have a disease, e.g., typhoid fever, that is manifested by a serial progression in temperature and yet is categorically different from the normal state. Similarly, the deviation in mood found in depression may be the manifestation of a disease process that is distinct from the normal state.

There is no general consensus among the authorities regarding the relation of depression to normal mood swings. Some writers, notably Kraepelin and his followers, consider depression a well-defined disease, quite distinct from normal mood. They postulate the presence of a profound biological derangement as the key factor in depression. This concept of a dichotomy between health and disease is generally shared by the *somatogenic school.* The *environmentalists* seem to favor the continuity hypothesis.

In their view, there is a continuous series of mood reactions ranging from a normal reaction to an extreme reaction in a particularly susceptible person. The psychobiological school founded by Adolph Meyer tends to favor this view.

The ultimate answer to the question as to whether there is a dichotomy or continuity between normal mood and depression will have to wait until the question of the etiology of depression is fully resolved.

Chapter 2.
Symptomatology of Depression

PREVIOUS SYSTEMATIC STUDIES

As stated in Chapter 1, there has been remarkable consistency in the descriptions of depression since ancient times. While there has been unanimity among the writers on many of the characteristics, however, there has been lack of agreement on many others. The core signs and symptoms such as low mood, pessimism, self-criticism, and retardation or agitation seem to have been universally accepted. Other signs and symptoms that have been regarded as intrinsic to the depressive syndrome include autonomic symptoms, constipation, difficulty in concentrating, slow thinking, and anxiety. Campbell (1953), e.g., listed 29 medical manifestations of autonomic disturbance, among which the most common in manic depressives were hot flashes, tachycardia, dyspnea, weakness, head pains, coldness and numbness of the extremities, frontal headaches, and dizziness.

There have been very few systematic studies designed to delineate the characteristic signs and symptoms of depression. Cassidy, Flanagan, and Spellman (1957) compared the symptomatology of 100 patients diagnosed as manic depressive with a control group of 50 patients with diagnoses of recognized medical diseases. The frequency of the specific symptoms was determined by having the patient complete a questionnaire of 199 items. Among the symptoms that were endorsed significantly more often by those in the psychiatric group were anorexia, sleep disturbance, low mood, suicidal thoughts, crying, irritability, fear of losing the mind, poor concentration, and delusions.

It is interesting to note that Cassidy and his coworkers found that only 25 per cent of the manic-depressive group thought that they would get well as compared with 61 per cent of those who were medically ill. This is indicative of the pessimism which is characteristic of manic depressives: Almost all could be expected to recover completely from their illness, in contrast to the number of incurably ill among the medical patients. Certain symptoms sometimes attributed to manic depressives, such as constipation, were found in similar proportions in the two groups.

Campbell reported a high frequency of medical symptoms, generally attributed to autonomic imbalance, among manic depressives. Cassidy's study, however, found that most of these medical symptoms occurred at least as frequently among the medically ill patients as among the manic-depressive patients. Moreover, many of these symptoms were found in a group of healthy control patients. Headaches, for instance, were reported by 49 per cent of the manic-depressive patients, 36 per cent of the medically-sick controls, and 25 per cent of the healthy controls. When the symptoms of manic-depressives, anxiety-neurotics, and hysteria patients were compared, it was found that autonomic symptoms occurred at least as frequently in the latter two groups as they did in the manic-depressive group. Palpitation, for instance, was reported by 56 per cent of the manic depressives, 94 per cent of the anxiety neurotics, and 76 per cent of the hysterics. It therefore seems clear that autonomic symptoms are not specifically characteristic of manic-depressive disorders.

Recent systematic investigations of the symptomatology of depressive disorders have been conducted to delineate the typical clinical picture, as well as to suggest typical subgroupings of depression (Grinker *et al.*, 1961; Friedman *et al.*, 1963). A major problem in interpreting the findings of these investigations is presented by the fact that the case material consisted primarily of depressed patients and did not include a control group of nondepressed psychiatric patients for comparison. It is not possible, therefore, to determine which symptom clusters might be characteristic of depression or its various subgroupings, and which might occur in any psychiatric patient or even in normals.

In this chapter, following a review of the chief complaints, the symptoms of depression are described under four major headings: emotional; cognitive; motivational; and physical and vegetative. This is followed by a section on delusions and hallucinations. Some of these divisions may appear arbitrary, and it is undoubtedly true that some of the symptoms described separately may simply be different facets of the same phenomenon. Nonetheless, I think it is desirable at this stage to present the symptomatology as broadly as possible, despite the inevitable overlap. Following the symptoms, a section on behavioral observation has been included. The descriptions in this latter section were obtained by direct observation of the patients' nonverbal as well as their verbal behavior.

CHIEF COMPLAINT

The chief complaint presented by depressed patients often points immediately to the diagnosis of depression; on the other hand, it sometimes

suggests a physical disturbance. Skillful questioning can generally determine whether the basic depressive symptomatology is present.

The chief complaint may take a variety of forms: (*1*) an unpleasant
emotional state; (*2*) a changed attitude towards life; (*3*) somatic symptoms of a specifically depressive nature; or (*4*) somatic symptoms not
typical of depression.

Among the most common subjective complaints (Lewis, 1934) are:
"I feel miserable." "I just feel hopeless." "I'm desperate." "I'm worried
about everything." Although depression is generally considered an affective
disorder, it should be emphasized that a subjective change in mood is not
reported by all depressed patients. As in many other disorders, the absence
of a significant clinical feature does not rule out the diagnosis of that disorder. In our series, for instance, only 53 per cent of the mildly depressed
patients acknowledged feeling sad or unhappy.

Sometimes the chief complaint is in the form of a change of one's
actions, reactions, or attitudes towards life. For example, a patient may
say, "I don't have any goals any more." "I don't care anymore what happens to me." "I don't see any point to living." Sometimes the major complaint is a sense of futility about life.

Often the chief complaint of the depressed patient centers around
some physical symptom that is characteristic of depression. The patient may
complain that he gets tired easily, that he has no pep, or that he has lost
his appetite. Sometimes he complains of some alteration in his appearance
or in his bodily functions. Women complain that they are beginning to
look old or are getting ugly. Other patients complain of some dramatic
physical symptom such as, "My bowels are blocked up."

Depressed patients attending medical clinics or consulting either in-
ternists or general practitioners frequently present some symptom suggestive of a physical disease (Watts, 1957). In many cases, the physical
examination fails to reveal any physical abnormality. In other cases, some
minor abnormality may be found but it is of insufficient severity to account
for the magnitude of the patient's discomfort. On further examination,
the patient may acknowledge a change in mood but is likely to attribute
this to his somatic symptoms.

Severe localized pain or generalized pain may often be the chief focus
of a patient's complaint. Bradley (1963) reported 35 cases of depression
in which the main complaint was severe, localized pain. In each case, feelings of depression were either spontaneously reported by the patient or
were elicited on interview. In those cases in which the pain was integrally
connected with the depression, the pain cleared up as the depression cleared

up. Kennedy (1944) and Von Hagen (1957) reported that pain associated with depression responded to electroconvulsive therapy (ECT).

In the study by Cassidy, Flanagan, and Spellman (1957), an analysis was made of the chief complaints of the manic-depressive patients. These complaints were divided into several categories which included (1) psychological; (2) localized medical; (3) generalized medical; (4) mixed medical and psychological; (5) medical, general and local; and (6) no clear information. Some of the typical complaints in each category are listed below:

(1) *Psychological (58 per cent)*: "depressed;" "I have nothing to look forward to;" "afraid to be alone;" "no interest;" "can't remember anything;" "get discouraged and hurt;" "black moods and blind rages;" "I'm doing such stupid things;" "I'm all mixed up;" "very unhappy at times;" "brooded around the house."

(2) *Localized medical (18 per cent)*: "head is heavy;" "pressure in my throat;" "headaches;" "urinating frequently;" "pain in head like a balloon that burst;" "upset stomach."

(3) *Generalized medical (11 per cent)*: "tired;" "I'm exhausted;" "I feel all in;" "tire easy;" "jumpy most at night;" "I can't do my work, I don't feel strong;" "I tremble like a leaf."

(4) *Medical and psychological (2 per cent)*: "I get scared to death and can't breathe;" "stiff neck and crying spells."

(5) *Medical, general and local (2 per cent)*: "breathing difficulty ... pain all over;" "I have no power. My arms are weak." "I can't work."

(6) *No information (9 per cent)*.

The authors tabulated the percentages of the various symptom types which were named by the manic-depressive patients and by the medically-

Table 2–1.
CHIEF COMPLAINTS OF 100 PATIENTS WITH MANIC-DEPRESSIVE
DIAGNOSIS AND 50 PATIENTS WITH MEDICAL DIAGNOSIS*

Type of complaint	Manic depressive (%)	Medical controls (%)
Psychological	58	0
Medical, localized	18	86
Medical, generalized	11	6
Medical, localized and generalized	2	0
Medical and psychological	2	6
No information	9	2

* Adapted from Cassidy, Flanagan, and Spellman, 1957.

sick controls (Table 2–1). It is worthy of note that a medical symptom, either localized or generalized, was reported by 33 per cent of the manic-depressive patients and by 92 per cent of the medically-sick controls.

SYMPTOMS

The decision as to which symptoms should be included here was made as the result of several steps: First, several textbooks of psychiatry and monographs on depression were studied to determine what symptoms have been attributed to depression by general consensus. Second, in an intensive study of 50 depressed patients and 30 nondepressed patients in psychotherapy, I attempted to tally which symptoms occurred significantly more often in the depressed than in the nondepressed group. On the basis of this tabulation, an inventory consisting of items relevant to depression was constructed and pretested on approximately 100 patients. Finally, this inventory was revised and presented to 966 psychiatric patients. Distributions of the symptoms reported in response to the inventory are presented in Tables 2–3 through 2–7.

One of the symptoms, namely *irritability*, did not occur significantly more frequently in the depressed than in the nondepressed patients. It, therefore, has been dropped from the list. Incidentally, Cassidy and his coworkers (1957) found that this symptom was more frequent in the anxiety-neurotic group than in the manic-depressive group.

Some of the symptoms often attributed to the manic-depressive syndrome are not included in the symptom descriptions in this chapter. For instance, *fear of death* was not included because it was not found to be any more common among the depressed patients than among the nondepressed in the preliminary clinical study. Cassidy, Flanagan, and Spellman found, in fact, that fear of death occurred in 42 per cent of patients with anxiety neurosis and only 35 per cent of the manic depressives. Similarly, constipation occurred in 60 per cent of the manic-depressive patients and 54 per cent of the patients with hysteria. Consequently, this particular symptom does not seem to be specific to depression.

Conventional nosological categories were not used in our analyses of the symptomatology. Instead of being classified according to their primary diagnoses, such as manic-depressive reaction, schizophrenia, anxiety reaction, etc., the patients were categorized according to the depth of depression which they exhibited, independently of their primary diagnoses. There were two major reasons for this: (*1*) In our own studies as well as in previous studies, it was found that the degree of interjudge reliability was relatively low in diagnoses made according to the standard nomenclature (see Chapter 11). Consequently, any findings based on diagnoses of such low reliability would be of relatively dubious value. The interpsychiatrist ratings of the depth of depression, on the other hand, showed a relatively high correlation (.87). (2) We found that the cluster of symptoms generally regarded as constituting the depressive syndrome occurs not only in disorders such as neurotic-depressive reaction and manic-depressive reaction, but also in patients whose primary diagnosis is anxiety reaction, schizophrenia, obsessional neurosis, etc. In fact, we have found that a patient with the primary diagnosis of one of the typical depressive categories may be less depressed than a patient whose primary diagnosis is schizophrenia, obsessional neurosis, etc. The sample, therefore, was divided into four groups according to the depth of depression: none, mild, moderate, and severe.

In addition to making the usual qualitative distinctions among the symptoms, I have attempted to provide a guide for assessing their severity. The symptoms are discussed in terms of how they are likely to appear in the mild, moderate, and severe states (or phases) of depression. This may serve as an aid to the clinician or investigator in making a quantitative estimate of the severity of depression. The tables may be used as a guide in diagnosing depression since they show the relative frequency of the symptoms in patients who were considered to be either nondepressed, mildly depressed, moderately depressed, or severely depressed.

Table 2–2.

DISTRIBUTION OF PATIENTS ACCORDING TO RACE, SEX, AND DEPTH OF DEPRESSION

Race and sex of patient	Depth of depression				
	None	Mild	Moderate	Severe	Total
White males	71	98	91	15	275
White females	51	90	137	40	318
Negro males	50	32	30	4	116
Negro females	52	77	102	26	257
Total Whites	122	188	228	55	593
Total Negroes	102	109	132	30	373
Total males	121	130	121	19	391
Total females	103	167	239	66	575
TOTAL	224	297	360	85	966

The method for collecting the data on which the tables are based is described in greater detail in Chapter 12. The description of the patient sample is found in Table 2–2.

EMOTIONAL MANIFESTATIONS

The term *emotional manifestations* refers to the changes in the patient's feelings or the changes in his overt behavior *directly* attributable to his feeling states (Table 2–3). In assessing emotional manifestations, it is im-

Table 2–3.
EMOTIONAL MANIFESTATIONS: FREQUENCY AMONG DEPRESSED AND
NONDEPRESSED PATIENTS

	Depth of depression			
	None (%) (n = 224)	*Mild* (%) (n = 288)	*Moderate* (%) (n = 377)	*Severe* (%) (n = 86)
Dejected mood	23	50	75	88
Self-dislike	37	64	81	86
Loss of gratification	35	65	86	92
Loss of attachments	16	37	60	64
Crying spells	29	44	63	83
Loss of mirth response	8	29	41	52

n = No. of patients.

portant to take into account the individual's premorbid mood level and behavior, as well as what the examiner might consider the *normal* range in the patient's particular age, sex, and social group. The occurrence of frequent crying spells in a patient who rarely or never cried before becoming depressed might indicate a greater level of depression than it would in a patient who habitually cried whether depressed or not.

Dejected Mood

The characteristic depression in mood is described differently by various clinically-depressed patients. Whatever term the patient uses to describe his subjective feelings should be further explored by the examiner. If the patient uses the word "depressed," for instance, the examiner should not take the word at its face value but should try to determine its connotation for the patient. Persons who are in no way clinically depressed may use this adjective to designate transient feelings of loneliness, boredom, or discouragement.

Sometimes the feeling is expressed predominantly in somatic terms, such as "a lump in my throat," or "I have an empty feeling in my stomach," or "I have a sad, heavy feeling in my chest." On further investigation, these feelings generally are found to be similar to the feelings expressed by other patients in terms of adjectives such as sad, unhappy, lonely, or bored.

The intensity of the mood deviation must be gauged by the examiner. Some of the rough criteria of the degree of depression are the relative degree of morbidity implied by the adjective chosen, the qualification by adverbs such as "slightly" or "very," and the degree of tolerance the patient expresses for the feeling (e.g., "I feel so miserable I can't stand it another minute.").

Among the adjectives used by depressed patients in answer to the question, "How do you feel?" are the following: miserable, hopeless, blue, sad, lonely, unhappy, downhearted, humiliated, ashamed, worried, useless, guilty. Eighty-eight per cent of the severely depressed patients reported some degree of sadness or unhappiness, as compared with 23 per cent of the nondepressed patients.

Mild: The patient indicates he feels blue or sad. The unpleasant feeling tends to fluctuate considerably during the day and at times may be absent, and the patient may even feel cheerful. Also the dysphoric feeling can be relieved partially or completely by outside stimuli, such as a compliment, a joke, or a favorable event. With a little effort or ingenuity the examiner can usually evoke a positive response. Patients at this level generally react with genuine amusement to jokes or humorous anecdotes.

Moderate: The dysphoria tends to be more pronounced and more persistent. The patient's feeling is less likely to be influenced by other people's attempts to cheer him up, and any relief of this nature is temporary. Also, a diurnal variation is frequently present: The dysphoria is often worse in the morning and tends to be alleviated as the day progresses.

Severe: In cases of severe depression, the patient is apt to state he feels "hopeless" or "miserable." Agitated patients frequently state they are "worried." In our series, 70 per cent of the severely-depressed patients indicated that they were sad all the time and "could not snap out of it," that they were so sad that it was very painful; or that they were so sad they could not stand it.

Negative Feelings Toward Self

Depressed patients often express negative feelings about themselves. These feelings may be related to the general dysphoric feelings just described, but they are different in that they are specifically directed toward the self.

The patients appear to distinguish feelings of dislike for themselves from negative attitudes about themselves such as, "I am worthless." The frequency of self-dislike ranged from 37 per cent in the nondepressed group to 86 per cent among the severely depressed.

Mild: The patient states that he feels disappointed in himself. This feeling is accompanied by ideas such as: "I've let everybody down . . . If I had tried harder, I could have made the grade."

Moderate: The feeling of self-dislike is stronger and may progress to a feeling of disgust with himself. This is generally accompanied by ideas such as: "I'm a weakling . . . I don't do anything right . . . I'm no good."

Severe: The feeling may progress to the point where the patient hates himself. This stage may be identified by statements such as: "I'm a terrible person . . . I don't deserve to live . . . I'm despicable . . . I loathe myself."

Reduction in Gratification

The loss of gratification is such a pervasive process among depressives that many patients regard it as the central feature of their illness. In our series, 92 per cent of the severely-depressed patients reported at least partial loss of satisfaction; this was the most common symptom among the depressed group as a whole.

Loss of gratification appears to start with a few activities and, as the depression progresses, spreads to practically everything the patient does. Even activities that are generally associated with biological needs or drives, such as eating or sexual experiences, are not spared. Experiences that are primarily psychosocial such as achieving fame, receiving expressions of love or friendship, or even engaging in conversations, are similarly stripped of their pleasurable properties.

The emphasis placed by some of the patients on loss of satisfaction gives the impression that they are especially oriented in their lives toward obtaining gratification. Whether or not this applies to the premorbid state cannot be stated with certainty, but it is true that in their manic states the feverish pursuit of gratification is a cardinal feature.

The initial loss of satisfaction from activities involving responsibility or obligation, such as those involved in the role of worker, housewife, or student, is often compensated for by increasing satisfaction from recreational activities. This observation has prompted Saul (1947) and others to suggest that, in depression, the "give-get" balance is upset; the patient, depleted psychologically over a period of time by activities predominantly *giving* in nature, experiences an accentuation of his passive needs, which are gratified by activities involving less of a sense of duty or responsibility (giving) and more of a tangible and easily obtained satisfaction. In the more advanced stages of the illness, however, even passive, regressive activities fail to bring any satisfaction.

Mild: The patient complains that some of the joy has gone out of his life. He no longer gets a "kick" or pleasure from his family, friends, or job. Characteristically, activities involving responsibility, obligation, or effort become less satisfying to him. Often, he finds greater satisfaction from *passive* activities involving recreation, relaxation, or rest. He may seek unusual types of activities in order to get some of his former thrill. One patient reported that he could always pull himself out of a mild depression by watching a performance of deviant sexual practices.

Moderate: He feels bored much of the time. He may try to enjoy some of his former favorite activities but they seem "flat" to him now. Business or professional activities which formerly excited him now fail to move him. He may obtain temporary relief from a change, such as a vacation, but the boredom returns upon resumption of his usual activities.

Severe: He experiences no enjoyment from activities that were formerly pleasurable. He may even feel an aversion for activities he once enjoyed. Popular acclaim or expressions of love or friendship no longer bring any degree of satisfaction. The patients almost uniformly complain that nothing gives them any degree of satisfaction.

Loss of Emotional Attachments

Loss of emotional involvement in other people or activities usually accompanies loss of satisfaction. This is manifested by a decline in his degree of interest in particular activities or in his affection or concern for other persons. Loss of affection for members of his family is often a cause for concern to the patient and occasionally is a major factor in his seeking medical attention. Sixty-four per cent of the severely-depressed patients reported loss of feeling for or interest in other people, whereas only 16 per cent of the nondepressed patients reported this symptom.

Mild: In mild cases, there is some decline in the degree of enthusiasm for, or absorption in, an activity. The patient sometimes reports that he does not experience the same intensity of love or affection for his spouse, children, or friends. On the other hand, he may feel more dependent on them.

Moderate: The loss of interest or of positive feeling may progress to indifference. A number of patients described this as a "wall" between themselves and other people. Sometimes a husband may complain that he no longer loves his wife, or a mother may be concerned that she does not seem to care about her children or what happens to them. A previously devoted employee may report he is no longer concerned about his job. A woman may no longer care about her appearance.

Severe: Loss of attachment to external objects may progress to apathy. The patient may not only lose any positive feeling for members of his family, but may be surprised to find that his only reaction is a negative one. In some cases, the patient experiences only a kind of cold hate which may be masked by dependency. A typical patient's report is, "I've been told I have love and can give love. But now I don't feel anything toward my family. I don't give a damn about them. I know this is terrible, but sometimes I hate them."

Crying Spells

Increased periods of crying are frequent among depressed patients. This is particularly true of the depressed women in our series. Of the severely-depressed patients, 83 per cent reported that they cried more frequently than they did before becoming depressed, or that they felt like crying even though the tears did not come.

Some patients who rarely cried when not depressed were able to diagnose the onset of depression by observing a strong desire to weep. One woman remarked, "I don't know whether I feel sad or not but I do feel like crying so I guess I am depressed." Further questioning elicited the rest of the cardinal symptoms of depression.

Mild: There is an increased tendency to weep or cry. Stimuli or situations that would ordinarily not affect the patient may now elicit tears. A mother, for example, might burst out crying during an argument with her children or if she feels her husband is not attentive. Although increased crying is frequent among mildly-depressed women, it is unusual for a mildly-depressed man to cry (Lewis, 1934).

Moderate: The patient may cry during the psychiatric interview, and references to his problems may elicit tears. Men who have not cried since childhood may cry while discussing their problems. Women patients may cry for no apparent reason: "It just comes over me like a wave and I can't help crying." Sometimes the patient feels relieved after crying but more often he feels more depressed.

Severe: By the time he has reached the severe stage, a patient who was easily moved to tears in the earlier phase may find that he no longer can cry even when he wants to. He may weep, but he has no tears ("dry depression"). Twenty-nine per cent of the severely-depressed patients reported that although they had previously been capable of crying when feeling sad, they no longer could cry—even though they wanted to do so.

Loss of Mirth Response

Depressed patients frequently volunteer the information that they have lost their sense of humor. The problem does not seem to be loss of the ability to perceive the point of the joke or even, when instructed, to construct a joke. The difficulty rather seems to be that the patient does not respond to humor in the usual way. He is not amused, does not feel like laughing, and does not get any feeling of satisfaction from a jesting remark, joke, or cartoon.

In our series, 52 per cent of the severely-depressed patients indicated that they had lost their sense of humor, as contrasted with 8 per cent of the nondepressed patients.

Nussbaum and Michaux (1963) studied the response to humor (in the form of riddles and jokes) in 18 women patients with severe neurotic and psychotic depressions. They found that improvements in response to humorous stimuli correlated well with clinical ratings of improvement of the depression.

Mild: Patients who frequently enjoy listening to jokes and telling jokes find that this is no longer such a ready source of gratification. They remark that jokes no longer seem funny to them. Furthermore, they do not handle kidding or joshing by their friends as well as previously.

Moderate: The patient may see the point of a joke and can even force a smile, but he is usually not amused. He cannot see the light side of events and tends to take everything seriously.

Severe: The patient does not respond at all to humorous sallies by other people. Where others may respond to the humorous element in a joke he is more likely to respond to the aggressive or hostile content and feel hurt or disgusted.

COGNITIVE MANIFESTATIONS

The cognitive manifestations of depression include a number of diverse phenomena (Table 2–4). One group is composed of the patient's distorted attitudes toward himself, his experience, and his future. This group includes low self-evaluations, distortions of the body image, and negative expectations. Another symptom, self-blame, expresses the patient's notion of causality: He is prone to hold himself responsible for any difficulties or problems that he encounters. A third kind of symptom involves the area of decision-making: The patient typically vacillates and is indecisive.

Table 2–4.
COGNITIVE AND MOTIVATIONAL MANIFESTATIONS: FREQUENCY AMONG
DEPRESSED AND NONDEPRESSED PATIENTS

| | *Depth of depression* | | | |
| | *None*
(%)
(n = 224) | *Mild*
(%)
(n = 288) | *Moderate*
(%)
(n = 377) | *Severe*
(%)
(n = 86) |
Manifestation				
Low self-evaluation	38	60	78	81
Negative expectation	22	55	72	87
Self-blame and self-criticism	43	67	80	80
Indecisiveness	23	48	67	76
Distorted self-image	12	33	50	66
Loss of motivation	33	65	83	86
Suicidal wishes	12	31	53	74

n = No. of patients.

Low Self-Evaluation

Low self-esteem is a characteristic feature of depression. Self-devaluation is apparently part of the depressed patient's pattern of viewing himself as deficient in those attributes that are specifically important to him: ability, performance, intelligence, health, strength, personal attractiveness, popularity, or financial resources. Often the sense of deficiency is expressed in terms such as "I am inferior" or "I am inadequate." This symptom was reported by 81 per cent of the severely-depressed patients and by 38 per cent of the nondepressed patients.

The sense of deficiency may also be reflected in complaints of deprivation of love or material possessions. This reaction is most apparent in patients who have had, respectively, an unhappy love affair or a financial reversal just prior to the depression.

Mild: The patient shows an excessive reaction to any of his errors or difficulties and is prone to regard them as a reflection of his inadequacy or as a defect in himself. He makes comparisons with other people and, more often than not, concludes he is inferior. It is possible, however, to correct his inaccurate self-evaluations, at least temporarily, by confronting him with appropriate evidence or by reasoning with him.

Moderate: Most of the patient's thought content revolves about his sense of deficiency, and he is prone to interpret neutral situations as indicative of this deficiency. He exaggerates the degree and significance of any errors. When he looks at his present and past life, he sees his failures as outstanding and his successes as faint by comparison. He complains that he has lost confidence in himself and his sense of inadequacy is such that when confronted with tasks he has easily handled in the past, his initial reaction is: "I can't do it."

The religious or moralistic patient tends to dwell on his sins or moral shortcomings. The patient who placed a premium on his personal attractiveness, intelligence, or business success tends to believe that he has slipped in these areas. Attempts to modify his distorted self-evaluations by reassuring the patient or by presenting contradictory evidence generally meet with considerable resistance; any increase in realistic thinking about himself is transient.

Severe: The patient's self-evaluations are at the lowest point. He drastically downgrades himself in terms of his personal attributes and his role as parent, spouse, employer, etc. He regards himself as worthless, completely inept, and a total failure. He claims that he is a burden to members of his family and that they would be better off without him. He may be preoccupied with ideas that he is the world's worst sinner, completely impoverished, or totally inadequate. Attempts to correct his erroneous ideas are generally fruitless.

Negative Expectations

A gloomy outlook and pessimism are closely related to the feelings of hopelessness mentioned previously. More than 78 per cent of the depressed patients reported a negative outlook, as compared with 22 per cent of the nondepressed group. This symptom showed the highest correlation with the clinical rating of depression (see Table 12–6).

The patient's pattern of expecting the worst and rejecting the possibility of any improvement poses formidable obstacles in attempts to engage him in a therapeutic program. His negative outlook is often a source of frustration to his friends, family, and physician when they try to help him. Not infrequently, for example, a patient may discard his antidepressant pills because he believes *a priori* that they "cannot do him good."

Unlike the anxious patient, who tempers his negative anticipations with the realization that the unpleasant events may be avoided or will pass in time, the depressed patient thinks in terms of a future in which his present deficient condition (financial, social, physical) will continue or will even get worse. This sense of permanence and irreversibility of his status or problems seems to form the basis for his consideration of suicide as a logical course of action. The relationship of hopelessness to suicide is indicated by the finding that, of all the symptoms that were correlated with suicide, the correlation coefficient of hopelessness: suicide was the highest.

Mild: The patient tends to expect a negative outcome in ambiguous or equivocal situations. When his associates and friends feel justified in anticipating favorable results, his expectations lean toward the negative or pessimistic. Whether the subject of his concern is his health, or his personal problems, or his economic problems, he has doubts as to whether any improvement will take place.

Moderate: He regards the future as unpromising and states he has nothing to which he can look forward. It is difficult to get him to do anything because his initial response is, "I won't like it" or "it won't do any good."

Severe: He views the future as black and hopeless. He states that he will never get over his troubles and that things cannot get better for him. He believes that none of his problems can be solved. The patient makes statements such as: "This is the end of the road. From now on I will look older and uglier." "There is nothing here for me any more. I have no place. There is no future." "I know I can't get better . . . It's all over for me."

Self-Blame and Self-Criticism

The depressive's perseverating self-blame and self-criticism appear to be related to his egocentric notions of causality and his penchant for criticizing himself for his alleged deficiencies. He is particularly prone to ascribe adverse occurrences to some deficiency in himself, and then to rebuke himself for having this alleged defect. In the more severe cases, the patient may blame himself for happenings that are in no way connected with him, and abuse himself in a savage manner. Eighty per cent of the severely-depressed patients reported this symptom.

Mild: In mild cases, the patient is prone to blame and criticize himself when he falls short of his rigid, perfectionist standards. If people seem less responsive to him, or he is slow at solving a problem, he is likely to berate himself for being dull or stupid. He seems to be intolerant of any shortcomings in himself and cannot accept the idea that it is human to err.

Moderate: The patient is likely to criticize himself harshly for any aspects of his personality or behavior which he judges to be substandard. He is likely to blame himself for mishaps that are obviously not his fault. His self-criticisms become more extreme.

Severe: In the severe state, the patient is even more extreme in his use of self-blame or self-criticism. He makes statements such as, "I'm responsible for the violence and suffering in the world. There's no way in which I can be punished enough for my sins. I wish you would take me out and hang me." He views himself as a social leper or criminal, and interprets various extraneous stimuli as signs of public disapproval.

Indecisiveness

Difficulty in making decisions, vacillating between alternatives, and changing decisions are depressive characteristics that are usually quite vexing to the patient's family and friends as well as to the patient himself. The frequency of indecisiveness ranged from 48 per cent in the mildly-depressed patients to 76 per cent in the severely-depressed group.

There appears to be at least two facets to this indecisiveness. The first is primarily in the cognitive sphere. The patient anticipates making the wrong decision: Each time he considers one of the various possibilities he tends to regard it as wrong and to think that he will regret making that choice. The second facet is primarily motivational and is related to "paralysis of the will," avoidance tendencies, and increased dependency. The patient has a lack of motivation to go through the mental operations that are required to arrive at a conclusion. Also, the idea of making a decision represents a burden to him; he desires to evade, or at least to get help with any situation that he perceives will be burdensome. Furthermore, he realizes that making a decision often commits him to a course of action and, since he desires to avoid action, he is prone to procrastinate.

Routine decisions which must be made in carrying out their occupational roles become major problems for the depressed patients. A professor could not decide what material to include in a lecture; a housewife could not decide what to cook for an evening meal; a student could not decide whether to spend the spring recess studying at college or whether to go home; an executive could not decide whether to hire a new secretary.

Mild: A patient who can ordinarily make rapid-fire decisions finds that solutions do not seem to occur to him so readily. Where in his normal state he reaches a decision "without even thinking about it," he now finds himself impelled to mull over the particular problem, review the possible consequences of the decision, and consider a variety of often irrelevant alternatives. His fear of making the wrong decision is reflected in a general sense of uncertainty. Frequently, he seeks confirmation from another person.

Moderate: Difficulty in making decisions spreads to almost every activity and involves such minor problems as what clothes to wear, what route to take to the office, and whether to have a haircut. Often it is of little practical importance which alternative is selected, but the vacillation and failure to arrive at some decision can have unfavorable consequences. A woman, for example, spent several weeks trying to choose between two shades of paint for her house. The two shades under consideration were hardly distinguishable, but her failure to reach a decision created a turmoil in the house, the painter having left his buckets of paint and scaffolding until a decision could be made.

Severe: The severely-depressed patients generally believe they are incapable of making a decision and, consequently, do not even try. When a housewife was prodded to make a shopping list or a list of clothes for her children to take to camp, she insisted she could not decide what to put down. The patient frequently has doubts about everything he does and says. One woman seriously doubted that she had given her correct name to the psychiatrist, or that she had enunciated it properly.

Distortion of Body Image

The patient's distorted picture of his physical appearance is often quite marked in depression. This occurs somewhat more frequently among women than among men. In our series, 66 per cent of the severely-depressed patients believed that they had become unattractive, as compared with 12 per cent of the nondepressed patients.

Mild: The patient begins to be excessively concerned with his physical appearance. A woman finds herself frowning at her reflection whenever she passes a mirror. She examines her face minutely for signs of blemishes. She becomes preoccupied with the thought that she looks plain or is getting fat.

Moderate: The concern about physical appearance is greater. The patient believes that there has been a change in his looks since the onset of the depression even though there is no objective evidence to support this idea. When he sees an ugly person, he thinks, "I look like that." As he becomes worried about his appearance, his brow becomes furrowed. When he observes his furrowed brow in the mirror, he thinks, "my whole face is wrinkled and the wrinkles will never disappear." Some patients seek plastic surgery to remedy the fancied or exaggerated facial changes.

Sometimes, the patient may believe that he has grown fat even though there is no objective evidence to support this. In fact, some patients have this notion even though they are losing weight.

Severe: The idea of personal unattractiveness becomes more fixed. The patient believes that he is ugly and repulsive looking. He expects other people to turn away from him in revulsion: One woman wore a veil and another turned her head whenever anybody approached her.

MOTIVATIONAL MANIFESTATIONS

Motivational manifestations include consciously experienced strivings, desires, and impulses that are prominent in depressions. These motivational patterns can often be inferred from observing the patient's behavior; however, direct questioning generally elicits a fairly precise and comprehensive description of his motivations (see Table 2–4).

A striking feature of the characteristic motivations of the depressed patient is their *regressive* nature. The term regressive is applicable in that the patient seems drawn to activities that are the least demanding for him either in terms of the degree of responsibility or initiative required, or the amount of energy to be expended. He turns away from activities that are specifically associated with the adult role and seeks activities that are more characteristic of the child's role. When confronted with a choice, he prefers passivity to activity and dependence to independence (autonomy); he avoids responsibility and escapes from his problems rather than trying to solve them; he seeks immediate, but transient, gratifications instead of delayed, but prolonged, satisfactions. The ultimate manifestation of the escapist trend is expressed in his desire to withdraw from life via suicide.

An important aspect of these motivations is that their fulfillment is generally incompatible with the individual's major premorbid goals and values. In essence, yielding to his passive impulses and his desires to retreat or commit suicide leads to abandonment of his family, friends, and vocation. Similarly, he defaults his chance to obtain personal satisfaction through accomplishment or interpersonal relations. By avoiding even the simplest problems, moreover, he finds that they accumulate until they seem overwhelming to him.

The specific motivational patterns to be described are presented as distinct phenomena although they are obviously interrelated and may, in fact, represent different facets of the same fundamental pattern. It is possible that certain phenomena are primary and the others are secondary or tertiary; for instance, it could be postulated that paralysis of the will is the result of escapist or passive wishes, a sense of futility, loss of external investments, or the sense of fatigue. Since these suggestions are purely speculative, it seems preferable at present to treat these phenomena separately, rather than prematurely to assign primacy to certain patterns.

Paralysis of the Will

The loss of positive motivation is often a striking feature of depression. The patient may have a major problem in mobilizing himself to perform even the most elemental and vital tasks such as eating, elimination, or taking medication to relieve his distress. The essence of the problem appears to be that, although he can define for himself what he should do, he does not experience any internal stimulus to do it. Even when urged, cajoled, or threatened, he does not seem able to arouse any desire to do these things. Loss of positive motivation ranged from 65 per cent of the mild cases to 86 per cent of the severe cases.

Occasionally an actual or impending shift in a patient's life situation may serve to mobilize his constructive motivations. One notably retarded and apathetic patient was suddenly aroused when her husband became ill and she experienced a strong desire to help him. Another patient experienced a return of positive motivation when informed she was going to be hospitalized, a prospect she viewed as extremely distasteful.

Mild: The patient finds that he no longer spontaneously desires to do certain specific things, especially those that do not bring any immediate gratification. An advertising executive observes a loss of drive and initiative in planning a special sales promotion; a college professor finds himself devoid of any desire to prepare his lectures; a medical student loses his desire to study. A housewife, who formerly felt driven to engage in a variety of domestic and community projects, described her loss of motivation in the following terms: "I have no desire to do anything. I just do things mechanically without any feeling for what I'm doing. I just go through the motions like a robot and when I run down I just stop."

Moderate: In moderate cases the loss of spontaneous desire spreads to almost all of the patient's usual activities. A woman complained, "There are certain things I know I have to do like eat, brush my teeth, and go to the bathroom, but I have no desire to do them." In contrast to the severely-depressed patient, the moderately-depressed patient finds he can "force" himself to do things. Also, he is responsive to pressure from other people or to potentially embarrassing situations. A woman, for instance, waited in front of an elevator for about 15 minutes because she could not mobilize any desire to press the button. When others approached the elevator, however, she rapidly pressed the button lest they think she was peculiar.

Severe: In severe cases, there often is complete paralysis of the will. The patient has no desire to do anything, even those things that are essential to life. Consequently, he may be relatively immobile unless prodded or pushed into activity by others. It is sometimes necessary to pull the patient out of bed, wash, dress, and feed him. In extreme cases, even communication may be blocked by the patient's inertia. One woman, who was unable to respond to questions during the worst part of her depression, remarked later that even though she "wanted" to answer she could not summon the "will power" to do so.

Avoidance, Escapist, and Withdrawal Wishes*

The wish to break out of the usual pattern or routine of life is a common manifestation of depression. The clerk wants to get away from his paper work, the student daydreams of faraway places, and the housewife yearns to leave her domestic duties. The depressed individual regards his duties as dull, meaningless, or burdensome and wants to escape to an activity that offers relaxation or refuge.

These escapist wishes resemble the attitudes described as paralysis of the will. A useful distinction is that the escapist wishes are experienced as definite motivations with specific goals, whereas paralysis of the will refers to the loss or absence of motivation.

Mild: The mildly depressed patient experiences a strong inclination to avoid or to postpone doing certain things that he regards as uninteresting or taxing. He tends to shy away from attending to details that he considers to be unimportant. He is likely to procrastinate or avoid entirely an activity that does not promise immediate gratification or which involves effort. Just as he is repelled by activities that involve effort or responsibility, he is attracted to more passive and less complex activities.

A depressed student expressed this as follows: "It's much easier to daydream in lectures than pay attention. It's easier to stay home and drink than call a girl for a date. . . . It's easier to mumble and not be heard than to talk clearly and distinctly. It's much easier to write sloppily than to make the effort to write legibly. It's much easier to lead a self-centered, passive life than to make the effort to change it."

Moderate: In moderate cases, avoidance wishes are stronger and spread to a much wider range of his usual activities. A depressed college professor described this as follows: "Escape seems to be my strongest desire. I feel as though I would feel better in almost any other occupation or profession. As I ride the bus to the university, I wish I were the bus driver instead of a teacher."

The patient thinks continually of ways of diversion or escape. He would like to indulge in passive recreation such as going to the movies, watching television, or getting drunk. He daydreams of going to a desert island or of becoming a hobo. At this stage, he may withdraw from most social contacts since interpersonal relations seem to be too demanding. At the same time, because of his loneliness and increased dependency, he may want to be with other people.

* This symptom had not been included in the inventory administered to the patients; hence, there are no data available regarding its relative frequency. On the basis of clinical observation, I believe it is a frequent symptom.

Severe: In severe cases, the wish to avoid or escape is manifested in marked seclusiveness. Not infrequently the patient stays in bed, and when people approach, he may hide under the covers. A patient said, "I just feel like getting away from everybody and everything. I don't want to see any-body or do anything. All I want to do is sleep." One form of escape that generally occurs to the severely-depressed patient is suicide. The patient feels a strong desire to end his life as a way of escaping from a situation he regards as intolerable.

Suicidal Wishes

Suicidal wishes have historically been associated with a depressed state. While suicidal wishes may occur in nondepressed individuals, they occur substantially more frequently in depressed patients. In our series this was the symptom reported least frequently (12 per cent) by the nondepressed patients, but it was reported frequently (74 per cent) by the severely de-pressed patients. This difference indicates the diagnostic value of this par-ticular symptom in the identification of severe depression. The intensity with which this symptom was expressed also showed one of the highest cor-relations with the intensity of depression (Table 12–6).

The patient's interest in suicide may take a variety of forms. It may be experienced as a passive wish ("I wish I were dead"); an active wish ("I want to kill myself"); as a repetitive, obsessive thought without any volitional quality; as a daydream; or as a meticulously conceived plan. In some patients, the suicidal wishes occur constantly throughout the illness and the patient may have to battle continually to ward them off. In other cases, the wish is sporadic and is characterized by a gradual build-up, then a slackening of intensity until it disappears temporarily. Patients often report, once the wish has been dissipated, that they are glad they did not succumb to it. It should be noted that the impulsive suicidal attempt may be just as dangerous as the deliberately planned attempt.

The importance of suicidal symptoms is obvious, since nowadays it is practically the only feature of depression that poses a reasonably high probability of fatal consequences. The incidence of suicide among manic depressives ranged from 2.8 per cent in one study with a 10-year follow-up (Stenstedt, 1952) to 5 per cent in a 25-year period of observation (Rennie, 1942).

Mild: Wishes to die were reported by about 31 per cent of the mildly depressed patients. Often these take the passive form such as, "I would be better off dead." Although the patient states he would not do anything to hasten his death, he may find the idea of dying attractive. One patient looked forward to an airplane trip because of the possibility the plane might crash.

Sometimes, the patient expresses an indifference towards living ("I don't care whether I live or die."). Other patients may show an ambivalence ("I would like to die but at the same time I'm afraid of dying.").

Moderate: In these cases, suicidal wishes are more direct, frequent, and compelling; there is a definite risk of either impulsive or premeditated suicidal attempts. The patient may express his desire in the passive form: "I hope I won't wake up in the morning;" or, "If I died, my family would be better off." The active expression of the wish may vary from ambivalent statement, "I'd like to kill myself but I don't have the guts," to the bald assertion, "If I could do it and not botch it up, I would go ahead and kill myself." The suicidal wish may be manifested by the patient's taking unnecessary risks. A number of patients drove their cars at excessive rates of speed in the hope that something might happen.

Severe: In severe cases, suicidal wishes tend to be intense although the patient may be too retarded to complete a suicidal attempt. Among the typical statements are the following: "I feel so hopeless. Why won't you let me die." "It's no use. All is lost. There is only one way out—to kill myself." "I must weep myself to death. I can't live and you won't let me die." "I can't bear to live through another day. Please put me out of my misery."

Increased Dependency*

The term dependency is used here to designate the *desire* to receive help, guidance, or direction rather than the actual process of relying on someone else. The accentuated wishes for dependency have only occasionally been included in clinical descriptions of depression; they have, however, been recognized and assigned a major etiological role in several psychodynamic explanations of depression (Abraham, 1911; Rado, 1928). The accentuated orality attributed to depressed patients by those authors includes the kinds of wishes that are generally regarded as "dependent."

Since increased dependency has been attributed to other conditions as well as to depression, the question could be raised whether dependency can be justifiably listed as a *specific* manifestation of depression. Increased-dependency wishes are seen in an overt form in people who have an acute or chronic physical illness; moreover, covert or repressed dependency has been regarded by many theoreticians as the central factor in certain psychosomatic conditions such as peptic ulcer, as well as in alcoholism and other

---

* In our study, the degree of dependency motivation was not included in the inventory.

addictions. However, it is my contention that frank, undisguised, and intensified desires for help, support, and encouragement are very prominent elements in the advanced stages of depression and belong in any clinical description of this syndrome. In other conditions, intensified dependency may be a variable and transient characteristic.

The desire for help seems to transcend the realistic *need* for help, i.e., the patient can often reach his objective without assistance. Receiving help, however, appears to carry special emotional meaning for the patient beyond its practical importance and is often satisfying—at least temporarily.

Mild: The patient who is ordinarily very self-sufficient and independent begins to express a desire to be helped, guided, or supported. A patient, for instance, who always had insisted on driving when he was in the car with his wife, asked her to drive. He felt that he was capable of driving, but the idea of her driving was more appealing to him at this time.

As the dependency wishes become stronger, they tend to supersede the individual's habitual independent drives. He now finds that he prefers to have somebody do things with him rather than do them alone. The dependent desire does not seem to be simply a by-product of the feelings of helplessness and inadequacy or fatigue. The patient feels a craving for help even though he recognizes that he does not need it and when the help is received, he generally experiences some gratification and lessening of his depression.

Moderate: The patient's desire to have things done for him, to receive instruction and reassurance is stronger. The patience who experiences a wish for help in the mild phase now experiences this as a *need*. Receiving help no longer is an optional luxury but is now conceived of as a necessity. A depressed woman, who was legally separated from her husband, begged him to come back to her. "I need you desperately," she said. It was not clear to her exactly what she needed him for, except that she wanted to have a strong person near her.

When confronted with a task or problem, the moderately-depressed patient feels impelled to seek help before attempting to undertake it himself. He not infrequently states that he wants to be told what to do. Some patients shop around for opinions about a certain course of action and seem to be more involved in the idea of getting advice than in using it. One woman would ask numerous questions about trivial problems but did not seem to pay much attention to the content of the answer—just so an answer was forthcoming.

Severe: The intensity of the desire to be helped is increased and the content of the wish has a predominantly passive cast. It is couched almost exclusively in terms of wanting someone to do everything for the patient and to take care of him. The patient is no longer concerned about getting direction or advice, or in sharing problems. He wants the other person to do the job and to solve the problem for him. A patient clung to the physician and pleaded, "Doctor, you must help me." Her desire was for the psychiatrist to do everything for her without her doing anything. She even wanted the psychiatrist to adopt her children.

The patient may show his dependency by not wanting to leave the doctor's office or not wanting him to leave. Terminating the interview often becomes a difficult and painful process.

VEGETATIVE AND PHYSICAL MANIFESTATIONS

The physical and vegetative manifestations are considered by some authors to be evidence for a basic autonomic or hypothalamic disturbance that is responsible for the depressive state (Campbell, 1953; Kraines, 1957). These symptoms, contrary to expectation, have a relatively low correlation with each other and with clinical ratings of the depth of depression. The intercorrelation matrix is shown in Table 2–5. The frequency of the symptoms among depressed and nondepressed patients is shown in Table 2–6.

Table 2–5.
INTERCORRELATION OF PHYSICAL AND VEGETATIVE
SYMPTOMS ($n = 606$) *

Symptom	*Fatigue*	*Loss of sleep*	*Loss of appetite*	*Loss of libido*
Depth of depression	.31	.30	.35	.27
Fatigability		.25	.20	.29
Sleep disturbance			.35	.29
Loss of appetite				.33

n = No. of patients.
* Pearson product-moment correlation coefficients.

Loss of Appetite

For many patients, loss of appetite is often the first sign of an incipient depression and return of appetite may be the first sign that it is beginning to lift. Some degree of appetite loss was reported by 72 per cent of the severely-depressed patients and only 21 per cent of the nondepressed patients.

Mild: The patient may find that he no longer eats his meals with the

Table 2–6.
VEGETATIVE AND PHYSICAL MANIFESTATIONS: INCIDENCE AMONG
DEPRESSED AND NONDEPRESSED PATIENTS

	Degree of depression			
Manifestation	*None (%)* (n = 224)	*Mild (%)* (n = 288)	*Moderate (%)* (n = 377)	*Severe (%)* (n = 86)
Loss of appetite	21	40	54	72
Sleep disturbance	40	60	76	87
Loss of libido	27	38	58	61
Fatigability	40	62	80	78

n = No. of patients.

customary degree of relish or enjoyment. There is also some dulling of his desire for food.

Moderate: The desire for food mostly may be gone and the patient may miss a meal without realizing it.

Severe: The patient may have to force himself—or be forced—to eat. There may even be an aversion for food. After several weeks of severe depression, the amount of weight loss may be considerable.

Sleep Disturbance

Difficulty in sleeping is one of the most notable symptoms of depression, although it occurs in a large proportion of nondepressed patients as well. Eighty-seven per cent of the severely-depressed patients reported some interference with sleep. Difficulty in sleeping was reported by 40 per cent of the nondepressed patients.

There have been a number of careful studies of the sleep of depressed patients (see Chapter 9). The investigators have presented solid evidence, based on direct observation of the patients and EEG recordings during the night, that depressed patients sleep less than do normal controls. In addition, the studies show an excessive degree of restlessness and movement during the night among the depressed patients.

Mild: The patient reports waking a few minutes to half an hour earlier than usual. In many cases, the patient may state that, although ordinarily he sleeps soundly until awakened by the alarm clock, he now awakens several minutes before the alarm goes off. In some cases, the sleep disturbance is in the reverse direction: The patient finds that he sleeps more than usual.

Moderate: The patient awakens one or two hours earlier than usual.

He frequently reports that his sleep is not restful. Moreover, he seems to spend a greater proportion of the time in light sleep. He also may awaken after three or four hours of sleep and require a hypnotic to return to sleep. In some cases, the patient manifests an excessive sleeping tendency and may sleep up to twelve hours a day.

Severe: The patient frequently awakens after only four or five hours of sleep and finds it impossible to return to sleep. In some cases, the patients claim that they have not slept at all during the night; they state that they can remember "thinking" continuously during the night. It is likely, however, as Oswald *et al* (1963) point out, that the patients are actually in a light sleep for a good part of the time.

Loss of Libido

Some loss of interest in sex, whether of an auto-erotic or heterosexual nature, was reported by 61 per cent of the depressed patients and by 27 per cent of the nondepressed patients. Loss of libido correlated most highly with loss of appetite, loss of interest in other people, and depressed mood (see Appendix).

Mild: There is generally a slight loss of spontaneous sexual desire and of responsiveness to sexual stimuli. In some cases, however, sexual desire seems to be heightened when the patient is mildly depressed.

Moderate: Sexual desire is markedly reduced and is aroused only with considerable stimulation.

Severe: Any responsiveness to sexual stimuli is lost and the patient may have a pronounced aversion for sex.

Fatigability

Increased tiredness was reported by 79 per cent of the depressed patients and only 33 per cent of the nondepressed. Some patients appear to experience this symptom as a purely physical phenomenon: The limbs feel heavy or the body feels as though it is weighted down. Others express fatigability as a loss of "pep" or energy. The patient complains of feeling "listless," "worn out," "too weak to move," or "run down."

It is sometimes difficult to distinguish fatigability from loss of motivation and avoidance wishes. It is interesting to note that fatigability correlates more highly with lack of satisfaction (.36) and with pessimistic outlook (.36) than with other physical or vegetative symptoms such as loss of appetite (.20) and sleep disturbance (.28) (see Appendix). The correlation with lack of satisfaction and pessimistic outlook suggests that the mental set may be a major factor in the patient's feeling of tiredness;

the converse, of course, should be considered as a possibility, viz., that tiredness influences the mental set.

Some authors have conceptualized depression as a "depletion syndrome" because of the prominence of fatigability; they postulate that the patient exhausts his available energy during the period prior to the onset of the depression and that the depressed state represents a kind of hibernation, during which the patient gradually builds up a new store of energy. Sometimes the fatigue is attributed to the sleep disturbance. Against this theory is the observation that even when the patients do get more sleep as a result of hypnotics, there is rarely any improvement in the feeling of fatigue. It is interesting to note, furthermore, that the correlation between sleep disturbance and fatigability is only .28. If the sleep disturbance were a major factor, a substantially higher correlation would be expected. As will be discussed in Chapter 17, fatigability may be a manifestation of loss of positive motivation.

There tends to be a diurnal variation in fatigability parallel to low mood and negative expectations. The patient tends to feel more tired upon awakening, but somewhat less tired as the day progresses.

Mild: The patient finds that he tires more easily than usual. If he has had a hypomanic period just prior to the depression, the contrast is marked: Whereas previously he could be very active for many hours without any feeling of tiredness, he now feels fatigued after a relatively short period of work. Not infrequently a diversion or a short nap may restore a feeling of vitality, but the improvement is transient.

Moderate: The patient is generally tired when he awakens in the morning. Almost any activity seems to accentuate his tiredness. Rest, relaxation, and recreation do not appear to alleviate this feeling and may, in fact, aggravate it. A patient who customarily walked great distances when well would feel exhausted after short walks when depressed. Not only physical activity, but focused mental activity such as reading, often increases the sense of tiredness.

Severe: The patient complains that he is too tired to do anything. Under external pressure he is sometimes able to perform tasks requiring a large expenditure of energy. Without such external stimulation, however, he does not seem to be able to mobilize his energy to perform even simple tasks such as dressing himself. He may complain for instance, that he does not have enough strength even to lift his arm.

DELUSIONS

Delusions in depression may be grouped into several categories: delusions of worthlessness; delusions of the "unpardonable" sin and of being punished or expecting punishment; nihilistic delusions; somatic delusions; and delusions of poverty. Any of the cognitive distortions described above may progress in intensity and achieve sufficient rigidity to warrant its being considered a delusion. A person with low self-esteem, for instance, may progress in his thinking to believing that he is the devil. A person with a tendency to blame himself may eventually begin to ascribe to himself certain crimes such as the assassination of the President.

To determine the frequency of the various delusions among psychotically depressed patients, a series of 280 psychotic patients were interviewed. The results are shown in Table 2–7.

Table 2–7.

FREQUENCY OF DELUSIONS WITH DEPRESSIVE CONTENT AMONG PSYCHOTIC PATIENTS VARYING IN DEPTH OF DEPRESSION ($n = 280$)

Delusion	Depth of depression			
	None (%) (n = 85)	*Mild (%)* (n = 68)	*Moderate (%)* (n = 77)	*Severe (%)* (n = 50)
Worthless	6	9	21	48
Sinner	11	19	29	46
Devil	3	4	3	14
Punishment	18	21	18	42
Dead	0	2	3	10
Body decaying	9	13	16	24
Fatal illness	5	6	14	20

n = No. of patients.

Delusions of Worthlessness

Delusions of worthlessness occurred in 48 per cent of the severely-depressed psychotics. This delusion was expressed in the following way by one patient: "I must weep myself to death. I cannot live. I cannot die. I have failed so. It would be better if I had not been born. My life has always been a burden. . . . I am the most inferior person in the world. . . . I am subhuman." Another patient said, "I am totally useless. I can't do anything. I have never done anything worthwhile."

Crime and Punishment

The patient believes he has committed a terrible crime for which he deserves or expects to be punished. Forty-six per cent of the severely-depressed, psychotic patients reported the delusion of being very bad sinners. In many cases, the patient feels that severe punishment such as torture or hanging is imminent. Forty-two per cent of the severely-depressed patients expected punishment of some type. Many other patients believed that they were being punished and that the hospital was a kind of penal institution. The patient wails, "Will God never give up?" "Why must I be singled out for punishment?" "My heart is gone. Can't He see this? Can't He let me alone?" In some cases the patient may believe that he is the devil; 14 per cent of the severely depressed psychotics had this delusion.

Nihilistic Delusions

Nihilistic delusions have traditionally been associated with depression. A typical nihilistic delusion is reflected in the following statement: "It's no use. All is lost. The world is empty. Everybody died last night." Sometimes the patient believes that he himself is dead; this occurred in 10 per cent of the severely-depressed patients.

Organ preoccupation is particularly common in nihilistic delusions. The patients complain that an organ is missing or that all their viscera have been removed. This was expressed in statements such as "My heart, my liver, my intestines are gone. I'm nothing but an empty shell."

Somatic Delusions

The patient believes that his body is deteriorating, or that he has some incurable disease. Twenty-four per cent of the severely depressed believed that their bodies were decaying. Twenty per cent believed that they had fatal illnesses. Somatic delusions are expressed in statements such as the following: "I can't eat. The taste in my mouth is terrible. My guts are diseased. They can't digest the food;" "I can't think. My brain is all blocked up;" "My intestines are blocked. The food can't get through." Allied to the idea of having a severe abnormality is a patient's statement, "I haven't slept at all in six months."

Delusion of Poverty

Delusions of poverty seem to be an outgrowth of the overconcern with finances manifested by depressed patients. A wealthy patient may complain bitterly, "All my money is gone. What will I live on? Who will buy food for my children?" Many authors have described the incongruity of a man of means who, dressed in rags, goes begging for alms or food.

In our study, delusions of poverty were not investigated. Because of the very high proportion of low-income patients in the series, it was difficult to distinguish a delusion of poverty from actual poverty.

In Rennie's study (1942), nearly half of the 99 cases had delusions as part of their psychoses. Forty-nine patients had ideas of persecution or of passivity. (The number of persons with each of these delusions is not given.) Typical depressive delusions were found in 25 patients: These dealt predominantly with self-blame and self-depreciation and with ideas of being dead, of their bodies being changed, or of immorality. Delusions were most common in the oldest age group (72 per cent). In patients more than 50 the content revolved predominantly around ideas of poverty, of being destroyed or tortured in some horrible manner, of being poisoned, or of being contaminated by feces.

HALLUCINATIONS

Rennie found that 25 per cent of the patients had hallucinations. This was most prominent in the recurrent depressive group. Samples of the types of hallucinations were as follows: "I conversed with God." "I heard the sentence, 'Your daughter is dead'." "I heard people talking through my stomach." "I saw a star on Christmas day." "I saw and heard my dead mother." "Voices told me not to eat." "Voices told me to walk backward." "Saw and heard God and angels." "Saw dead father." "Animal faces in the food." "Saw and heard animals." "Saw dead people." "Heard brother's and dead people's voices." "Saw husband in his coffin." "A voice said, 'Do not stay with your husband'." "Saw snakes and Negroes." "Saw two men digging a grave."

In our study, we found that 13 per cent of the severely-depressed, psychotic patients acknowledged hearing voices that condemned them. This was the most frequent type of hallucination reported.

CLINICAL EXAMINATION

APPEARANCE

The psychiatrists in our study made ratings of the intensity of certain clinical features in the depressed and nondepressed patients. Many of these features would be considered *signs*; i.e., they are abstracted from observable behaviors rather than from the patients' self-descriptions. Other features were evaluated on the basis of the patients' verbal reports as well as on the observation of their behavior. Some of the clinical features overlap those described in the previous section. This particular study provides an opportunity to compare the frequency of symptoms elicited in response to the inventory with the frequency of symptoms derived from a clinical examination.

The sample consisted of the last 486 patients of the 966 patients previously described in Table 2–2. The distribution of the clinical features among the nondepressed, mildly depressed, moderately depressed, and severely depressed are found in Table 2–8.

Table 2–8.
FREQUENCY OF CLINICAL FEATURES OF PATIENTS VARYING IN
DEPTH OF DEPRESSION ($n = 486$)

Clinical feature	Depth of depression			
	None (%)	Mild (%)	Moderate (%)	Severe (%)
Sad facies	18	72	94	98
Stooped posture	6	32	70	87
Crying in interview	3	11	29	28
Speech: slow, etc.	25	53	72	75
Low mood	16	72	94	94
Diurnal variation of mood	6	13	37	37
Suicidal wishes	13	47	73	94
Indecisiveness	18	42	68	83
Hopelessness	14	58	85	86
Feeling inadequate	25	56	75	90
Conscious guilt	27	46	64	60
Loss of interest	14	56	83	92
Loss of motivation	23	54	88	88
Fatigability	39	62	89	84
Sleep disturbance	31	55	73	88
Loss of appetite	17	33	61	88
Constipation	19	26	38	52

n = No. of patients.

Most cases of depression can be diagnosed by inspection (Lehmann, 1959). The sad, melancholic expression combined with either retardation or agitation are practically pathognomonic of depression. On the other hand, many patients conceal their unpleasant feelings behind a cheerful facade ("smiling depression") and it may require careful interviewing to bring out a pained facial expression.

The facies show typical characteristics that are associated with sadness. The corners of the mouth are turned down, the brow is furrowed, the lines and wrinkles are deepened, and the eyes are often red from crying. Among the descriptions used by clinicians are glum, forlorn, gloomy, dejected, unsmiling, solemn, wearily resigned (Lewis, 1934). Lewis reported weeping occurred in most of the women, but in only one-sixth of the men in his sample.

In severe cases, the facies may appear to be frozen in a gloomy expression. Most patients, however, show some lability of expression, especially when their attention is diverted away from their feelings. Genuine smiles may be elicited at times even in the severe cases, but they are generally transient. Some patients present a forced or social smile, which may be deceiving. The so-called mirthless smile, which indicates a lack of any genuine amusement, is easily recognized. This type of smile may be elicited in response to a humorous remark by the examiner and indicates the patient's intellectual awareness of the humor but without any emotional response to it.

A sad facies was observed in 85 per cent of the depressed group (including mild, moderate, and severe cases) and in 18 per cent of the non-depressed group. In the severely depressed group, 98 per cent showed this characteristic.

RETARDATION

The most striking sign of a retarded depression is reduction in spontaneous activity. The patient tends to stay in one position longer than usual and to use a minimum of gestures. His movements are slow and deliberate as though his body and limbs are weighted down. He walks slowly, frequently hunched over, and with a shuffling gait. These postural characteristics were observed in 87 per cent of the severely-depressed patients in our sample.

The speech shows decreased spontaneity and the verbal output is reduced. The patient does not initiate a conversation or volunteer statements and, when questioned, responds in a few words. Sometimes, speaking is decreased only when a painful subject is being discussed. The pitch of the patient's voice is often lowered and he tends to speak in a monotone. These vocal characteristics were observed in 75 per cent of the severely-depressed patients.

The more retarded patients may start sentences but not complete them. They may answer questions with grunts or groans. The most severe cases may be mute. As Lewis points out, it is sometimes difficult to distinguish the scanty talk of a depressive from that of a well-preserved, suspicious, paranoid schizophrenic. In both conditions, there may be pauses, hesitations, evasion, breaking-off, and brevity. The diagnosis must rest on other observations—of content and behavior.

In severe depressions the patient may manifest signs of a syndrome that has been labelled *stupor* or *semi-stupor*. (Hoch, 1921). If left alone, he may remain practically motionless whether standing, sitting, or lying in bed. There is rarely, if ever, any waxy flexibility as seen in catatonia or any apparent clouding of consciousness. The patients vary in the degree to which they respond to stimulation. Some respond to sustained efforts by the examiner to establish rapport; others appear oblivious. I questioned several patients in the latter category after they recovered from their depression and they reported that they had experienced feelings and thoughts during clinical examination but had felt incapable of expressing them in any way.

In extreme cases, the patient does not eat or drink even with urging. Food placed in his mouth may remain there until removed and under such circumstances tube feeding becomes necessary as a life-preserving measure. Sometimes, the patient does not move his bowels and digital removal of feces or enemas are necessary. Saliva accumulates and drools out of his mouth. He blinks infrequently and may develop corneal ulcers. A more complete description of these extreme cases will be found in the section on Benign Stupors in Chapter 8.

Bleuler (1911, p. 209) described the melancholic triad consisting of depressive affect, inhibition of action, and inhibition of thinking. The first two characteristics are certainly typical of retarded depression. There is, however, a strong question as to whether there is an inhibition of the thought process. Lewis (1934) believes that thinking is active—or even hyperactive—even though speech is inhibited. Refined psychological tests, furthermore, have failed to show significant interference with thought processes (Chapter 10).

AGITATION

The chief characteristic of the agitated patient is his ceaseless activity. He cannot sit still but moves about constantly in the chair. He conveys a sense of restlessness and disturbance in wringing his hands or handkerchief, tearing his clothing, picking at his skin, and clenching and unclenching his fingers. He may rub his scalp or other parts of his body until the skin is worn away.

He may get out of his chair many times in the course of an interview and pace the floor. At night, he may get out of bed frequently and walk incessantly back and forth. It is just as difficult for him to engage in constructive activity as it is for him to stay still. His agitation is also manifested by frequent moans and groans. He approaches the doctors, nurses, and other patients and besieges them with requests or pleas for reassurance.

The emotions of frenzy and anguish are congruent with his thought content. He wails, "Why did I do it. Oh, God, what is to become of me.

Please have mercy on me." He believes that he is about to be butchered or buried alive. He moans, "My bowels are gone. It's intolerable." He screams, "I can't stand the pain. Please put me out of my misery." He groans, "My home is gone. My family is gone. I just want to die. Please let me die."

The thought content of the retarded patient appears to revolve around passive resignation to his fate. The agitated patient, on the other hand, cannot accept or tolerate the torture he envisions. The agitated behavior appears to represent desperate attempts to fight off his impending doom.

Chapter 3.
Course and Prognosis

DEPRESSION AS A CLINICAL ENTITY

In the previous chapter, depression was treated as a psychopathological dimension or syndrome. The clinical features of depression were examined in cross-section, i.e., in terms of the cluster of pathological phenomena exhibited at a given point in time. In this chapter, depression is treated as a discrete clinical entity (such as manic-depressive reaction or neurotic-depressive reaction) that has certain specific characteristics occurring over time: in terms of onset, recovery, and recurrence. As a clinical entity or reaction type, depression has many salient characteristics that distinguish it from other clinical types such as schizophrenia, even though these other types may have depressive elements associated with them. The depressive constellation as a concomitant of other nosological entities will not be described in this chapter but will be considered later in terms of its association with schizophrenic symptomatology in the schizo-affective category (Chapter 8).

Among the important characteristics of the clinical entity of depression are the following: There is generally a well-defined onset, a progression in the severity of the symptoms until the condition bottoms out, and then a steady regression (improvement) of the symptoms until the episode is over; the remissions are spontaneous; there is a tendency toward recurrence; the intervals between attacks are free of depressive symptoms.

IMPORTANCE OF COURSE AND OUTCOME

The *longitudinal* aspects of depression have been the subject of many investigations since the time of Kraepelin. Adequate information regarding the short-term and long-term course of depression is important, not only for practical management, but also for an understanding of the psychopathology, and for evaluation of specific forms of treatment. Considerable data on the life histories of depressed patients were accumulated before the advent of the specific therapeutic agents—electroconvulsive therapy (ECT) and drugs. These data are generally regarded as reflecting the natural history of the disorder, although it is difficult to separate out the effects of hospitalization.

The physician charged with making a determination of the prognosis in a given case is confronted with a number of questions.

1. In the case of a first episode of depression, what are the prospects for complete recovery, and what is the likelihood of residual symptoms or of a chronic, unrecovered state?

2. What is the probable duration of the first attack?

3. What is the likelihood of recurrence, and what is the probable duration of any multiple attacks?

4. How long must one wait following a patient's recovery from a given attack before ruling out the likelihood of recurrence?

5. What is the risk of death through suicide?

Answers to these questions can be provided by reference to cases diagnosed as manic-depressive psychoses. A number of fairly well-designed studies have been conducted to determine the fate of such patients. It should be emphasized that the available data applies primarily to hospitalized patients.

In the case of affective disorders other than manic depressive, the available data is either too unreliable or too scanty to allow definite conclusions. The diagnosis of involutional melancholia (Chapter 7) is subject to so much variation that the findings of any particular study cannot be generalized in any scientific sense. A particular sample diagnosed as involutional depression at one hospital would inevitably include a high proportion of cases that would be diagnosed as manic depressive or schizophrenic at hospitals deemphasizing the use of the label of involutional melancholia.

It is even more difficult to arrive at any conclusions regarding the duration, outcome, and relapse rate of the newer splinter groups, such as neurotic-depressive reactions and psychotic-depressive reactions. There are several reasons for this. First, since these nosological categories have come into use only recently, there has not been sufficient time for long-term observation. Second, the preponderance of the neurotic-depressive cases have been treated in private practice or in outpatient clinics; statistical surveys are more difficult to carry out under such circumstances. Third, since most patients in these two groups have received modern psychiatric management—psychotherapy, drugs, or electroconvulsive therapy—it is difficult to picture clearly the spontaneous ebb and flow of these conditions. It will probably be possible to obtain some relevant data from drug studies using a group of such patients as placebo-controls. A series described by Paskind as "manic depressive" in 1930 undoubtedly contained a preponderance of cases that would currently be diagnosed as "neurotic-depressive reactions." Since this study antedated the modern somatic therapies, the findings may be assumed to be relevant to the natural history of neurotic depressive reactions.

SYSTEMATIC STUDIES

Kraepelin (1913) studied the general course of 899 cases of manic-depressive phychosis. The period of observation varied considerably; some patients were followed for brief periods and others for as long as 40 years. Moreover, since the follow-up depended largely on readmission to the hospital, the information on patients who were not readmitted is scanty. Despite these limitations, his study is of great value in providing solid facts regarding recurrent episodes; frequency and duration of the attacks, and duration of the intervals between attacks.

His sample is as follows: single depression, 263; recurrent depression, 177; biphasic* single episode, 106; combined, recurrent, 214; single manic episode, 102; and recurrent manic, 47.

A study of Paskind (1929, 1930a, 1930b) of cases of depression seen in private practice presents the most complete data available on the course of depressions observed outside the hospital. Although there are many serious methodological deficiencies in this study, the data presented are relevant to milder episodes of depression. Paskind reviewed the records of 633 cases of depression in the private practice of Dr. Q. T. Patrick. Although all of these cases had been placed in the all-inclusive category of manic-depressive phychosis, a review of the case histories presented in the articles leaves little doubt that these cases would be diagnosed as neurotic-depressive reactions according to the new nomenclature. In reviewing the tabulated data presented by the author, it is apparent that his findings are based on 248 cases abstracted from the original group. The cases were collected over a period of 32 years, but there is no mention of the average period of observation nor of any systematic attempt to obtain follow-up material on these patients. Paskind noted that 88 cases (32 per cent of the 248) could be classified as "brief attacks of manic-depressive

---

* The term biphasic is used to denote cases in which both manic and depressive episodes occurred. These cases have been designated by a variety of terms: compound, mixed, combined, double-form, cyclothymic, and cyclical. The alternating and circular types refer to cases in which one phase follows immediately after the opposite phase without any free interval. The "closed circular type" refers to uninterrupted cycles of manic and depressive phases.

psychosis," since the average duration of the episodes ranged from a few hours to a few days.

Paskind describes the symptoms of the short attacks as being exactly like those of longer attacks: profound sadness and unhappiness without obvious cause; self-reproach; self-blame; self-derogation; lack of initiative; lack of response to usual interests accompanied by a keen awareness of this lack; avoidance of friends; a feeling of hopelessness; death wishes; and inclinations or desire to commit suicide. Paskind states that the well-known antidotes for depression, such as a philosophic outlook, the company of friends, amusements, diversions, rest, change of scene, and good news do not cause the attacks to disappear. "Instead one finds a person in a normal mood who without apparent cause becomes within a brief period profoundly sad and unhappy; in spite of all attempts to cheer him, the attack remains for from a few hours to a few days; when it does disappear it does so as abruptly and mysteriously as it came."

Rennie (1942) did a follow-up study of 208 patients with manic-depressive reactions admitted to the Henry Phipps Psychiatric Clinic between 1913 and 1916. Atypical cases were not included because the author wanted to study only clear-cut, manic-depressive reactions. Several patients having what seemed to be manic excitements at the time of admission developed schizophrenic reactions on long-term observation. These cases were excluded, as were cases of depression that had lost the preponderant depressive affect and had, in the course of years, evolved slowly into more automatic and schizophrenic-like behavior. Also excluded were depressive patients with hypochondriasis who had lost most of their depressive affect and who had sunk into a state of chronic invalidism with little depressive content. The material, consequently, can be regarded as following reasonably stringent criteria for diagnosing the manic-depressive syndrome.

Follow-up on these patients was obtained by letter, by social service interview, by physician's interview, by newspaper notices of suicide, and by records from other hospitals. In only one case was no follow-up data obtained. The follow-up period evidently ranged from 35 to 39 years.

In Rennie's study, the following clinical groups were described in order of frequency: (1) recurrent depression: 102 patients—15 had symptom-free intervals of at least 20 years between attacks, and 52 had remissions of at least 10 years; (2) Cyclothymic (biphasic), 49 patients in whom all combinations were observed, with elation and depression sometimes following each other in closed cycles; (3) single attacks of depression, recovered—26 patients; (4) single attacks of depression, unrecovered—14 patients, of whom 9 committed suicide; (5) recurrent manic attacks, 14 cases; (6) single manic attacks—two patients (These remained well for over 20 years after the attack. A third patient became manic for the first time at age 40 and was still hospitalized at age 64).

A comparison of the relative frequency of depressed, biphasic, and manic patients observed in various studies is presented in Chapter 6.

Lundquist (1945) made a longitudinal study of 319 manic-depressive patients whose first hospitalization for this disorder was at the Langbrö Hospital in the years 1912–1931. The investigator reviewed the records and checked the appropriateness of the diagnoses to "satisfy all reasonable demands in regard to reliability." His sample consisted of 123 men (38 per cent) and 196 women (62 per cent).

After locating the discharged patients, follow-up was conducted by a personal examination of the patient at the hospital, by a home visit by a social worker if the patient lived in Stockholm, by a detailed questionnaire mailed to the patient living outside of Stockholm, and by a review of the hospital record of the patient currently hospitalized elsewhere.

The period of observation varied considerably: between 20–30 years, 42 per cent; 10–20 years, 38 per cent; and less than 10 years, 20 per cent.

The duration of an episode was defined as the time that elapsed between the patient's recognition of his symptoms and his return to his former occupation. Recovery was based on the rough gauge of the patient's ability to resume his work and his ordinary mode of life.

Onset of Episodes

The relative frequency of an insidious onset, as compared with an acute onset, was studied by Hopkinson (1963). One hundred consecutive inpatients diagnosed as having an affective illness were investigated. All were more than 50 years of age on admission, and 39 had suffered previous attacks before the age of 50. Eighty patients were examined personally by the author, and in the remaining 20 cases, the pertinent data were abstracted from the case histories.

When the onset of the illness was studied, it was found that 26 per cent of the cases exhibited a well-defined prodromal period; the remaining 74 per cent of the cases were considered of acute onset. Complaints made by these patients in the prodromal period were vague and nonspecific. Tension and anxiety occurred in all to some extent. The duration of the prodromal period before the onset of a clear-cut depressive psychosis ranged from 8 months to 10 years; the mean duration was 33.5 months.

In a later study (1965), Hopkinson investigated the prodromal phase in 43 younger patients (ages 16–48). Thirteen (30.2 per cent) showed a prodromal phase of 2 months to 7 years (mean = 23 months). The clinical

features of the prodromal period were chiefly tension, anxiety, and indecision.

In summary, 70–75 per cent of the patients, in both studies, with an
affective disorder had an acute onset.

The relationship of acuteness of onset to prognosis has been studied by
several investigators. Steen (1933) found, in a study of 493 patients, that
the recovery rate was higher among manic depressives who showed an acute
onset than among those with a protracted onset. On the other hand,
Strecker *et al.* (1931), in a comparison of 50 recovered manic depressives
and 50 nonrecovered, found that an acute onset ocurred no more frequently in the recovered group than in the chronic group. More recently,
in a study of 96 cases grossly diagnosed as manic depressive, Astrup,
Fossum, and Holmboe (1959) found that an acute onset favored recovery.

Hopkinson (1965) found a significantly higher *frequency* of attacks
per patient among his cases with an acute onset (mean = 2.8) than among
those patients with a prodromal phase (mean = 1.3).

Lundquist (1945) reported that patients over 30 with an acute onset
(less than a month) had a significantly shorter *duration* of their episodes
than those with a gradual onset. In the age group of 30–39 years, the mean
duration of the acute onset cases was 5.1 months and of the gradual onset
cases, 27.2 months.

The average age of onset of depression varies so widely from study to
study that no definite conclusions can be made. The following statistics
for the decade of peak incidence may serve as a rough guide: 20–30,
Kraepelin (1913); 30–39, Stenstedt (1952), Cassidy, Flanagan, and
Spellman (1957), and Ayd (1961); 45–55, Rennie (1942); and 50 and
older, Lundquist (1945).

Recovery and Chronicity

There is considerable variation among the authors on the proportion
of patients remaining chronically ill following the onset of depressive illness. It is difficult to make comparisons among the various studies because
different diagnostic criteria are used, the definition of chronicity varies,
the periods of observation vary, and in many studies, no distinction is
made between those who became chronic after the first attack and those
who became chronic only after multiple attacks.

The relatively well-designed, retrospective study by Rennie indicated
that approximately 3 per cent were found on long-term follow-up to be
chronically ill. Kraepelin reported that 5 per cent of his cases became
chronic. Lundquist reported that 79.6 per cent of the depressives recovered

completely from the first attack. Age of onset was a factor: The recovery rate ranged from 92 per cent for patients less than 30 years old to 75 per cent in the 30–40 age group. It is probable that his percentages are lower than those of the others because of his more stringent definition of complete recovery.

Astrup, Fossum, and Holmboe (1959) divided their group of manic-depressive patients into the categories of "chronic," "improved," and "recovered." Of the 70 "pure" manic depressives, 6 (8.6 per cent) were still chronically ill at the time of follow-up. The majority had recovered completely, and a minority showed residual "instability" and were classified as improved.* The follow-up period was five years or more.

It is noteworthy that a patient may have an initial manic or depressive episode from which he recovers completely and, after a long symptom-free interval, he may relapse into a chronic state. Rennie reports the case of a patient who had an initial episode of mania followed by depression, the entire cycle lasting about a year. He was symptom-free for 23 years afterward and then he lapsed into a state of manic excitement lasting 22 years.

Kraepelin (1913) indicates that a patient may have chronic depression of many years' duration and still have a complete remission. He presents an illustrative case (p. 143) with a single attack lasting 15 years, from which the patient made a complete recovery.

DURATION

Some idea of the average or expected duration of an episode of depression is obviously important so that the physician can adequately prepare the patient and family psychologically and give them a basis for making decisions about the business affairs of the patient as well as appropriate financial arrangements for his care.

One aspect of the usual depressive episode that is of importance in treatment is the fact that the episode tends to follow a curve, i.e., tends to progressively worsen, then bottoms out, and then progressively improves until the patient returns to his premorbid state. By determining the time of onset of the depression, the physician can make a rough estimate as to when an upward turn in the cycle may be expected. It is particularly important when assessing the efficacy of specific forms of treatment to take into account the spontaneous start of the upward swing.

There is some variation in the findings of the numerous studies relevant to duration. Undoubtedly, these variations may be attributed to dif-

* The precise figures for the improved and recovered categories are not available from Astrup's monograph because of the lumping together of the manic-depressive and schizo-affective patients.

ferent methods of observation and to different criteria for making diagnoses and judging improvement. In general, the relatively unrefined clinical studies (which will be discussed presently) indicate a longer duration than do the systematic studies.

Lundquist (1945) found that the median duration of the attack of depression in patients younger than 30 was 6.3 months, and for those older than 30, 8.7 months. This difference was statistically significant. There was no significant difference between men and women in regard to duration. (As noted previously, he also found acute onset associated with shorter duration). Paskind (1930b) also found in his outpatient group a shorter duration of attacks occurring before age 30 than after age 30. Rennie's study yielded similar results, the first episode lasting on the average 6.5 months. He found, incidentally, that the average duration of hospitalization was 2.5 months. In Paskind's series of non-hospitalized depressives, the median duration was 3 months. He found that 14 per cent of the episodes lasted one month or less, and that almost 80 per cent were completed in six months or less.

The earlier, less refined studies predominantly report a period of 6–18 months as the average duration of the first attack: Kraepelin (1913), 6–8 months; Pollack (1931), 1.1 years; Strecker *et al.* (1931), 1.5 years. The clinical impression of the recent writers of monographs on depression shows similar variation. Kraines (1957) states that the average depressive episode lasts about 18 months. Ayd (1961) reports that prior to age 30, the attacks average 6–12 months; between the ages of 30 and 50, they average 9–18 months; and after 50, they tend to persist longer, with many patients remaining ill from three to five years.

In regard to the *duration of multiple episodes* of depression, there has been a prevalent opinion among clinicians that there is a trend towards prolongation of the episodes with each recurrence (Kraepelin, 1913). Lundquist, however, performed a statistical analysis of the duration of multiple episodes and found there was no significant increase in duration with successive attacks. Paskind's (1930b) study of outpatient cases similarly showed that the attacks do not become longer as the disease recurs. The median duration for first attacks was four months, and for second, third, or subsequent attacks three months.

The differences in the findings between the rough clinical studies and the statistical studies may reflect a difference in samples and/or different criteria for recovery from the depression. It is probable that certain biases influenced the selection of cases in the less refined studies and, therefore, the samples cannot be considered representative.

Lundquist found a significant association between prolonged duration and the presence of delusions in younger but not older patients. The presence of confusion, on the other hand, favored a shorter duration.

Brief Attacks of Manic-Depressive Psychosis

Paskind (1929) described 88 cases of depression of very brief duration; viz., from a few hours to a few days. These patients had essentially the same symptoms as those in his other extramural cases of longer duration and constituted 13.9 per cent of his large series of cases diagnosed as manic-depressive disorder. The case histories he presents leave little doubt that they would currently be diagnosed as neurotic-depressive reaction.

Most of these patients with brief attacks also experienced longer episodes of depression. In 51, the brief attacks came first, and were followed from months to decades later by longer attacks lasting from several weeks to several years. In 18, longer attacks occurred first, and were followed by the transient episodes. In nine, there were brief episodes only.

RECURRENCE

There is considerable variation in the literature relevant to the frequency of relapses among depressed patients. Except as indicated, the statistics for manic-depressive psychosis include some manic patients in addition to the depressed patients. In the earlier studies, German authors reported a substantially higher incidence of recurrence than American investigators (Lundquist, 1945). These differences may be attributed to more stringent diagnostic criteria and to longer periods of observation by the German authors.

Of the more refined studies, Rennie's reported relapse rate is closer to that of the German writers than to the other American investigators. He found that 97 of 123 patients (79 per cent) initially admitted to the hospital in a depressed state subsequently had a recurrence of depression. (These figures do not include 14 patients who committed suicide after the first admission or who remained chronically ill.) When the cyclothymic cases (i.e., patients who had at least one manic attack in addition to the depression) are added to this group, the proportion of relapse is 142 patients of 170 (84 per cent).

The Scandinavian investigators Lundquist (1945) and Stenstedt (1952) reported, respectively, a 49 per cent and a 47 per cent incidence of relapse. In comparing their studies with Rennie's, one can reasonably conclude that the more stringent diagnostic criteria employed by Rennie and the longer period of observation of his sample may account for the higher percentage of relapses in his report.

The differences in relapse rate are reflected in a striking difference in the rate of multiple recurrences. In Rennie's series more than half of the depressed patients had three or more recurrences (see Table 3–1).

Table 3–1.
FREQUENCY OF SINGLE AND MULTIPLE ATTACKS OF DEPRESSION

Frequency of depression	Rennie		Lundquist	
	No. of patients	(%)	No. of patients	(%)
1 attack	26	21.0	105	61.0
2 attacks	33	27.0	45	26.0
3 attacks	28	23.0	11	6.5
4 + attacks	36	29.0	11	6.5
TOTAL	123	100	172	100

The frequency of multiple recurrences in the cyclothymic cases was particularly high in Rennie's series. Thirty-seven of the 47 patients in the group had four or more episodes. In Kraepelin's series, 204 out of 310 cases of this type (67 per cent) had one or more recurrences, with more than half having three or more attacks.

Another important aspect of the recurrent attacks is their duration. The opinion has frequently been expressed that the episodes become progressively longer with each recurrence. Rennie, however, in analyzing his data, found that the second episode had the same duration as the initial episode in 20 per cent, was longer in 35 per cent, and was shorter in 45 per cent. Paskind found that the median duration decreased with successive attacks.

INTERVALS BETWEEN ATTACKS

In examining the literature on the intervals between episodes of depression, one is struck by the fact that recurrences may occur after years, or even decades, of apparent good health. The systematic studies offer little encouragement for the notion of a permanent cure analogous to five year cures reported for cancer treatment. Recurrences have been reported as long as 40 years after recovery from an initial depression (Kraepelin).

The findings presented by Rennie, in particular, are noteworthy in that the highest proportion of relapses occurred 10–20 years after the initial episode of depression. His follow-up showed the following relapse rate for his 97 cases of recurrent depressions: Recurrence less than 10 years after the first attack of depression in 35 per cent; 10–20 years, 52 per cent; more than 20 years, 13 per cent. It should be emphasized that 65 per cent had recurrences after remissions of 10–30 years.

In an earlier study, Kraepelin had tabulated the symptom-free intervals between 703 episodes of depression. Unlike Rennie's study, Kraepelin's included intervals after the second and later attacks (as well as intervals between the first and second episodes). He found that with each successive attack the intervals tended to become shorter. Since his series consisted of hospitalized patients, it is interesting to note the same trend among the extramural patients in Paskind's study. A comparison of the distribution of intervals in ten-year categories is shown in Table 3–2. For the purposes of comparison, Rennie's results are also included. It should be emphasized that his findings apply only to the *first* interval. The tendency for his intervals to be longer than Kraepelin's and Paskind's may be explained by the fact that the later intervals included in their study are shorter than the first intervals.

Table 3–2.

COMPARISON OF DISTRIBUTION OF TIME INTERVALS BETWEEN
MANIC-DEPRESSIVE EPISODES IN INPATIENT AND OUTPATIENTS

Source	No. of intervals	Duration of time intervals (%)				
		0–9 yrs.	10–19 yrs.	20–29 yrs.	30–39 yrs.	More than 40 yrs.
Kraepelin (1913) (inpatients)	703	80.5	13.5	4.8	1.1	.14
Paskind (1930b) (outpatients)	438	64.0	27.8	5.7	1.6	.92
Rennie (1942) (inpatients)	97*	35.0	52.0	15.0		

* Includes only *first* interval (i.e. between first and second episodes).

Kraepelin and Paskind show a somewhat similar distribution of the intervals, with Paskind's outpatient cases having longer periods of remission than Kraepelin's hospitalized cases.

Another way of expressing the duration of the intervals is in terms of the median duration of the specific intervals. Table 3–3 shows that the median interval is longer in the outpatient cases of Paskind, and also that in both outpatient and hospitalized cases the median intervals tend to be shorter with successive attacks.

Table 3–3.

COMPARISON OF MEDIAN INTERVALS FOR INPATIENTS AND OUTPATIENTS

	No. of cases	First interval (yrs.)	Second interval (yrs.)	Third and subsequent intervals (yrs.)
Inpatients (Kraepelin 1913)	167	6	2.8	2
Outpatients (Paskind 1930b)	248	8	5	4

In Kraepelin's study, the biphasic cases showed consistently shorter symptom-free intervals than the simple depressions.

Further support for the observation that after the first recurrence the interval tends to become shorter is found in Lundquist's study. In the age group older than 30, the mean duration of the first interval was about seven years, and the second interval three years. This difference was statistically significant.

Lundquist's data, classified according to three-year intervals, showed that the overwhelming preponderance of relapses occurred in the first nine years. It should be pointed out, that his follow-up period was as short as 10 years in some cases, as compared to 25–30 years in Rennie's series. Hence, it is probable that many of the cases in Lundquist's series would have shown a relapse if they had been followed for a longer period than 10 years. Lundquist computed the *probability* of a relapse after a patient has recovered from an initial episode of depression (Table 3–4). These findings were

Table 3–4.

PROBABILITY OF RECURRENCE AFTER RECOVERY FROM FIRST ATTACK*

	Years after first depression				
Age at first attack	3	6	9	12	15
Age < 30 years	12%	13%	4%	—	—
Age 30 + years	10%	12%	9%	8%	6%

* From Lundquist (1945).

tabulated separately for the young depressives and older depressives, but no significant difference was found between the two groups. It may be noted that the highest probability of recurrence was in the 3–6-year interval.

SCHIZOPHRENIC OUTCOME

In Rennie's sample of 208 cases of manic-depressive psychosis, four cases changed their character sufficiently to justify the conclusion of an ultimate schizophrenic development. A review of these cases suggested that there was a strong component of schizophrenic symptomatology at the time of the diagnosis of manic-depressive psychosis.

Hoch and Rachlin (1941) reviewed the records of 5,799 cases of schizophrenia admitted to the Manhattan State Hospital, New York City. They found 7.1 per cent of these patients had been diagnosed as manic depressive during previous admissions. Whether there was an alteration in the nature of the disorder, an initial misclassification, or a change in diagnostic criteria, was not established by these writers.

Lewis and Piotrowski (1954) found that 38 (54 per cent) of 70 patients, originally diagnosed as manic depressives, had their diagnoses changed to schizophrenia in a 3–20 year follow-up. In reviewing the original records, the authors demonstrated that the patients whose diagnoses were changed were misclassified initially, i.e., they showed clear-cut schizophrenic signs at the time of their first admission. Because of the very loose criteria used in diagnosing manic depressive disorder in the early decades of this century, it is difficult to determine what proportion, if any, of the clear-cut manic depressives had a schizophrenic outcome.

Lundquist reported that about 7 per cent of his manic-depressive cases eventually developed a schizophrenic picture.

Astrup, Fossum, and Holmboe (1959) isolated 70 cases of "pure" manic-depressive disorder and followed these from 7–19 years after the onset of the disorder. They found that none had a schizophrenic outcome. In contrast, 13 (50 per cent) of a group of 26 cases diagnosed as schizo-affective phychosis showed schizophrenic symptomatology on follow-up.

SUICIDE

At the present time, the only important cause of death in depression is suicide.* Previously, inanition due to lack of food and secondary infection were occasional causes of death but with modern hospital treatment such complications are unusual.

The actual suicide risk among depressed patients is difficult to assess because of the incomplete follow-ups and difficulties in establishing the cause of death. Long term follow-ups by Rennie (1942) and by Lundquist

---

* In this section, the discussion will deal primarily with studies of suicide among depressed patients. The topic of suicide is broad and many excellent monographs are available (for example, Farberow and Schneidman, 1961; Meerloo, 1962).

(1945) indicated that approximately 5 per cent of the patients initially diagnosed in a hospital as manic depressive (or as having one of the other depressive disorders) subsequently committed suicide. Since the national rate is about .01 per cent (Vital Statistics of the United States, 1960), their findings suggest that the risk of suicide in a patient hospitalized at some time in his life for depression is about 500 times the national average. The more recent studies, however, show a lower suicidal rate among depressed patients.

Pokorny (1964) investigated the suicide rate among former patients in a psychiatric service of a Texas veterans' hospital over a 15-year period. Using a complex actuarial system, he calculated the suicide rates per 100,000 per year as follows: depression, 566; schizophrenia, 167; neurosis, 119; personality disorder, 130; alcoholism, 133; and organic, 78. He then calculated the age-adjusted suicide rate for male Texas veterans as 22.7 per 100,000. The suicide rate for depressed patients, therefore, was 25 times the expected rate and substantially higher than that of other psychiatric patients.

Temoche, Pugh, and MacMahon (1964), studying the suicide rates among current and former mental institution patients in Massachusetts, found a substantially higher rate of suicide among depressed patients than nondepressed patients. The computed ratio for depressives was 36 times as high as for the general population and about three times as high as for either schizophrenics or alcoholics.

The suicide rate among patients who are known to be suicidal risks is apparently high. Moss and Hamilton (1956) conducted a follow-up study for periods of two months to 20 years of 50 patients who had been considered "seriously suicidal" during their previous hospitalization (average 4 years). Eleven (22 per cent) of the 50 later committed suicide. In a retrospective study of 134 suicides, Robins *et al.* (1959) found that 68 per cent had previously communicated suicidal ideas and that 41 per cent had specifically stated they intended to commit suicide.

The available figures clearly indicate that the suicidal risk is greatest during weekend leaves from the hospital and shortly after discharge from the hospital. Wheat (1960), surveying suicides among psychiatric hospital patients, found that 30 per cent committed suicide during the period of hospitalization. Sixty-three per cent of the suicides among the discharged patients occurred within one month after discharge. Temoche, Pugh, and MacMahon (1964) calculated that the suicidal risk in the first six months after discharge is 34 times greater than in the general population and in the second six months about nine times greater. About half of the suicides occurred within 11 months of release.

Many studies have reported the observation that women depressives attempt suicide more frequently than men but that men are more often successful. Kraines (1957) reported that, in his series of manic-depressive patients, twice as many women as men attempted suicide and three times as many men as women were successful suicides.

Although no data are available regarding the suicidal methods employed by depressives, the statistics for the general population may be relevant. In 1961 (Statistical Abstract of the United States, 1963), the most common method employed by men was firearms, followed by poisoning, and hanging. Poisoning was most frequently used by women (44 per cent of the women used this method as compared with 18 per cent of the men). Barbiturate overdosage accounts for 6 per cent of all suicides and 18 per cent of all accidental deaths (*Medical Tribune*, August 1962, p. 24); it is probable that many of these "accidental" deaths are unreported suicides.

There is evidence that the number of suicides each year is greater than the official report of 19,450 in the United States in 1960. Many accidental deaths actually represent concealed suicides. MacDonald (1964), for instance, collected 37 cases of attempted suicide by automobile. Some writers believe that the actual rate of suicide is three or four times as great as the official rate. The number of attempted suicides is believed to be seven or eight times the number of successful suicides (Stengel, 1962).

Homicide may occur in association with suicide among depressed patients (Campbell, 1953). Reports, for example, of a mother killing her children and then herself are not rare. One woman, who was convinced by her psychotherapist that her children needed her even though she believed herself worthless, decided to kill them as well as herself to "spare them the agony of growing up without a mother." She subsequently followed through with her plan.

The best indication of a suicidal risk is the communication of suicidal intent (Robins, *et al*. 1959). As Stengel (1962) points out, the notion that the person who talks about suicide will never carry it out is fallacious. Also, a previous unsuccessful suicidal attempt greatly increases the probability of a subsequent successful suicidal attempt (Motto, 1965).

In addition to trying to elicit suicidal wishes from the depressed patient, the clinician should look for signs of hopelessness. In our studies we found that suicidal wishes had a higher correlation with hopelessness than with any other symptom of depression (see Appendix). Furthermore, Pichot and Lempérière (1964), in a factor analysis of the Depression Inventory, extracted a factor containing only two variables, pessimism (hopelessness) and suicidal wishes (see Chapter 12).

CONCLUSIONS

1. Complete recovery from an episode of depression occurs in 70–95 per cent of the cases. About 95 per cent of the younger patients recover completely.

2. The median duration of the attacks is approximately 6.3 months among inpatients and approximately 3 months among outpatients. The more severe cases (i.e., those requiring hospitalization), therefore, have a longer duration than the milder cases.

3. When the initial attack occurs before age 30, it tends to be shorter than when it occurs after 30. Acute onset also favors shorter duration.

4. Contrary to prevalent opinion, there is *not* a trend towards prolongation of the attacks with each recurrence, the later attacks lasting about as long as the earlier attacks.

5. After an initial attack of depression, 47–79 per cent of the patients will have a recurrence at some time in their lives. The correct figure is probably closer to 79 per cent, because this is based on a longer follow-up period.

6. The likelihood of frequent recurrences is greater in the biphasic cases than in cases of depression without a manic phase.

7. After the first attack of depression, most patients have a symptom-free interval of more than three years before the next attack.

8. Although the duration of multiple episodes remains about the same, the symptom-free interval tends to decrease with each successive attack. In the biphasic cases the intervals are consistently shorter than in the simple depressions.

9. Whether any of the cases of pure depression have a schizophrenic outcome cannot be determined as yet, because of the relatively high percentage of incorrect diagnoses at the time of the initial episode. At most, only 5 per cent become schizophrenic after repeated attacks.

10. Approximately 5 per cent of hospitalized manic-depressive patients subsequently commit suicide. The suicidal risk is especially high on weekend leaves from the hospital and during the month following hospitalization and remains high for six months after discharge.

11. The notion that a person who threatens suicide will not carry out the threat is fallacious. The communication of suicidal intent is the best single predictor of a successful suicidal attempt. Previously unsuccessful suicidal attempts are followed by successful suicides in a substantial proportion of the cases.

Chapter 4.
Classification of the
Affective Disorders

THE OFFICIAL NOMENCLATURE

To find the various types of depression in the nomenclature of the American Psychiatric Association (APA), it is necessary to hunt through many sections. This scattering of the affective disorders contrasts with the consolidation found in other classification systems [e.g., the British Classification (Fleming, 1933)]. It is a reflection of several historical trends, including the dissolution of Kraepelin's grand union of all affective disorders into the manic-depressive category, the isolation of new entities such as neurotic depressive reaction, and the attempt to separate the disorders on the basis of presumed etiological differences.

In the major division of "psychotic disorders" in the APA nomenclature, the heading "Disorders due to disturbance of metabolism, growth, nutrition, or endocrine function" embraces a single category, *involutional psychotic reaction*. This etiological heading is misleading because it suggests an organic basis for involutional depressions, although there is no more evidence of organicity in this form of depression than in any other. There is no provision moreover, for the coding of the two types, melancholic and paranoid, found in the previous edition of the nomenclature (Cheney, 1934). This change may have unfortunate consequences, since it fuses two syndromes of later life that may be etiologically, as well as phenomenologically, distinct (see Chapter 7).

Under the title, "Disorders of psychogenic origin or without clearly defined tangible cause or structural change" we find the *manic-depressive reaction* and the new category, *psychotic depressive reaction*. The inclusion of these depressive reactions under this etiological title is questionable, since there is no more evidence of psychogenicity in these disorders than in any other affective disorder.

The *schizo-affective disorder*, which has salient affective features, is currently listed as a subtype of the schizophrenic reaction. The appropriateness of this placement is also open to question. In terms of its historical conceptualization, its course, and its prognosis, this disorder may be more closely allied to manic-depressive reaction (see Chapter 8).

The *depressive reaction*, the current form of the reactive depression, previously considered an offshoot of manic-depressive psychosis (Cheney, 1934), gains complete autonomy under the "psychoneurotic reactions."

DERIVATION OF SYSTEM OF CLASSIFICATION

The present system of classification represents a composite of the ideas of three schools of thought; those of Emil Kraepelin, Adolph Meyer, and Sigmund Freud. The division of the various nosological categories, particularly of the psychoses, reflects the original boundaries drawn by Kraepelin. The major modification in the terminology reflects the Meyerian influence. Meyer rejected the Kraepelinian concept of disease entities, and formulated in its place a theory of "reaction types." The reaction types were conceived by him to be the result of the interaction between the specific hereditary endowment and the matrix of psychological and social forces impinging on the organism. The term reaction in the nomenclature reflects the Meyerian view.

Freud's influence is seen in the descriptions of the specific categories in the glossary section of the APA Manual. Here the syndromes are outlined according to the psychoanalytic theories; the various affective disorders are presented in terms of the concepts of guilt, retroflected hostility, and defense against anxiety.

RELIABILITY AND VALIDITY OF CLASSIFICATION

Many recent studies in the United States and the United Kingdom have cast doubt on the reliability of the official nomenclatures. Some investigators, however, suggest that the essential problem may be in the *application* of the nomenclature, rather than in its construction (Kreitman *et al.*, 1961; Beck *et al.*, 1962; Ward *et al.*, 1962). In our studies, for instance, we found that there were substantial discrepancies among diagnosticians concurrently interviewing the same patients. We also found, however, that we could improve diagnostic agreement considerably by formulating operational definitions of the categories in the official nomenclature (see Chapter 11).

The validity of a nomenclature refers to the accuracy with which the diagnostic terms designate veridical entities. Unfortunately, in the case of the so-called functional psychiatric disorders, there has been no known pathology or physiological abnormality to provide guidelines in the construction of the nomenclature. The basic definition of the nosological categories has rested entirely on clinical criteria.

In assessing the validity of a medical or psychiatric classification, it is appropriate to ask whether the specific groups or syndromes isolated from each other are different in ways that are of medical or psychiatric significance, that is, in terms of symptoms, duration, outcome, tendency to recur, and response to treatment. In general, the studies made seem to justify the isolation of the group of depressive disorders from other psychiatric disorders; in addition, there is some support for the separation within the affective group of the *endogenous* depressions from the *reactive* depressions.

Clark and Mallet (1963) conducted a follow-up study of cases of depression and schizophrenia in young adults. Seventy-four cases were diagnosed as manic-depressive psychosis or reactive depression and 76 patients who were initially diagnosed as schizophrenics were followed for three years. During the follow-up period, 70 per cent of the schizophrenics were readmitted, as were 20 percent of the depressives. Thirteen (17 per cent) of the schizophrenics became chronic, as compared with only 1 (1.3 per cent) of the depressives. Of the 15 depressed patients requiring readmission to the hospital, four were considered to have schizophrenia at that time. Of the 76 patients initially diagnosed as schizophrenic, none was considered to have a depressive disorder on readmission.

Treatment responses have recently been correlated with the major diagnostic categories. It has been found that patients diagnosed as schizophrenic tend to respond favorably to the administration of phenothiazines, whereas patients who are primarily depressed tend to improve with either electroconvulsive treatment (ECT) or the so-called antidepressant drugs (see Chapter 19).

Several inferences may be drawn from the clinical studies. Two major categories are distinguishable (as Kraepelin suggested) when rate of recovery and chronicity are examined as parts of the clinical picture. These are (1) depressive disorders having a relatively high rate of complete recovery, a low rate of relapse within three years of the initial diagnosis, and a low rate of chronicity; and (2) Schizophrenia having a high rate of relapse and a high rate of chronicity. Some cases that initially evince the clinical picture of depression, ultimately develop symptoms of schizophrenia. But it is rare for a patient who has symptoms of schizophrenia to develop manic-depressive symptoms later. Lewis and Piotrowski (1954) suggest that many cases are diagnosed incorrectly as manic depressives because of insufficient recognition of certain signs of schizophrenia. The major division between these two disorders is further upheld by the differential effectiveness of certain treatments.

There is much less evidence in support of the subcategories within the group of affective disorders. Considerable doubt remains regarding the validity of dividing Kraepelin's aggregate category, manic-depressive psychosis, into involutional psychotic reaction, neurotic depressive reaction, and psychotic depressive reaction. If these subcategories can be justified, then provision must be made in the nomenclature for classifying mild manic states, such as a "hypomanic reaction," which would be analogous to neurotic depressive reaction.

DICHOTOMIES AND DUALISMS

Many authorities such as Aubrey Lewis (1938) and Paul Hoch (1953) regard depression as essentially a single entity, while others slice the syndrome along various planes to produce several dichotomies. This controversy reflects fundamental differences between the unitary and the separatist schools (Partridge, 1949). The unitary school (gradualists) maintains that depression is a single clinical disorder that can express itself in a variety of forms; the separatists state that there are several distinguishable types.

ENDOGENOUS VS. EXOGENOUS

This division attempts to establish the basic etiology of depression. Cases of depression are divided into those caused essentially by internal factors (endogenous), and those caused by external factors (exogenous). Although originally the exogenous group included such environmental agents as toxins and bacteria, recent writers have equated exogenous with psychogenic factors. This dichotomy will be discussed at greater length below.

AUTONOMOUS VS. REACTIVE

Some writers have made a distinction between types of depression on the basis of their degree of reactivity to external events. Gillespie (1929) described several groups of depressed patients that differed in their responsiveness to external influences. He labelled those cases that followed a relentless course irrespective of any favorable environmental influences as "autonomous." Those that responded favorably to encouragement and understanding were labelled "reactive."

Agitated vs. Retarded

Depression has often been characterized in terms of the predominant activity level. Many authors consider agitation as characteristic of depressions of the involutional period and retardation as characteristic of earlier depressions. Recent studies (see Chapter 7) have discounted this hypothesis.

Psychotic vs. Neurotic

Most contemporary authors draw a sharp line between psychotic and neurotic depressions. The gradualists, however, (Lewis, 1938; Hoch, 1953) believe that this distinction is artificial, and that the differences are primarily quantitative. They assert that the reported distinctions are based entirely on differences in the severity of the illness.

ENDOGENOUS AND EXOGENOUS DEPRESSIONS

The focus of the controversy between the separatists and the gradualists has been primarily on the etiological concepts of depression. The separatists favor two distinct entities. One category consists of cases that are *endogenous,* i.e., caused primarily by some biological derangement in the human organism. The second category, viz., *reactive depressions,* consists of cases caused primarily by some external stress (bereavement, financial reverses, loss of employment). The former includes manic-depressive psychosis and involutional melancholia; the latter consists of reactive, psychogenic, or neurotic, depression. The unitary school considers these distinctions artificial and does not recognize the validity of labelling some cases endogenous and others reactive.

The concept of two etiologically different types of depression is not new. In 1586 Timothy Bright, a physician, wrote a monograph, *Melancholy and the Conscience of Sinne,* in which he distinguished two different types of depression. He described one type "where the perill is not of the body" and requires "cure of the minde" (i.e., psychotherapy). In the second type, "the melancholy humour, deluding the organical actions, abuseth the minde;" this type requires physical treatment.

Origin of Endogenous-Exogenous Model

The words "endogen" and "exogen" were coined by the Swiss botanist Augustin de Candolle (1816). The concept was introduced into psychiatry toward the end of the nineteenth century by the German neuropsychiatrist P. J. Moebius.* Moebius attached the label of "endogenous" to the group

---

* For a more complete discussion of the evolution of the concept, see Heron (1965).

of mental disorders considered at that time to be due to degeneration or hereditary factors (internal causes). He further distinguished another group of mental disorders that he considered to be produced by bacterial, chemical, and other toxins (external causes); this group was given the label of "exogenous." The endogenous-exogenous view of psychiatric disorders was a completely organic dichotomy that left no room for a different order of causative agents, namely the social or psychogenic. The exclusiveness of this doctrine caused semantic difficulties when the concept later had to be adapted to include social determinants of abnormal behavior.

The dualism inherent in the endogenous-exogenous concept is apparent in the writing of Kraepelin (1913). He accepted Moebius's classification and stated that the principal demarcation of etiology of mental disorders is between *internal* and *external* causes. He proposed that there was a natural division between the two major groups of diseases, exogenous and endogenous: In manic-depressive illness, "the real causes of the malady must be sought in permanent internal changes which very often, perhaps always, are innate." Environment could at most be a precipitant of manic-depressive disease, because by definition an endogenous illness could not at the same time be an exogenous illness.

"THE GREAT DEBATES"

The controversy regarding the endogenous-exogenous concept has been most prominent in Great Britain, and a number of outstanding authorities have taken part on both sides of the argument (Partridge, 1949). Earlier, Kraepelin had endeavored to include almost all forms of depression under one label, manic-depressive disorder. Later, German writers, with their tendency to formalism and categorization, almost uniformly split depressions into endogenous and exogenous. The British, however, have been sharply divided on this point, and as a result of the clash of opinions in a series of great debates, the concepts of depression have been considerably refined (although unanimity has not as yet been attained).

The first of the debates was touched off by Mapother in 1926, when he attacked the notion of a clinical distinction between neurotic depressions and psychotic depressions. (This argument later shaded into the controversy of endogenous versus reactive depression.) He held that the only reason for making a distinction was the practical difficulties connected with commitment procedures. He claimed that he could "find no other basis for the distinction; neither insight, nor cooperation in treatment, nor susceptibility to psychotherapy." He attacked the notion that there are neurotic conditions that are purely psychogenic and psychotic conditions that are dependent on structural change. His view was that all depressions, whether ostensibly psychogenic or seemingly endogenous, are mediated by essentially the same means.

Mapother's concept is an interesting statement of the phenomenon of depression: "The essence of an attack is the clinical fact that the emotions for the time have lost enduring relation to current experience and whatever their origin and intensity they have achieved a sort of autonomy." There were a number of rebuttals in the discussion of Mapother's paper, and then another debate in 1930, which touched off another series of discussions and papers (see Partridge).

DISTINCTION BETWEEN ENDOGENOUS AND REACTIVE DEPRESSIONS

From the various conflicting as well as complimentary opinions regarding the validity of differentiating endogenous from reactive or neurotic depressions, it is possible to make a composite picture of endogenous depression as it emerged from the debates. This may be helpful in understanding the referents of the term endogenous, which is widely used in the literature, although it is not included in any official nomenclature.

In general, there are two major defining characteristics of the category *endogenous depression*. First, it is generally equated with psychosis and is consequently distinguished from neurotic depressions. Second, it is regarded as arising primarily from internal (physiological) factors and can thus be contrasted with reactive depressions produced by external stress. To complicate the distinctions, however, reactive depressions, although often equated with neurotic depressions, are sometimes distinguished from them.

The *etiology* of endogenous depression has been ascribed to a toxic chemical agent, to a hormonal factor, or to a metabolic disturbance (Crichton-Miller, 1930; Boyle, 1930). The autonomy from external environmental stimuli was considered an essential feature. Crichton-Miller likened the mood variation to the swinging of a pendulum, completely independent of the environment. Neurotic variations in mood, in contrast, were compared to the motion of a boat with insufficient keel, subject to the oscillations in its milieu.

The specific *symptomatology* has been characterized as a diffuse coloring of the whole outlook, phasic morning-evening variation, continuity, detachment from reality, loss of affection, and loss of power to grieve (Buzzard, 1930). To this should be added Gillespie's observation that the symptoms seem alien to the individual and not congruent with his premorbid personality.

The role of *heredity* in endogenous depressions has been stressed by a number of writers. Gillespie (1929) reported that a family history of psychosis is common in this group, and Buzzard (1930) suggested that suicide and alcoholism are frequent in the family background. *Constitutional factors* as reflected in body build were emphasized by Strauss.

Reactive depressions are distinguished from endogenous depressions because they fluctuate according to ascertainable psychological factors (Gillespie, 1929). In terms of the symptomatology, the distinguishing features are a tendency to blame the environment, and insight into the abnormal nature of the condition.

SYSTEMATIC STUDIES

Several investigations in recent years have employed modern statistical techniques in an effort to determine whether depressive illnesses are simply drawn from different points along a single continuum, or whether a number of qualitatively distinct entities exist. Two of the most sophisticated research studies in the current psychiatric literature have addressed themselves to this question.

Kiloh and Garside (1963) reported a study designed to differentiate between endogenous and neurotic (exogenous) depression. Their article reviews the historical development of the controversy and the experimental literature and presents data collected by the authors.

They studied the records of 143 depressed outpatients, and abstracted data relevant to their investigation. Thirty-one of the patients had been diagnosed as having endogenous depression, 61 as having neurotic depression, and 51 as being doubtful. Thirty-five clinical features of the illness were selected for additional study. A factor analysis was carried out, and two factors were extracted. The first factor was a general factor; the bipolar second factor was considered by the authors to differentiate between neurotic and endogenous depression. The second factor accounted for a greater part of the total variance than the general factor and was therefore more important in producing the correlations among the 35 clinical features analyzed.

Kiloh and Garside found significant correlation between certain clinical features and each of the diagnostic categories. The clinical features that correlated significantly ($p < .05$) with the diagnosis of neurotic depression were, in decreasing order of the magnitude of their correlations: reactivity of depression; precipitation; self-pity; variability of illness; hysterical features; inadequacy; initial insomnia; reactive depression; depression worse in evening; sudden onset; irritability; hypochondriasis; obsessionality. The features that correlated significantly with endogenous depression were: early awakening; depression worse in morning; quality of depression; retardation;

duration one year or less; age 40 or older; depth of depression; failure of concentration; weight loss of seven or more pounds; previous attacks.

A subsequent study by Carney, Roth, and Garside (1965) extended to inpatients the overall approach used by Kiloh and Garside in their study of outpatients. Carney and his coworkers studied 129 inpatient depressives treated with ECT. All patients were followed up for three months, and 108 patients were followed for six months. Initially, all were scored for the presence or absence of 35 features considered to discriminate between endogenous and neurotic depressions. Diagnoses were made before or shortly after treatment was started. Improvement was rated on a four-point scale at the termination of ECT, at three months, and at six months. At three months, only 12 of 63 neurotic depressives (19 per cent) were found to have responded well to ECT, whereas 44 of 53 endogenous depressives (83 per cent) had responded well.

A factor analysis of the clinical features produced three significant factors: a bipolar factor, "corresponding to the distinction between endogenous and neurotic depression"; a general factor with high loadings for many features common to all the depressive cases studied; and a "paranoid psychotic factor." The bipolar factor closely resembled that which was extracted in the study by Kiloh and Garside. Among features with high positive loadings on the first factor, and thus corresponding to a diagnosis of endogenous depression, were: adequate premorbid personality; absence of adequate phychogenic factors in relation to illness; a distinct quality to the depression; weight loss; pyknic body build; occurrence of previous depressive episode; early morning awakening; depressive psychomotor activity; nihilistic, somatic, and paranoid delusions; and ideas of guilt. Among features with a negative loading, corresponding to a diagnosis of neurotic depression, were anxiety; aggravation of symptoms in the evening; self-pity; a tendency to blame others; and hysterical features.

By means of multiple regression analysis, three series of 18 weighted coefficients for the differential diagnosis between the two varieties of depression and for the prediction of ECT response at three and six months were calculated. The multiple correlations between the summed features, on the one hand, and diagnosis and outcome at three and six months, on the other, were 0.91, 0.72, and 0.74 respectively. It was found that ECT response could be better predicted by the direct use of the weights for ECT response than from the diagnostic weights alone. The weights based on the 18 clinical features were complex, and therefore a table was constructed giving simplified weights based on ten features of diagnosis. When the weighted scores for each patient were computed, it was found that, of the patients with a score of six or higher, 52 had been diagnosed clinically as endogenous and three as neurotic. Those patients scoring below six included one endogenous and 60 neurotic depressives. The amount of overlap, consequently, was small, and the findings supported the two-type hypothesis.

Methodological Problems

Several methodological questions may be raised in connection with these studies. First, the reliability of the ratings of the clinical material is not reported. As has been pointed out in many papers, interjudge agreement tends to be relatively low when applied to clinical material; low reliability automatically imposes a limit on the validity of any findings based on these ratings. Furthermore, since the psychiatrists making the ratings were cognizant of the underlying hypotheses, the possibility of bias in making their judgments cannot be excluded.

The second methodological problem is concerned with differences between the two groups studied, with respect to uncontrolled variables of importance, such as age and sex. For example, relative sleeplessness and loss of appetite are characteristic of older patients. (We found a relatively high correlation between age and loss of appetite among our psychiatric patients.) There is also evidence that females react differently to stress than do males. Since these studies did not control adequately for either age or sex (or for other demographic variables), we cannot be certain that the salient differences between the two groups are explained by the dualistic hypothesis.

A problem is also presented in the interpretation of the factor analysis. The authors extracted a bipolar factor which seemed to indicate a division of the patient sample into two independent groupings. In order to prove that these groupings apply to different kinds of patients rather than simply to different clusters of signs and symptoms, it is necessary to show that there is a clear-cut splitting of the patient sample into two independent groups. Kiloh and Garside did not present any information regarding the distribution of the cases. In the study by Carney, Roth and Garside, however, a separation of the endogenous and neurotic groups was achieved by weighting items based on the statistical analysis.

Both studies represent important contributions to the study of clinical forms of depression. The differential response to ECT in the Carney study, furthermore, not only supports the concept of independent groups, but has important therapeutic application. Replication of these studies is indicated to validate the findings.

Kiloh and Garside reviewed the experimental literature relevant to the differentiation between endogenous and neurotic depression. The main points of their review are summarized and evaluated in the following discussion.

Genetic Studies

Kiloh and Garside cite the work of several investigators (Kallmann, 1952; Shields and Slater, 1960). These authors had gathered data that indicate that "a single dominant autosomal gene showing incomplete penetrance is an essential prerequisite to the development of endogenous depression."

Stenstedt's study (1959) of 307 cases of involutional melancholia is also cited. He found that patients fell into two sharply delimited groups, one consisting of cases of manic-depressive illness and the other of exogenous depression, characterized by a low genetic loading for manic-depressive illness and an onset relating to stress.

Studies of Symptomatology

Hamilton and White (1959) performed a factor analysis on data obtained from 64 severely depressed patients who had been evaluated with the use of Hamilton's rating scale (1960a). The first of the four factors obtained included such clinical features as depressed mood, guilt, retardation, loss of insight, suicidal attempt, and loss of interest. It proved, according to the authors, to be correlated with a clinical diagnosis of retarded depression. Significantly different mean scores between the endogenous and reactive groups were obtained for this first factor. It should be emphasized, however, that this finding does not specify whether the difference is qualitative or merely quantitative.

Unfortunately, the so-called precipitating factors given to justify the diagnosis of reactive depression seem unconvincing. In the three cases of reactive depression presented, the authors refer to the following as the psychological precipitating factors: one patient was left alone for prolonged periods while his wife went to look after their sick daughter; another was put in charge of a program that was beyond his capabilities; the third patient learned that the pulmonary tuberculosis which he had had for nine years was bilateral.

Findings contradictory to those reported by Hamilton and White are contained in a study by Rose (1963). This investigator used the same clinical rating scale in studying 50 depressed patients. The patients were divided into endogenous, reactive, and doubtful groups. In contrast to Hamilton and White, Rose found no significant differences in symptoms among the three groups.

Physiological Responses and Tests

Kiloh and Garside refer to the work on sedation threshold by Shagass and Jones (1958), which indicates that cases of endogenous depression have lower sedation thresholds than those of neurotic depression. They also cite the work of Ackner and Pampiglione (1959), and Roberts (1959), which fail to confirm the results of Shagass. These studies will be discussed in greater detail in Chapter 9, but it should be mentioned here that endogenous depressives tend to be older than reactive or neurotic depressives. If the samples are controlled for age, it is likely that the distinction in sedation threshold will vanish.

The work of Shagass and Schwartz (1962) on cortical excitability following electrical stimulation of the ulnar nerve is also cited. They found that in 21 patients with psychotic depression, the mean recovery time was significantly increased. Again, age was not properly controlled; more refined studies are necessary to establish the validity of these findings.

The Funkenstein test is cited by the authors as additional evidence supporting the distinction between these two types of depression (Sloane, Lewis, and Slater, 1957). Again, most of the recent, better designed studies have failed to substantiate these findings (see Chapter 9).

A number of studies of salivation in depression are referred to by the author. The study by Busfield, Wechsler, and Barnum (1961), for example, showed a significantly lower salivation rate in the endogenous than in the exogenous group. However, when the patient group was subdivided according to age, the differences were not only not significant, but in the oldest age group the exogenous patients had a lower salivation rate than the endogenous.

Body Build

Kiloh and Garside quote a study by Rees (1960) that demonstrated an association between neurotic depression and leptomorphic physique, and between eurymorphic physique and manic-depressive disorder. Here again, the mean age of the manic-depressive group was significantly higher than that of the neurotic-depressive group. As will be indicated in Chapter 9, body build becomes more eurymorphic with increasing age.

Response to Treatment

Kiloh and Garside cite several studies that suggest that exogenous depression reacts poorly to electroconvulsive therapy, and endogenous depression reacts favorably. Some evidence to support this claim is contained in a study by Rose (1963), who found that better response was obtained only for the women who had endogenous depression. There was no difference in treatment response among the men in this study. [The study by Carney and his coworkers (1965) described in detail above tends to substantiate the claim of a differential response.]

Summary

The studies cited by Kiloh and Garside lend slight support to the endogenous-exogenous hypothesis. Further investigations with better control of variables such as age and sex are required before any definite conclusions can be made.

DEPRESSIVE EQUIVALENTS

Many writers have attempted to spread the umbrella of depression to cover cases showing clinical symptoms or behaviors different from those generally indicative of depression. The term *depressive equivalents* was introduced by Kennedy and Wiesel (1946) to describe patients who had various somatic complaints but who did not show any apparent mood depression. They reported three cases characterized by somatic pain, sleep disturbance, and weight loss, all of whom recovered completely after a course of ECT.

A number of other terms have been applied to designate such cases of concealed depression. These include: incomplete depression, latent depression, atypical depression, and masked depression. Various psychosomatic disorders, hypochondriacal reactions, anxiety reactions, phobic reactions, and obsessive-compulsive reactions have also been implicated as masking the typical picture of depressive reactions (Kral, 1958).

The use of such a term as depressive equivalents raises many difficult conceptual, semantic, and diagnostic problems: (1) How can a syndrome substitute for a depressive reaction? (2) Since the usual indices of depression are lacking, how can the diagnosis of masked depression, etc. be made? (3) Since the concept of depressive equivalent is so loose, it could be stretched to encompass practically any psychiatric or somatic syndrome.

One of the main criteria for diagnosing a depressive equivalent has been the response of patients with formerly intractable symptoms to ECT (Kennedy and Wiesel). Denison and Yaskin (1944), in a report on "Medical and surgical masquerades of the depressed state," list several criteria for the diagnosis of an underlying depression. These include: previous attacks of somatic complaints similar to the present attack, with complete recovery after several months, disturbance of sleep cycle, loss of appetite, loss of energy disproportionate to the somatic complaints, diurnal variation in intensity of somatic symptoms, and feeling of unreality.

It is apparent that more systematic work must be done in describing the phenomenology of these states and in defining their similarities to and differences from manifest depression.

In the consideration of disguised depressions, it is worth emphasizing the truism that depression may mask organic disease as well as vice versa. This subject is discussed in detail by Sandler (1948).

DEPRESSIONS SECONDARY TO SOMATIC DISORDERS

Depressions have been observed in association with a wide variety of nonpsychiatric disorders. In some instances, the depression appears to be a manifestation of the physiological disturbance caused by structural disease or toxic agents. In other instances, the depression seems to be a psychological reaction to being acutely or chronically ill, i.e., the illness is a nonspecific precipitating factor. In either event, the depressive symptomatology *per se,* is not distinguishable from that observed in primary depressions (Lewis, 1934).

Conditions that specifically impair the normal functioning of the nervous system may produce depression (Castelnuovo-Tedesco, 1961). These conditions may be acute (the acute brain syndromes) such as those associated with alcohol, drugs, head trauma, or post-ictal states. Or the conditions may be chronic (chronic brain syndromes) such as those associated with cerebral arteriosclerosis, senile dementia, neurosyphilis, multiple sclerosis, malnutrition, and various vitamin deficiency syndromes.

Depression as a complication of the use of the tranquilizing drugs has frequently been reported. Early reports of the use of reserpine in the treatment of hypertension implicated this drug as a causative agent in many depressions. More recently, the phenothiazines have been suspected. Simonson (1964), for instance, interviewed 480 patients who were having their first acknowledged depression. He found that 146 (30 per cent) had been taking a phenothiazine prior to the depression. Ayd (1958) on the other hand, is skeptical of the role of the tranquilizers in producing a depression. He studied 47 cases of so-called *drug-induced depression,* and concluded that each case presented a history of predisposition to psychic disturbance and of physical and psychological stresses which helped to precipitate the depression.

Depressive symptomatology has been found in a substantial proportion of patients hospitalized for medical disorders (Schwab *et al.*, 1965; 1966). Yaskin (1931) and Yaskin, Weisenberg, and Pleasants (1931) reported a high frequency in patients with organic disease of the abdominal organs, particularly carcinoma of the pancreas. Dovenmuehle and Verwoerdt (1962) reported that 64 per cent of 62 patients hospitalized for definitely diagnosed cardiac disease had depressive symptoms of moderate or severe degree.

Other types of generalized somatic disorders that, according to Castelnuovo-Tedesco, are likely to be complicated by depression are: (*1*) certain infectious diseases—especially infectious hepatitis, influenza, infectious mononucleosis, atypical pneumonia, rheumatic fever, and tuberculosis; (*2*) so-called psychosomatic disorders such as ulcerative colitis, asthma, neurodermatitis, and rheumatoid arthritis; (*3*) anemias; (*4*) malignancies; and (*5*) endocrine disturbances.

In view of the popular theory that primary depression is caused by an endocrine disturbance, it is interesting that certain diseases of the endocrine glands are associated with a high frequency of depression. Michael and Gibbons (1963) point out that the adrenocortical hyperfunction of Cushing's syndrome is almost always accompanied by mood change. The alteration in mood is generally depressive, but it may also be characterized by emotional lability and over-reactiveness. In their review of the reports of psychiatric disturbance related to Cushing's syndrome, Michael and Gibbons state that the incident of psychiatric disturbance generally exceeds 50 per cent. Severe mental disturbance, extreme enough to warrant the label *psychotic,* is found in 15–20 per cent of the cases. In one series, 12 out of 13 patients with Cushing's syndrome were reported to be consistently or intermittently depressed. There was, however, no close correlation between the symptoms of depression and the steroid output.

Michael and Gibbons also reviewed the incidence of depression in Addison's disease. They noted that depression occurred in 25 per cent of the cases, and, somewhat surprisingly, euphoria occurred in 50 per cent. Psychiatric disturbances have also been reported in cases of hypopituitarism. In longstanding untreated cases, the symptoms may appear in an extreme form. The most prominent symptom tends to be apathy and inactivity. Mild depression, occasionally interrupted by brief episodes of irritability and quarrelsomeness, is also prominent.

Chapter 5.
Neurotic and Psychotic Depressive Reactions

There is considerable controversy among authorities regarding the separation of psychotic and neurotic depressions. Although this cleavage has been part of the official nomenclature for many years, authorities such as Paul Hoch (1953) question the distinction. Hoch states:

> The dynamic manifestations, the orality, the super-ego structure, etc., are the same in both, and usually the differentiation is made arbitrarily. If the patient has had some previous depressive attacks, he would probably be placed in the psychotic group; if not, he would be placed in the neurotic one. If the patient's depression is developed as a reaction to an outside precipitating factor, then he is often judged as having a neurotic depression. If such factors are not demonstrated, he is classified then as an endogenous depression. Actually there is no difference between a so-called psychotic or a so-called neurotic depression. The difference is only a matter of degree.

Hoch's statement epitomizes the point of view of the *gradualists* as opposed to the concept of the *separatists,* who make a dichotomy between neurotic and psychotic depression. The historical precedent for the gradualist concept is found in Kraepelin's statement (1913):

"We include in the manic-depressive group certain slight and slightest colorings of mood, some of them periodic, some of them continuously morbid, which on the one hand are to be regarded as the rudiment of more severe disorders; on the other hand, passing over without sharp boundary into the domain of personal predisposition."

Paskind (1930b) also believed that the psychotic depressions are simply severe forms of the manic-depressive syndrome. They differ from the milder forms in terms of the dramatic symptoms, but not in terms of any fundamental factors. He stated (p. 789):

"The situation is somewhat similar, for example, to what descriptions of diabetes would be if only hospital cases were described. Almost every case of diabetes would then show acidosis, coma, gangrene, and massive infection."

Separating depression into two distinct disorders would, according to Paskind, be analogous to separating diabetes into two distinct entities on the basis of severity.

The preponderant opinion in the contemporary literature, however, favors the separation of the neurotic and psychotic depressions. Some support for the two-disease concept is provided by the studies of Kiloh and Garside (1963), and Carney, Roth, and Garside (1965). These authors demonstrated, through the use of factor analysis, a bipolar factor, the poles corresponding to neurotic depression and endogenous depression, respectively (see Chapter 4). Sandifer, Wilson, and Green (1966) obtained a bimodal distribution of scores on their rating scale, which they interpreted as representing two types of depression. The bimodal distribution, however, may depend on the type of instrument employed. Schwab *et al* (1967), for instance, found a bimodal distribution of scores on the Hamilton Rating Scale but not on the Beck Depression Inventory.

PSYCHONEUROTIC DEPRESSIVE REACTION

DEFINITION

In the American Psychiatric Association diagnostic manual (1952), this syndrome is characterized as follows:

The reaction is precipitated by a current situation, frequently by some loss sustained by the patient, and is often associated with a feeling of guilt for past failures or deeds. . . . The term is synonymous with 'reactive depression' and is to be differentiated from the corresponding psychotic reaction. In this differentiation, points to be considered are (1) life history of patient, with special reference to mood swings (suggestive of psychotic reaction), to the personality structure (neurotic or cyclothymic), and to precipitating environmental factors, and (2) absence of malignant symptoms (hypochrondriacal preoccupation, agitation, delusions, particularly somatic, hallucinations, severe guilt feelings, intractable insomnia, suicidal ruminations, severe psychomotor retardation, profound retardation of thought, stupor).

In addition to this statement regarding the manifest characteristics of this condition, the following psychodynamic formulation is included in the manual: "The anxiety in this reaction is allayed, and hence partially relieved, by depression and self-depreciation. . . . The degree of the reaction in such cases is dependent upon the intensity of the patient's ambivalent feeling towards his loss (love, possession) as well as upon the realistic circumstances of the loss." The value of this formulation will be discussed presently.

Although not specified in the manual, the defining characteristics of psychoneurotic depressive reaction may be assumed to be the generally accepted features of depression. The more *malignant* symptoms indicative of a psychotic depression are mentioned above. It is noteworthy that the authors consider the presence of suicidal ruminations to exclude a diagnosis of neurotic depression. This notion is contradicted by the finding that this symptom was found in 58 per cent of patients diagnosed as neurotic depressive reaction (Table 5–1). A patient with a low mood such as dejection, low self-esteem, indecisiveness, and, possibly, some of the physical and vegetative symptoms mentioned in Chapter 2, may be considered to have a neurotic-depressive reaction.

In addition to the brief description of the manifest symptoms, the glossary also introduces two etiologic concepts. The first, viz., that the depression is precipitated by a current situation, is a derivative of the concept of reactive depression, the development of which will be discussed. The second etiologic concept is that the depression is a defense against anxiety (pp. 12 and 32), and that the ambivalent feelings towards the presumed lost object determine the intensity of the reaction.

This specific psychodynamic formulation represents an attempt by the authors of the manual to provide a psychological explanation for this condition. It is not clear whether the psychodynamic formulation is intended to be a defining characteristic of the category. It would seem that the attempt should be regarded as *experimental*, and the validity of the category should not depend on the validity of the psychodynamic formulation or on whether it is possible to discern this particular configuration in a given case. Reports of investigators trying to apply the psychodynamic formulation have questioned its usefulness in making the diagnosis (Ascher, 1952; Ward *et al.*, 1962). The concept that neurotic depressive reaction is *reactive*, seems to be more integral to the definition of this syndrome and it may be considered, at least by some, that if some external stress cannot be demonstrated in a particular case, then the use of this diagnosis is not justified in that case.

Despite the inclusion of this category in many nomenclatures, it is by no means generally accepted. In fact, a large number of writers on depression seem to accept the *gradualist* or *unitary concept*, viz., that the difference between neurotic and psychotic depression is one of degree, and that there is no more justification in constructing separate categories than there is for dividing scarlet fever into two groups such as mild and severe. Proponents of this point of view include the authors who have written most extensively about depression, such as Mapother (1926) and Lewis (1934) in England, and Ascher (1952), Cassidy, Flanagan, and Spellman (1957), Campbell (1953), Kraines (1957), Robins *et al.* (1959), and Winokur and Pitts (1965) in the United States.

EVOLUTION OF THE CONCEPT

In order to evaluate the clinical and conceptual basis for this nosological category, it might be helpful first to trace its development. In the gradual evolution of the concept, there have been a number of radical twists and turns so that there is little resemblance between the term as it is now understood and its original conception.

In the earlier classifications, the reactive-depressive category was not fused with neurotic depression as it is today. Kraepelin recognized a condition similar to the current notion of neurotic. depressions and allocated it to the category of congenital neurasthenia which he listed under constitutional psychopathic states. He also referred to a group of "psychogenic depressions" that he considered to differ from the manic-depressive psychosis. Patients with psychogenic depressions showed a high degree of reactivity to external situations and their depression tended to improve when the external situation improved. The manic-depressive attack, in contrast, was not primarily the result of an external stress situation and, once started, it continued independent of the precipitating circumstances and ran its own course.

Bleuler (1924) evidently allocated the milder depressions to the manic-depressive category, as indicated by his statement that "probably everything designated as periodic neurasthenia, recurrent dyspepsia, and neurasthenic melancholias belong entirely to manic-depressive insanity." He also conceded the existence of psychogenic depressions: "Simple psychogenic depressions, occurring in psychopaths not of the manic-depressive group and reaching the intensity of a mental disease, are rare."

The most definite precursor of the concept of neurotic-depressive reaction was that of reactive depression. In 1926, Lange listed psychogenic and reactive depression separately in his classification of depression. He differentiated psychogenic depressions from the endogenous variety on the basis of greater aggressiveness, egocentricity, stubbornness, and overt hostility. In addition, he stated that there were no discernible variations in mood in the psychogenic depressions. Changes in the milieu influenced this condition, and it became better when the personality conflict was solved. Wexberg (1928) described seven different groups of "mild depressive states." He included a "reactive group," but made no distinction between neurotic and psychotic in his classification.

Paskind (1929) described 663 cases of mild manic-depressive disorder seen in outpatient practice. Harrowes (1933) defined six groups of depression which included separate categories for the reactive and psychoneurotic types. Patients classified as psychoneurotic depressions showed "psychopathy, neuropathy, anxiety attacks, feelings of failure in life, sex trauma, unreality feelings and a greater subjectively than objectively depressed mood." This condition occurred in the third decade of life and, while mild, tended toward chronicity.

Aubrey Lewis (1934), in his classic paper on depression, stated that a careful analysis of 61 cases indicated that the neurotic symptoms appeared with equal frequency among the reactive and the endogenous forms of depression. He stressed that no sharp line could be drawn between psychotic and neurotic depressions.

It is apparent that despite the objections of authorities such as Lewis, there was a dominant tendency among nosographers to separate reactive and neurotic depressions from other types of depressions. The concepts of reactive and of neurotic depressions gradually converged. The fusion of these categories occurred officially in 1934. At that time, the American Psychiatric Association approved a new classification in which reactive depression was subsumed under the psychoneuroses. This concept did not attain wide currency in the decade that followed, however, as indicated by the failure of most American textbooks and reference books on psychiatry to include a category of depression among the psychoneuroses.

The new category, reactive depression, was defined in Cheney's *Outlines for Psychiatric Examinations* (1934) as follows:

"Here are to be classified those cases which show depression in reaction to obvious external causes which might naturally produce sadness, such as bereavement, sickness, and financial and other worries. The reaction of a more marked degree and of longer duration than normal sadness, may be looked upon as pathological. The deep depression with motor and mental retardation are not present, but these reactions *may be more closely related in fact to the manic-depressive reactions than to the psychoneuroses.*" [My italics]

At this stage in its development, the concept of neurotic depression was still closely allied to the all-embracing category of manic-depressive disorder.

The next step in the evolution of the current concept was a major thrust in the direction of the current etiologic concept. In the United States War Department classification, adopted in 1945, the term *neurotic depressive reaction* was used. The term *reaction* represented a clearcut deviation from the Kraepelinian notion of a defined disease entity, and incorporated Adolph Meyer's psychobiological concept of an interaction of a particular type of personality with the environment. Since the presence of a specific external stress was more salient in an army at war than in civilian practice, the emphasis on reaction to stress seemed to gain increased plausibility.

The other significant departure in the definition in the Army nomenclature was the introduction of two psychoanalytic hypotheses, viz., (1) that depression represents an attempt to allay anxiety through the mechanism of introjection, and (2) that depression is related to *repressed aggression*. It states:

"The anxiety in this reaction is allayed, and, hence, partially relieved by self-depreciation through the mental mechanism of introjection. It is often associated with guilt for past failure or deeds. . . . This reaction is a nonpsychotic response precipitated by a current situation—frequently some loss sustained by the patient—although dynamically the depression is usually related to a repressed (unconscious) aggression."

The United States War Department classification received an extensive trial in the armed forces and was subsequently adopted in a slightly revised form by the Veterans Administration. The opinion of psychiatrists using the nomenclature, both in the army and at Veterans Administration clinics and hospitals, was evidently favorable, because this classification was subsequently used as the basis for the 1952 *Diagnostic Manual* of the American Psychiatric Association. The new categories of neurotic-depressive reaction and psychotic-depressive reaction had become firmly established.

CRITIQUE OF CONCEPT

The preponderant evidence seems to favor the usefulness and validity of the category of neurotic-depressive reaction when used as a descriptive concept. Despite Ascher's criticisms (1952), the group seems to be relatively homogeneous. The recent systematic studies by Kiloh and Garside (1962) and by Carney, Roth, and Garside (1965) provide statistical evidence that a number of clinical features distinguish the syndrome from endogenous depression. It has also been demonstrated many times that patients diagnosed as neurotic-depressive reaction tend to respond poorly to electroconvulsive therapy, but cases of psychotic or endogenous depression tend to have a favorable response (see Chapter 18).

One observation that deserves further consideration is that some patients who experience one or more typical episodes of neurotic-depressive reaction later develop psychotic-depressive reactions and/or manic reactions (Paskind, 1930b). In such cases, the early neurotic attacks seem to be mild or abortive forms of manic-depressive psychosis. In specific episodes, furthermore, a patient may initially show a typical clinical picture of neurotic depression but, as the illness progresses, will begin to show increasingly more signs of a psychotic depressive reaction.

Case Example

The patient was a 25-year-old engineer, who gave the following spontaneous description of his problem: "I am feeling very depressed. I feel as though I'm dragging myself down as well as my family. I have caused my parents no end of aggravation. The best thing would be if I dug a hole and buried myself in it. If I would get rid of myself, everybody would be upset for a time but then they would get over it. They would be better off without me."

The immediate life situation related to his depression was a job he had taken three months before. After graduating from college, he had had a succession of jobs and had started a small business that failed. He was not doing well in his current position and was certain that he would be fired within a few days. He experienced a gradual loss of self-confidence as his work did not seem to measure up to the expectations of his employer. Two days before his psychiatric consultation he received notice that he would be fired. He became very discouraged and experienced a complete loss of appetite and considerable difficulty in sleeping. He thought of various ways of killing himself, such as taking an overdose of pills or throwing himself from a high building.

A day before his consultation with me, he called his older brother to inform him that he was leaving town. His intention as that time was to commit suicide in a distant city. His brother suspected that something was wrong, so he came over to visit and to talk to him. After discussing the problem with his brother, the patient began to feel better. His brother told him he would lend him money to tide him over until he could get another position and he also made arrangements for the patient to start psychotherapy. The patient went to a football game that afternoon and began to feel better since his favorite team won.

When I saw him the following day, he looked dejected and moderately depressed. He did not show any retardation or agitation. I administered the Depression Inventory (see Chapter 12). His cumulative score of 20 indicated a moderate depression. He acknowledged having the following symptoms: continual unremitting sadness; discouragement; feelings of being a failure; lack of satisfaction; guilt feelings for "having let everybody down"; self-dislike; self-reproach; suicidal wishes; some loss of interest in other people; indecisiveness; insomnia; anorexia; and easy fatigability.

After the initial interview, which consisted of supportive psychotherapy in addition to history taking, the patient said he felt much better. During the next two or three days he was practically symptom free, and then he had a mild recurrence of his symptoms. He was seen in psychotherapy twice more at weekly intervals, and his depression cleared up completely and did not return. During this period of time, moreover, arrangements were made for him to obtain another job that was more in keeping with his particular abilities.

There are several noteworthy features about this case that are relevant to the definition of *neurotic depression*. (1) The patient developed the depression in response to certain stressful external situations. (2) The intensity of the feeling was considerably alleviated by interpersonal factors. (3) When there was a change in the external situation, the depression cleared up completely. (4) The content of the depressed thinking revolved around the precipitating event.

PSYCHOTIC DEPRESSIVE REACTION

The term *psychotic depressive reaction* does not appear in any of the official American or European classifications prior to the end of World War II. In 1951, the standard Veterans Administration classification included this term. In 1952, it was included in the official classification of the American Psychiatric Association. In the glossary accompanying this nomenclature, psychotic depressive reaction was characterized as including patients who are severely depressed and who give evidence of gross misinterpretation of reality, including at times delusions and hallucinations.

The nomenclature distinguishes this reaction from the manic-depressive reaction, depressed type, on the basis of the following features: absence of a history of repeated depressions or of marked psychothymic mood swing, and presence of environmental precipitating factors. This category evidently is considered to be the analogue of the neurotic-depressive reaction and a present day counterpart of the reactive psychotic depressions described in the German literature in the 1920's. There are several features relevant to this diagnostic category that have troubled some authorities in the field, many of whom do not accept the distinction between neurotic depressive reaction and psychotic depressive reaction. The first depressive episode of a typical manic-depressive disorder may very well appear in reaction to some environmental stress (Kraepelin, 1913). On the basis of symptomatology, there are no criteria to distinguish the psychotic-depressive reaction from the depressed phase of the manic-depressive reaction.

The characteristics of psychotic-depressive reaction are illustrated in the following cases,* selected from a group of soldiers who experienced psychotic-depressive reaction after accidentally killing their buddies during the Korean War. The cases had the following common features relevant to the concept of psychotic-depressive reaction: (1) The psychosis followed a specific event that was highly disturbing to the patient; (2) there were clear-cut psychotic symptoms such as delusions and hallucinations; (3) the content of the patients' preoccupations, delusions, and hallucinations revolved around the dead buddy; (4) the typical symptoms of depression were present—depressed mood, hopelessness, suicidal wishes, and

* From Beck and Valin (1953).

self-recriminations; (5) the patients recovered completely after a course of ECT or psychotherapy; and (6) there was no previous history of depression or mood swings.

Case 1.

A 21-year-old soldier was referred to Valley Forge Army Hospital from a disciplinary barracks to which he had been confined for "culpable negligence." While near the line in Korea, he and his best buddy, Buck, had been working very hard laying wire. They paused to take a break and started "fooling around" and throwing water at each other. Buck threw a loaded carbine to him, and he accidentally discharged it into Buck's mouth and killed him. Buck and he had been best friends for a long time and had worked together as a solitary pair for several weeks. He had a clinging attachment to Buck, who was a very self-sufficient and adequate person. He subsequently stated, "Buck was the only person who ever understood or loved me."

Because of the negligence involved in the careless handling of a loaded gun, the patient had a general court martial 3 months later and was sentenced to confinement at hard labor for 3 years. At the time of the court martial he seemed to be struggling to contain his guilt feeling and had only a vague recollection of the details of the accident. However, he was able to maintain good contact with reality until nine months later. At that time he began to ruminate constantly about his offense. Within a few days, he experienced an acute psychotic break. He was transferred to Valley Forge Army Hospital in a very disturbed state. He was crying violently, attempted to strangle himself with his pajamas and then to slash his wrist on the window screen, and was extremely combative. He had visual hallucinations of Buck and carried on long conversations with him. He revealed that at times Buck told him "bad things" and at other times "good things." The "bad things" were that he should kill himself and the "good things" were that he should keep on living. He was given a series of 20 electroconvulsive treatments and experienced a complete remission of his psychosis.

Case 2.

While examining a revolver behind the line in Korea, a 20-year-old soldier accidentally discharged the gun, shooting another soldier through the chest and killing him. He was sentenced to two years of hard labor for "culpable negligence." Eight months after the accident, while serving his term, he became increasingly upset and had to be hospitalized. He began to engage in obsessive rumination about the accident and in fantasies that would magically undo the deed. Within a few weeks, he became openly psychotic, suicidal, and violent. He had visual and auditory hallucinations involving the dead soldier. He saw the latter coming to him sitting on a cloud and holding a revolver in his left hand. The soldier would upbraid him for what he had done and would then "take off" in reverse. In the course of 20 electroconvulsive treatments, there was complete remission of symptoms.

Case 3.

A 22-year-old rifleman accidentaly shot his platoon sergeant while on patrol in Korea. He tried to conceal his emotional reaction to the event but a month later he began to hear voices saying, "This is it . . . take a rifle and put a clip in and kill yourself." Another voice then said, "Don't do it, it won't do any good. Then there will be two of you [dead]." At the time of his transfer to Valley Forge Army Hospital he showed moderate agitation, depression, and tremendous anxiety. He frequently expressed the fear of losing his genitalia. In the course of psychotherapy, his symptoms largely abated.

DIFFERENTIAL DIAGNOSIS

In trying to make a distinction between neurotic and psychotic depression, the best guide is to designate as psychotic depressive all cases that show definite signs of psychosis, such as loss of reality, delusions and hallucinations.

Foulds (1960) conducted a systematic study to determine what symptoms differentiated neurotic and psychotic depressives. He administered an inventory of 86 items to 20 neurotic depressives and 20 psychotic depressives, all under 60 years of age. He found that 14 items occurred at least 25 per cent more frequently among the psychotic than among the neurotic group. Using those 14 items as a scale, he was able to sort out correctly 90 per cent of the patients diagnosed clinically as psychotic depressives and 80 per cent of the neurotic depressives. In the list below, the frequency among the psychotics is stated first in the parentheses after each item and that among neurotics is second.

1. He is an unworthy person in his own eyes (12–3).
2. He is a condemned person because of his sins (12–3).
3. People are talking about him and criticizing him because of things he has done wrong (10–1).
4. He is afraid to go out alone (13–4).
5. He has said things that have injured others (9–2).
6. He is so "worked-up" that he paces about wringing his hands (11–4).
7. He cannot communicate with others because he doesn't seem to be on the same "wave-length" (10–3).
8. There is something unusual about his body, with one side being different from the other, or meaning something different (6–0).
9. The future is pointless (12–7).
10. He might do away with himself because he is no longer able to cope with his difficulties (8–3).
11. Other people regard him as very odd (8–3).
12. He is often bothered with pains over his heart, in his chest, or in his back (8–3).

13. He is so low in spirits that he just sits for hours on end (12–7).
14. When he goes to bed, he wouldn't care if he "never woke up again" (10–5).

Ideas or delusions relevant to being unworthy, condemned, and criticized, and the delusion of being physically altered, are the best differentiators between the two groups.

Aside from delusions, the typical signs and symptoms of depression are found in a large proportion of both neurotic and psychotic depressives. As shown in Table 5–1, the features appear with relatively high frequency in both conditions. This frequency distribution was obtained by abstracting the ratings and diagnoses made by our psychiatrists on a random sample of psychiatric inpatients and outpatients (see Chapter 12). Each clinical feature was rated according to its severity as: absent, mild, moderate, or severe. The records of 50 patients diagnosed as psychotic depressive reaction and of 50 diagnosed as neurotic depressive reaction were used in this analysis.

Table 5–1.

FREQUENCY OF CLINICAL FEATURES IN NEUROTIC DEPRESSIVE REACTION (NDR) AND PSYCHOTIC DEPRESSIVE REACTION (PDR)

Clinical feature	Feature present		Present to severe degree	
	NDR (%) (n = 50)	PDR (%) (n = 50)	NDR (%) (n = 50)	PDR (%) (n = 50)
Sad facies	86	94	4	24
Stooped posture	58	76	4	20
Speech: slow, etc.	66	70	8	22
Low mood	84	80	8	44
Diurnal variation of mood	22	48	2	10
Hopelessness	78	68	6	34
Conscious guilt	64	44	6	12
Feeling inadequate	68	70	10	42
Somatic preoccupation	58	66	6	24
Suicidal wishes	58	76	14	40
Indecisiveness	56	70	6	28
Loss of motivation	70	82	8	48
Loss of interest	64	78	10	44
Fatigability	80	74	8	48
Loss of appetite	48	76	2	40
Sleep disturbance	66	80	12	52
Constipation	28	56	2	16

n = No. of patients.

It is apparent that in almost all instances the signs and symptoms of depression were observed in the majority of both neurotic and psychotic depressives. Diurnal variation of mood occurred substantially more frequently among the psychotic depressives, but it was present in only a minority of these cases. Constipation occurred twice as frequently in the psychotic depressive group as might be expected because the patients in this group were generally in the older age category. Although almost all the clinical features were observed more frequently in the psychotic depressed group, the disparity in their relative frequency was not marked (with the exception of the two just mentioned).

Since each clinical feature was evaluated not only in terms of presence and absence but also in terms of severity, it was possible to ascertain the relative severity of the specific signs and symptoms in the two groups. It was found that the psychotic depressives tended to show a greater degree of intensity or severity on each of these signs and symptoms. This was expected, since the global rating of depth of depression was substantially higher in the psychotic depressive group. The frequency of *severe* ratings in the two groups is shown in Table 5–1. In every instance, the psychotic depressive group received substantially more severe ratings than the neurotic group.

It may be concluded that there are no specific signs or symptoms, aside from delusions, that distinguish psychotic from neurotic depressives; and the more severe the symptoms, the more likely a patient is to be diagnosed as psychotic depressed. These findings tend to support the thesis that, so far as specific depressive symptoms are concerned, the difference between the neurotic and the psychotic depressive reactions is quantitative rather than qualitative.

Chapter 6.
Manic-Depressive Reaction

DEFINITION

The contemporary clinical concept of manic-depressive disorder stems directly from the work of Kraepelin. When he started his ventures into the classification of the mental disorders, he was confronted with a collection of brilliantly described syndromes that were apparently unrelated. He consolidated the various disorders into two major categories: dementia praecox and manic-depressive insanity. He regarded dementia praecox as a progressive disorder leading eventually to a chronic state of intellectual deterioration; manic-depressive insanity was viewed as episodic (i.e., characterized by remissions and recurrences) and nondeteriorating. The new manic-depressive category ultimately was extended to almost all the recognized syndromes that included salient affective features. He stated (1913), "Manic-depressive insanity comprehends on the one hand, the entire domain of so-called periodic and circular insanity, and on the other, simple mania, usually distinguished from the above. In the course of years I have become more and more convinced that all the pictures mentioned are merely forms of one single disease process. . . . Manic-depressive insanity, as its name indicates, takes its course in single attacks, which either present the signs of so-called manic excitement (flight of ideas, exaltation, and over-activity), or those of a peculiar phychic depression with psychomotor inhibition, or a mixture of the two states."

Kraepelin attempted to define his nosological groups according to the model of general paresis that had been shown to be due to syphilis of the nervous system. His model of manic-depressive disorder may be expressed in terms of the following hypotheses:

1. It is a definite disease entity. The concept of disease entity was challenged by a number of contemporary German writers and was attacked in the United States by Adolf Meyer (1908), who substituted the concept of "reaction-types" for "disease entities." Meyer's ascendancy in this respect is reflected in the current official American nomenclature (APA, 1952).

2. It has a specific neuropathology and etiology. Kraepelin suggested that the basic cause was probably a metabolic instability that accounted for the affective symptoms and fluctuations. To the present time no definite neuropathological lesions have been found, and knowledge of the basic causes has not advanced much further than in Kraepelin's day.

3. It has a definite prognosis. He regarded complete recovery from a particular episode as characteristic of this disease. Unlike dementia praecox, there is no intellectual deterioration. The view of complete recovery in all cases has been disputed by many authors, and Kraepelin himself conceded that about 10 per cent of the cases become chronic.

4. It has a definite symptomatology. This consisted of the classic depressive and manic symptoms.

5. It is recurrent. The tendency to recurrence led Kraepelin to the concept of a chronic instability that makes the patient vulnerable to repeated attacks; recurrences were observed in only half of his cases, however.

6. The manic and depressive attacks were viewed as opposite poles of the same underlying process.

If Kraepelin's concept had been supported by subsequent experience, there would be little problem of classification today. Each of the hypotheses listed above has been attacked by subsequent writers on the basis of either formal logical grounds, clincial experience, or experimental evidence. On the other hand, the major outlines of his descriptive model conform sufficiently to observable clinical behaviors to ensure its longevity until a better scheme is evolved on the basis of positive research findings.

An example of the attacks on the validity of the manic-depressive category is found in statements by authorities such as Zilboorg (1933), who asserted, "On the basis of my clinical experience I am under the definite impression that manic-depressive psychoses despite their age-long existence do not actually represent a separate clinical entity, but they are a pure culture, as it were, of that cyclical rhythm which is easily observed in hysterics, compulsive neuroses, and even in various forms of schizophrenia." It is possible, according to Zilboorg, that these alternations of manic and depressive are but extreme expressions of a number of mental illnesses.

In the definition of terms in the American Psychiatric Association diagnostic manual (1952), manic-depressive reactions are described as follows: "These groups comprise the psychotic reactions which fundamentally are marked by severe mood swings, and a tendency to remission and recurrence. Various accessory symptoms such as illusions, delusions, and hallucinations may be added to the fundamental affective alteration."

It appears from this definition that the manic-depressive label has been limited to those cases having a manic (or hypomanic) as well as a depressive phase. Thus, Kraepelin's great synthesis of the affective disorders under the manic-depressive label has been splintered into the neurotic and psychotic depressive reactions, involutional reactions, and schizo-affective type of schizophrenia. Only the hard core of the original manic-depressive category still remains. This splitting is reflected in the notable drop in the frequency of the use of this diagnosis for first admissions to state hospitals throughout the United States from 12 per cent in 1933 to 3 per cent in 1953 (Loftus, 1960).

RELATIONSHIP OF MANIC TO DEPRESSIVE EPISODES

The observation that manic episodes may occur in people who have had depressions (or vice versa) was noted two thousand years ago (Chapter 1). Despite the long history of this observation, there is still considerable uncertainty about the relationship of these two forms of mental illness. Kraepelin lumped together single depressions, multiple depressions, single manias, multiple manias, and cases of depression alternating with manias (the circular cases). This attempt to bring together all the diverse clinical pictures under the same rubric is still a subject of controversy. It is frequently argued that the biphasic cases are sufficiently different from the pure depressions to warrant the completely separate categorization found in the current APA nomenclature. On the other hand, Kraepelin's integration of all the affective disorders may ultimately prove to be analogous to the final crystallization of the concept of tuberculosis or syphilis, both of which displayed a wide variety of clinical features but were eventually shown to be caused by a specific pathogenic agent.

As Cameron (1944) has pointed out, there is a question as to how long after a depression a manic attack may occur and still be considered part of a manic-depressive cycle. Although the majority opinion holds that there is no time limit, a minority of psychiatrists feel that sporadic depressive and manic attacks simply indicate separate affective disorders occurring in a susceptible person.

Another problem is raised by the fact that a large proportion of depressed patients show a mild hypomanic tendency after recovering from their depressions. Psychiatrists who advocate the notion of a cyclical disorder would classify these cases as manic depressive. Others consider this transient hypomanic phase merely a compensatory phenomenon related to the depression and not a manifestation of a manic phase (Loftus, 1960).

A third problem is raised by the fact that although the polarization of symptoms seems to support the two-phase concept, there is no evidence as yet that these two conditions are opposite in their biological substrates. Such physiological differences as have been observed appear to be secondary to the difference in activity level rather than any primary difference in the underlying disorder (Cameron, 1942).

The relative frequency of depressed, manic, and circular cases depends to a large extent on the definition of the manic-depressive syndrome. In Kraepelin's series (1921) the relative frequency was: depression only, 49 per cent; manic only, 17 per cent; and circular or combined, 34 per cent. Rennie (1942) reported the following proportions: depression only, 67 per cent; manic only, 9 per cent; and combined, 24 per cent. Clayton, Pitts, and Winokur, (1965) reported that of 366 patients diagnosed as having affective reaction, 31 (9 per cent) had the diagnosis of mania.

The signs and symptoms of the depressed phase have been described in Chapter 2. The characteristics of the manic phase will now be described.

SYMPTOMATOLOGY OF MANIC PHASE

The symptomatology of the manic disorder presents a striking contrast to that of the depressive disorder. In fact, when one considers each of the symptoms they seem to be at opposite end points of a bipolar dimension. As is shown in Table 6–1, in which the various symptoms are categorized as primarily emotional, cognitive, motivational, or vegetative, in almost every instance the manic reactions are directly opposite to those of the depressive reactions. The major exception to this is the difficulty in sleeping, which is encountered in both conditions.

Emotional Manifestations

Elation

Most manic patients convey a picture of complete lightness of heart and gaiety. They make statements such as, "I feel I am floating on air;" "I'm bursting with happiness;" "I've never felt so wonderfully happy in my life;" "I am bursting with joy." Some manic patients are aware of a false sense of well-being and may even feel uncomfortable with such an exaltation of spirit.

The euphoria of the manic patients is sharply contrasted with the feelings of the depressed patient who is sad, morose, and unhappy: The difference may be expressed in terms of the contrast of pleasure and pain.

Table 6–1.

COMPARISON OF MANIC AND DEPRESSIVE SYMPTOMS

Manic	*Depressive*
EMOTIONAL MANIFESTATIONS	
Elated	Depressed
Increased gratification	Loss of gratification
Likes self	Dislikes self
Increased attachments	Loss of attachments
Increased mirth response	Loss of mirth response
COGNITIVE MANIFESTATIONS	
Positive self-image	Negative self-image
Positive expectations	Negative expectations
Blames others	Blames self
Denial of problems	Exaggeration of problems
Arbitrary decision-making	Indecisive
Delusions: self-enhancing	Delusions: self-degrading
MOTIVATIONAL MANIFESTATIONS	
Driven and impulsive	Paralysis of the will
Action-oriented wishes	Wishes to escape
Drive for independence	Increased dependent wishes
Desire for self-enhancement	Desire for death
PHYSICAL AND VEGETATIVE MANIFESTATIONS	
Hyperactivity	Retardation/agitation
Indefatigable	Easily fatigued
Appetite variable	Loss of appetite
Increased libido	Loss of libido
Insomnia	Insomnia

Increased Gratification

The manic patient, in contrast to the depressed patient, is capable of getting gratification from a wide variety of experiences and the intensity of his gratification far exceeds that of his normal phase. A leaf falling from a tree may cause feelings of ecstasy or an interesting advertisement may produce a great thrill. In contrast, the depressed patient gets little or no gratification. Even activities that in a normal state could arouse great feelings of pleasure now "leave him cold." When he moves into the manic phase, however, he not only responds to such experiences but reacts excessively to them.

Apparently only the pure manics experience consistent gratification. Those manics who have mild paranoid trends generally experience irritation. This irritation is apt to be stimulated whenever the patient encounters any disagreement, criticism, or obstacle to his goals.

Self-Love

Whereas the depressed patient often dwells on how much he dislikes himself, even to the extent of loathing or hating himself, the manic patient experiences a feeling of affection or love for himself. He has the same type of intense amorous feeling towards himself as a person romantically involved with somebody else. He experiences a sense of thrill when he thinks about himself or talks about himself and is very pleased and satisfied with all his attributes. In contrast to the self-depreciation of the depressed patient, he tends to idealize himself. He proclaims his great virtues and deeds and constantly congratulates himself for them.

Increased Attachment to People and Activities

Whereas the depressed patient complains that he no longer has any feelings for members of his family or friends and that he has lost interest in his work and his various favorite pastimes, the manic patient often experiences a surplus of fondness for other people and plunges into his various interests with abundant zest. He experiences a broadening as well as an intensification of the interests. Some manics are so stimulated that they jump from one activity to another. They are often extremely successful in pursuing a number of projects during the manic phase. I have observed a number of successful scientists, artists, and businessmen who reached their peak performance during hypomanic or manic phases.

The manic patient tends to reach out to other people and enjoy their company. He strikes up conversations with strangers and may influence a large number of people to his way of thinking. A manic patient is often a disruptive influence on a psychiatric ward because of his ability to stimulate the other patients towards a particular goal of his own—for example, rebellion against hospital authority. On the other hand, some manic patients are unusually successful in breaking through the autistic barrier of withdrawn schizophrenics.

Increased Mirth Response

The depressed patient characteristically manifests a loss of a sense of humor but the manic patient is full of fun. He tells jokes, composes rhymes and jingles, relates stories in an amusing way, and sings. He is often very witty and his good humor has an infectious quality. When presented at a case conference a manic patient can readily move the entire audience to laughter.

In contrast to the depressed patient's tendency to weep, cry, or moan, the manic patient laughs and exudes happiness.

Cognitive Manifestations

Positive Self-Image

It is immediately apparent in conversation with a manic patient that he has a highly positive view of himself. He not only overestimates the degree or significance of his physical attractiveness, but he claims many other outstanding attributes; this is apparent in his use of superlatives. Some manics assert that they are the most beautiful people who ever lived and proclaim that they have great talents, ingenuity, insight, and understanding. This positive self-concept is in marked contrast to the depressed patient who sees himself as utterly devoid of any positive attributes and as possessing only weaknesses and vices.

Positive Expectations

The manic patient is optimistic about the outcome of anything he undertakes. Even when confronted with an insoluble problem he is confident that he will find a solution. This attitude contrasts with that of the depressed patient who attaches a low probability of success to any of his attempts. With his tendency to overestimate his prospects, the manic patient often gets involved in very risky business ventures and as a result may lose a considerable amount of money.

Assignment of Blame

In contrast to the depressed patient who tends to blame himself for almost anything that goes wrong, the manic patient tends to allocate the fault to other people even though a particular error may be obviously the result of his own decisions or actions. The tendency to blame his difficulties on others often makes it hard for other people to work with a manic patient.

Denial

The manic patient tends to deny the possibility of any personal weaknesses, deficiencies, or problems. He generally rejects suggestions that his behavior is excessive or that he may have some psychiatric disorder. When he is confronted with difficult problems he tends to gloss over them. He is likely to deny any obvious mistake he has made. The depressed patient, in contrast, tends to maximize problems and to see weaknesses and deficiencies in himself where they do not exist.

Arbitrariness

The manic patient differs sharply from the depressed patient who is plagued by indecisiveness and vacillation. The manic patient tends to make decisions rapidly—often without any solid foundation. The quickness in making decisions is related to impulsivity. One woman would go off on buying sprees, for instance, whenever she was in the manic phase; when depressed, she would return all the purchases to the stores.

Delusions

The delusions of the manic patient tend to be of the self-enhancing type. He firmly believes he is the most handsome man who ever lived, or the world's greatest genius, or possessed of prodigious physical abilities. He may regard himself as superman or as the reincarnation of God. He may believe he has billions of dollars and a vast empire. These delusions contrast with those of the depressed patient, which are concerned with ideas of unworthiness, poverty, deterioration, and sinfulness.

MOTIVATIONAL MANIFESTATIONS

Impulse-Driven

The manic patient conveys the impression of being driven by impulses over which he has little or no control. Even though he claims that he does what he wants to do, it is generally obvious that it is difficult for him to stop his activities. In general, he appears to be overstimulated and to have an extraordinarily strong drive in a multitude of directions. The depressed patient, in contrast, experiences paralysis of the will. He seems unable to mobilize spontaneously enough motivation to attend to even the basic amenities of living.

Action-Oriented

The wishes of the manic patient generally have some objective that would provide a prospect of personal fulfillment. He wants to impress people, to help them, to create something new or to be successful at a given task. The types of goal he has are similar to those of his contemporaries, even though more extravagant and backed up by a compulsive drive. He wants to move into life. The depressed patient, in contrast, desires to escape from life.

Drive for Independence

The patient in the manic phase sheds the dependency that was manifest during the depressed phase. He no longer feels that he needs help from other people and often assumes the role of the benefactor and helper. He wants to assume responsibilities by himself and to demonstrate his self-sufficiency.

Drive for Self-Enhancement

The desires of the manic patient center around the wish to increase his prestige, his popularity, and his possessions. In his expansive way he wishes to take in everything that life has to offer, and at the same time demonstrate to an increasingly greater extent his superior attributes. This is in contrast to the depressed patient who is driven to increasingly greater constriction of his sphere of experience and of his self-esteem.

PHYSICAL AND VEGETATIVE MANIFESTATIONS

Hyperactivity

The manic patient engages in a much higher level of activity than in his normal period. He often talks endlessly, to the point that his voice becomes hoarse. Unlike the agitated patient, however, whose activity is aimless, the manic patient has specific goals. The overactivity, both in speech and action, is in marked contrast to the slowing down in speech and action exhibited by the depressed patient.

High Tolerance for Fatigue

The manic patient seems to have a very high threshold for subjective fatigue. He claims he has endless energy and can go for many hours or even days, without rest. Some manic patients seem to maintain a high level of activity for weeks on end, with only a few hours' sleep at night. This is in marked contrast to the conspicuous fatigability of the depressed patient.

Appetite

The appetite of the manic patients is variable. In a case reported in 1911, Karl Abraham described the increased "orality" of manic patients. Although in some cases of mania the appetite may be voracious, in other cases, it may be diminished. The depressed patient generally has a loss of appetite and may skip a meal without being aware of it.

Increased Libido

The sexual drive is generally increased in the manic patient. The patients tend to be rather reckless and may be quite promiscuous during the manic phase. This characteristic of course is in marked contrast to the loss of libido experienced during a depressive episode.

Insomnia

As mentioned previously, the manic has a tendency to have less than the average amount of sleep. There is no fixed pattern to his sleeping. In many cases he feels so charged up that he is unable to go to sleep. In other cases he may awaken three or four hours earlier than usual. An interesting feature of his subjective reactions to his insomnia is the statement, "I woke up completely refreshed even though I had only two hours sleep." Insomnia is also characteristic of depressives but usually follows the pattern of early morning wakening rather than great difficulty in falling asleep.

BEHAVIORAL OBSERVATIONS OF MANIC PHASE

During the manic phase the behavior, speech, and temperament of the patient are so typical of this condition that it is generally easy to identify a manic patient upon entering a ward. He tends to be energetic, aggressive, animated, and overactive. He presents a demeanor of impulsivity, boldness, and lack of inhibition. He is generally sociable, genial and exhibitionistic. One of the striking features is the contagiousness of his humor and good spirits. The people in contact with him often remark on how they can empathize very readily with him because of his free emotional expression.

When frustrated, however, the manic patient may show a good deal of hostility and may launch vulgar tirades against the people he regards as his frustrators; at times he may be violent or assaultive. Some may show a dramatic alternation between a cheerful, outgoing manner and a withdrawn, suspicious, paranoid behavior. One patient had cycles of manic behavior alternating with paranoid behavior, each of about four to six hours' duration.

The spontaneous speech of the patient is usually increased and he generally finds it difficult to stop talking. He may continue to talk or sing until he becomes hoarse or he may lose his voice entirely. He frequently shows a flight of ideas by moving rapidly from one subject to another. In contrast to the disconnected flight of ideas of the schizophrenic, the manic usually demonstrates some unifying theme underlying his tangential associations.

The patient conveys the impression of being extremely susceptible to stimuli rising from within himself or within his environment. He is prone to associate or to respond rapidly to any external stimulus or to any thought that may arise. He frequently resorts to joking, making puns, rhyming, and humming or singing.

The manic patient often poses serious problems on the ward. He is not only difficult to control but he may mobilize other patients to join him in rebellious behavior. On the other hand, a manic patient may have a notable effect in arousing the interest and activity of a withdrawn, mute, schizophrenic patient.

The manic patients do not show any intellectual deterioration. In the more advanced stages, however, there tends to be an increased tendency towards errors because of the distractability.

Because of the decreased controls and impulsiveness, manic patients often get themselves into difficult situations and require hospitalization to prevent them from giving away all their money, embarking on unwise financial schemes, or engaging in other forms of self-destructive behavior.

Clayton, Pitts, and Winokur (1965) enumerated the frequency of 13 clinical features in 31 cases of mania. The results are presented in Table 6–2. It is notable that hyperactivity, flight of ideas, and push of speech occurred in all cases.

Table 6–2.
FREQUENCY OF CLINICAL FEATURES IN MANIA ($N = 31$) *

Symptom	Percentage of patients with symptom recorded as positive
Hyperactivity	100
Flight of ideas	100
Push of speech	100
Euphoria	97
Distractibility	97
Circumstantiality	96
Decreased sleep	94
Grandiosity and/or religiosity	79
Ideas of reference	77
Increased sexuality	74
Delusions	73
Passivity	47
Depersonalization and/or derealization	43

N = No. of patients.
* Modified from Clayton, Pitts, and Winokur (1965).

PERIODICITY OF MANIC-DEPRESSIVE BEHAVIOR

Many authors have noted a regularity or rhythm (periodicity) in the behavior of some manic-depressive patients. This has been most notable in the consistant diurnal variations in mood and in the regularity of the recurrence of manic and depressive phases.

Richter (1965) reviewed a number of case reports of patients who showed recurrences of their symptoms at relatively fixed time intervals. He postulated the existence of "biological clocks" to account for the regularities of the cycles. The timing of the cycles may vary from 24 hours to 10 years. He refers, for example, to a case reported by Kraepelin of a patient who experienced attacks of depression at the age of 30, 40, 50 and 60. Recently Bunney and Hartmann (1965) found 10 cases in the literature showing a regular cycle of 24 hours of mania alternating with 24 hours of depression, and added a complete description of an additional case.

Richter also reports some interesting experiments to demonstrate biological clocks in animals with specific brain lesions. He was able to produce cyclic changes in rats through incision of the pituitary gland. He also showed that by bringing the animals almost to the point of complete physical exhaustion, he could induce marked cyclical changes in their activity level.

Unfortunately, neither the reports of periodicity in the manic-depressive patients nor the experiments cast much light on the nature of the disturbance. Only a very small percentage of the cases show a fixed cycle; in fact, wide variation in the interval between recurrences is the rule. Even the diurnal mood variation attributed to depression is not found with great frequency (see Chapter 2). At this time it seems premature to stretch the concept of a biological clock beyond the very few cases that do show periodicity. Many of the latter cases have been studied thoroughly, however, and do show interesting biochemical fluctuations (see Chapter 9).

PREMORBID PERSONALITY OF MANIC-DEPRESSIVE PATIENTS

Many writers have emphasized the existence of a specific type of premorbid personality in patients who subsequently develop a manic depressive reaction. The particular premorbid personality is alleged to be characterized by traits such as gregariousness, joviality, and cheerfulness. Despite the widespread acceptance of this concept of a characteristic premorbid personality there have been no systematic studies that support this notion. Titley (1936) rated manic depressives and normals for the relative strengths of traits such as interests, sociability, and friendliness. He failed to find any differences between the two groups of subjects.

Further evidence against the notion of a specific type of premorbid personality in manic-depressive disorder is provided by a study by Kohn and Clausen (1955). The authors found that manic depressives were as likely as schizophrenics to have been socially isolated in early adolescence. The proportion of social isolates in both groups was close to one-third while in a normal control group the proportion of social isolates was close to zero. These results contradict the conception that manic depressives are extraverted in their younger years and that schizophrenics are predominently isolated.

Chapter 7.
Involutional Psychotic Reaction

The concept of a depression that is specific for the involutional period is embodied in the current term *involutional psychotic reaction* in the APA nomenclature (1952). The diagnostic manual specifies five criteria, each of which, as will be seen, is subject to question. The *etiology* is definitely indicated by listing this condition under the heading, "Disorders due to disturbance of metabolism, growth, nutrition or endocrine function." The *age of onset* is specified as the "involutional period." The *symptomatology* consists of "worry, intractable insomnia, guilt, anxiety, agitation, and somatic concerns." This nosological category includes a primary paranoid type as well as the depressive type that is our principal interest in this discussion. The *course* is described as "prolonged" and the *premorbid personality* as "compulsive." Some of the questions regarding the validity of this class-designation, as well as its defining characteristics, will be discussed in this chapter.

Although previous versions of the nomenclature listed two types (the melancholic and the paranoid) for coding purposes, there is no longer a separate code for each of these types. This omission may prove to be unfortunate in view of the gathering evidence that the involutional reaction consists of either late-occurring schizophrenia or late-occurring psychotic depressive reactions.

HISTORY OF THE CONCEPT

In his original formulation of the two great divisions of mental illness, dementia praecox and manic-depressive psychosis, Kraepelin conceived of the agitated depression of middle life as a completely independent entity with a variable prognosis. Other clinicians, however, were not convinced of the validity of this distinction. Thalbitzer (1905) contended that the so-called involutional melancholia properly belonged with the manic-depressive syndrome, and this point of view was buttressed by Dreyfus (1907) who made a detailed study of a series of 81 patients diagnosed by

Kraepelin as involutional melancholics. In reviewing this clinical material, Dreyfus decided that six cases were of questionable diagnosis and that the other 75 were manic depressives. He concluded that the overwhelming majority of cases of agitated depressions in the involutional period correspond to mixed states of manic-depressive psychosis and that there is no justification for considering involutional melancholia a separate entity. He was evidently impressed by the relatively high frequency of recovery in these patients (66 per cent) and, applying Kraepelin's criterion of prognosis, he reasoned that these cases belonged with other depressions of good prognosis that occurred in the earlier age group. He observed, furthermore, that 54 per cent had had previous psychotic episodes.

Kraepelin accepted Dreyfus's findings and ultimately yielded to his point of view: In the Eighth Edition of his text, he included involutional melancholia in the category of manic-depressive psychosis.

The controversy was hardly settled, however. In the United States, Kirby (1908), having reviewed Dreyfus's monograph, commented, "In a number of cases, the manic-depressive symptoms were plainly in evidence, the cases having been improperly placed with the melancholias. In a considerable number of other cases the author's conclusions that manic-depressive symptoms were present is based on extremely meager data." He consequently refused to accept Dreyfus's conclusions.

In another attack on Dreyfus's position, Hoch and MacCurdy (1922) disputed the assertion that involutional melancholics almost always recovered. They demonstrated in their series of patients a group that did not improve. They separated two groups of cases: one, allied with manic-depressive psychosis, which generally improved; and one allied with schizophrenia, which did not improve.

The outcome of the controversy was that although the official nomenclature in the United States followed the Kraepelinian system in its major outlines (Cheney, 1934), it departed from Kraepelin's taxonomy in listing involutional melancholia as a distinct diagnostic entity. Also, in England, despite the protestations of writers such as Aubrey Lewis, involutional melancholia is classified separately from manic-depressive psychosis (Henderson and Gillespie, 1963). This distinction is also made in the international classification of diseases of the World Health Organization, the Canadian nomenclature, the German classification (*Wurzberg Scheme*), the Danish nosology, the Russian classification, the Japanese classification, and the French standard classification (Stengel, 1959). It is apparent, on the other hand, from a perusal of recent publications, that the term is seldom used in systematic studies.

ETIOLOGY

The occurrence of this condition during the menopausal period in women (but presumably at a later age in men) has led some authors to attribute a major factor to hormonal or biochemical changes at this time of life. This thesis received temporary support from some uncontrolled studies suggesting that this condition responded to estrogenic therapy. These findings were later contradicted by a better-designed study by Palmer, Hastings, and Sherman (1941), who found estrogenic therapy less effective than electroconvulsive therapy. The final blow to the hope of estrogenic therapy was delivered by Ripley, a clinical psychiatrist, Shorr, an internist, and Papanicolaou, an endocrinologist, who combined their skills in a study (1940) of depressions in the involutional period. They found that estrogenic therapy did not directly modify the patient's depression, although it did provide some relief of the typical vasomotor symptoms associated with the menopause. At the present time, estrogens are rarely used for depressions in the involutional period.

There has been no solid experimental evidence linking abnormalities of growth, metabolism, or endocrine function to the occurrence of involutional depressions. Henderson and Gillespie (1963) reported that in their series at the Glasgow Royal Mental Hospital, 57 per cent of the women and 70 per cent of the men broke down as the result of psychic factors, whereas physical factors were of importance in only 21 per cent of the women and 6 per cent of the men.

It is apparent that the etiology of the depressions in the involutional period has not as yet been demonstrated and is still largely a matter of conjecture. It is, therefore, difficult to justify the listing of this condition under the heading of "disorders due to disturbance of metabolism, etc.," whereas the manic-depressive condition, for which there is some evidence of a genetic factor, is listed under the heading of "disorders of psychogenic origin or without clearly defined tangible cause or structural change."

The main basis for ascribing an organic etiology to the involutional depressions has been their occurrence during the involutional period. The same fact, however, can be used as evidence of psychogenicity as stated by Cameron (1944): "There is a gradual decline in physical vigor and health. Chronic illnesses in oneself, or in one's kin and friends, grow commoner and call one's attention to the passage of time. The realization of ambitions becomes obviously less likely. There is apt to be less personal plasticity and less interest in new friends and new adventures. In women the loss of youth and the end of child-bearing, and in men the prospect of diminished powers and of retirement, undoubtedly operate as etiologic factors."

AGE

There is no general agreement on the age range for involutional depression beyond vague terms such as the "involutional period," or "climacterium." For reasons not completely clear, moreover, this period is assumed to occur about ten years later in men than in women. Henderson and Gillespie state that this syndrome occurs between ages 40–55 in women and between 50–65 in men (1963). In another place, however, they concede that "a very similar syndrome may occur at an earlier age, in the twenties and thirties in women, and before the fifth decade in men" (1963, p. 233). Other writers have stretched the age limits so far in both directions as to attenuate the claim for a depressive syndrome that is specific for the involutional period.

Another question relevant to the specified age period is whether there is any valid difference between involutional depressions and depressive episodes of manic-depressive syndrome occurring in the same age period. There has been an assumption among nosographers that the onset of manic-depressive disorder is earlier than that of involutional depression. Hence, the diagnosis is often decided on the basis of age. When one examines the tabulated frequencies of the cases diagnosed in the state hospitals in New York, it is apparent that diagnostic fashion may have been a factor. The tables in the *Annual Report* show that as the diagnosis of involutional melancholia has increased, there has been a corresponding drop in the diagnosis of manic-depressive disorder (State of New York Department of Mental Hygiene, 1960).

Several studies of depressions occurring during the climacterium, furthermore, have indicated that in a large majority of the cases a depressive episode had occurred earlier in life. Berger (1908) found, in a study of 140 cases of climacteric psychosis, that only 14 of the patients were in their first psychosis, and he concluded that there is no specific phychosis of the climacterium. Driess (1942), in a study of 163 depressions in this age group, found there were only 17 patients who were experiencing their first depression.

SYMPTOMATOLOGY

The symptomatology generally ascribed to involutional depression is essentially that of an agitated depression. A number of authors have attempted to define various forms of this syndrome based on symptom variations but, as Henderson and Gillespie point out, these groups appear to be largely artificial.

Since agitation is the main symptom that would tend to differentiate involutional depressions from other depressions, certain questions naturally follow:

1. What proportion of all *agitated* depressions have their onset during the climacterium? Also, what proportion of depressions during the climacterium are characterized by agitation, and what proportion show retardation?

2. Is there any essential difference in symptomatology between cases diagnosed as involutional depression and cases of manic depression that have their onset early in life and that recur in the involutional period? In other words, is there a change in their symptomatology from retardation to agitation?

When the relative frequency of agitation and retardation in depressed patients in the involutional period is compared, the significance of agitation as a distinguishing characteristic is vitiated. Malamud, Sands, and Malamud (1941) reported, in a study of 47 cases diagnosed as involutional psychosis, that 17 (36 per cent) showed retardation and 24 (52 per cent) showed agitation. The remainder presumably showed neither retardation nor agitation.

Cassidy, Flanagan, and Spellman (1957) addressed themselves directly to the question of whether involutional patients could be distinguished from younger depressed patients on the basis of their symptomatology. They compared the relative frequency of 66 medical and psychiatric symptoms in two groups—20 female depressed patients aged 45 and older (with no previous episodes of depression), and 46 younger depressed females. There was no significant difference in the frequency of the symptoms. Retardation of thought, for instance, occurred with similar frequency in each group. Unfortunately, no data was presented regarding the relative frequency of agitation.

The most relevant—and crucial—study in the literature has been reported by Hopkinson (1964). He investigated the characteristics of 100 consecutive cases of affective illness in patients aged 50 or more at the University Clinic of the University of Glasgow. He studied the 61 cases experiencing their first affective illness, who, consequently, would be diagnosed as involutional, and compared these with the 39 who having had previous attacks, consequently, would be considered manic depressive. Contrary to the prevalent conception, he found that agitation occurred significantly more frequently in the manic-depressive group than in the involutional-depression group (61.5 per cent vs. 36.0 per cent; p < .02). This finding is strong evidence against the notion of a specific, involutional syndrome distinguishable from other depressions on the basis of the symptomatology.

In the course of our systematic investigation of depression (which will be discussed further in Chapter 11), we collected data relevant to the question of the relationship of agitation to involutional depression. We found that of 482 patients rated by the psychiatrists as to the degree of agitation, 47 per cent showed some degree of agitation (mild, moderate, or severe). The incidence of agitation among the various nosological categories was: neurotic-depressive reaction (95 cases) 57 per cent; psychotic-depressive reaction (27 cases) 70 per cent; involutional reaction (21 cases) 52 per cent; manic depressive, depressed phase (6 cases) 17 per cent; schizophrenic reaction (161 cases) 42 per cent; and all other nosological categories (172 cases) 44 per cent.

It is notable that agitation was a common symptom that occurred among the nondepressed patients, such as the schizophrenics, as well as among the depressed. Also, agitation was more frequently observed in patients diagnosed as psychotic depressive reaction and neurotic depressive reaction than in those diagnosed as involutional reaction. This seems to support the thesis that agitation is not specifically found among involutional depressions.

Another way of approaching the data is to determine whether agitation might be related to the involutional age period, irrespective of the specific diagnosis. When all the cases of the psychotic depressives were analyzed, it was found that there were 52 cases of agitated depression. Of these, 25 patients were younger than 45, and 27 patients were 45 or older, indicating that agitated depression occurs no more frequently among older psychotic depressives than among younger psychotic depressives. Similarly, among the 95 cases of agitation in the neurotic-depressive category, 72 occurred before age 45.

PREMORBID PERSONALITY

Several studies have attempted to define the premorbid personalities of patients with involutional depressions. The first study by Titley (1936) was methodologically superior to some of the later studies, and will be described in greater detail. On the basis of histories obtained by other psychiatrists, he compared the relative strength of various traits such as over-conscientiousness, meticulousness, and stubbornness in three groups of individuals: 10 involutional melancholics, 10 manic depressives, and 10 normal controls. Each was rated on a five point scale for each trait, and a trait score for each of the three groups was obtained by summing up the combined ratings of all the members of each group.

Titley found that the group scores of the involutionals were higher than those of the other two groups for the following traits: ethical code, saving, reticence, sensitivity, stubborness, over-conscientiousness, meticulousness about work, and meticulousness about person. The involutionals scored lower on the following: interests, adjustability, sociability, friendliness, tolerance, and sex adjustment.

Several limitations are apparent in this study, and these prevent ready acceptance of the findings. First, summing up the scores instead of presenting the median score in each group actually distorts the data in studies where there is no evidence of a normal distribution in the population. One or two extreme cases, particularly in such small groups, can radically alter the group score. Second, the normals scored slightly higher than the manic depressives on traits that have been generally described as indicative of the premorbid personality of manic depressives (interest, friendliness, sociability). This suggests either that the study disproves the hypothesis of a prevalent personality type among manic depressives or that this study is invalid. Third, there is a marked disparity in the mean age of the involutionals compared with the other two groups: involutional, 56.2 years; manic depressive, 29.2 years; and normal, 34.0 years. This finding suggests the possibility that the differences in premorbid personality may be a function of the age of the patients rather than of the type of illness. Fourth, the diagnostic categories used have a high degree of unreliability (see Chapter 11). Furthermore, the kind of patient characteristics assessed are notoriously difficult to rate and generally have a high degree of interjudge unreliability.

Finally, the number of each group (10) was relatively small, and in the absence of any tests of statistical significance there is no reason to ascribe the obtained differences to anything but chance.

Several other studies purportedly supported Titley's hypothesis of a typical premorbid personality in involutionals. Palmer and Sherman (1938) reached this conclusion on the basis of a comparison of the protocols of 50 involutionals with those of 50 manic depressives. They did not, however, present any tabulation or statistical analysis of their data, so the validity of their conclusions cannot be evaluated.

Malamud, Sands, and Malamud (1941) similarly endorsed Titley's profile of involutional traits, on the basis of a study of 47 involutional patients. An examination of their data indicates that the typical traits (conscientious, prudish, stubborn) occurred in only a minority of the cases, and the characteristic of outgoingness occurred just as often as the most frequent of the other traits. In decreasing order of frequency, the traits ascribed to the involutionals were: outgoing (15), introverted (15), sensitive (15), conscientious (9), prudish (7), stubborn (5), and frugal (3). Their own findings appear to contradict the contention of a specific personality organization in melancholics.

In summary, the studies do not settle the problem of a specific premorbid personality in melancholia. The investigations were too loosely designed to permit any definite conclusions, and in at least one instance (Malamud, Sands, and Malamud) the findings, if taken at their face value, appear to invalidate the notion of a specific premorbid personality.

CONCLUSION

A survey of the systematic studies of involutional depression raises strong doubt regarding the usefulness of this nosological category. The widespread belief that involutional depression may be distinguished from other types of psychotic depression on the basis of symptoms (such as agitation) has not been supported by controlled studies. Furthermore, there is no evidence that hormonal changes during the climacterium are in any way responsible for the depressions occurring during this period.

In the light of the currently available evidence, there is no more justification for allocating a special diagnostic label to depressions in the involutional period than there is for setting up other age-specific categories such as adolescent depressions or middle-age depressions. Moreover, the listing of the depressive and paranoid reactions of later life under the rubric of involutional reactions artificially binds together two clinically distinct disorders simply on the basis of the age of the patient.

Chapter 8.
Schizo-Affective Reaction

DEFINITION

The frequent association of prominent schizophrenic and affective symptoms, having engaged the interest of psychiatric nosographers for over a century, has led to the inclusion of schizo-affective reaction as a new category in the most recent American Psychiatric Association nomenclature (1952). This category is listed as a subtype of schizophrenic reaction along with the more traditional subtypes such as hebephrenic, catatonic, and paranoid, and its distinguishing characteristic is the occurrence of affective features (either pronounced depression or elation) in a setting of typical schizophrenic thinking and behavior.

As Clark and Mallet (1963) have pointed out, a large proportion of psychotic patients show an admixture of schizophrenic and affective features, and it is difficult to decide whether a given case should be regarded as "schizophrenia with affective features," or as "affective disorder with schizophrenia." In the United States it has been customary to assign these cases to the schizophrenic group. This practice is in keeping with the dictum of Lewis and Piotrowski (1954) that ". . . even a trace of schizophrenia is schizophrenia."

Two important questions are evoked by this innovation in the nosology: (1) Is this group properly placed in the schizophrenia hierarchy, does it belong with the manic-depressive group, or should it be classified as an independent entity? and (2) Is the prognosis for complete remission comparable to the affective disorders, or is it likely to be poorer, as in schizophrenia?

EVOLUTION OF CONCEPT

A review of the older literature indicates that three mainstreams converged to produce the current concept of schizo-affective reaction. The first consists of *new* subcategories of manic-depressive reactions; it includes

Kirby's description of a "catatonic syndrome allied to manic-depressive insanity" (1913) and August Hoch's delineation of "benign stupors" (1921). The second encompasses a number of syndromes with a symptomatology similar to schizophrenia but with a good prognosis; included here are Kasanin's "schizo-affective disorder" (1933) and many other syndromes with common features but with different names (Vaillant, 1964a). The third consists of studies of cases initially diagnosed as manic-depressive psychosis but that later showed the typical symptomatology of chronic schizophrenia (Hoch and Rachlin, 1941).

Catatonia and Manic-Depressive Psychosis (Kirby, 1913)

Kirby attempted to isolate from the dementia praecox category a group of cases showing catatonic symptoms that seemed to him to be more closely allied to the manic-depressive syndrome than to dementia praecox. In the introduction to his article he pointed out that Kraepelin's conception of catatonia as part of the dementia praecox group, and as sharing its poor prognosis, was contrary to Kahlbaum's previous formulation. Kahlbaum had stated that in catatonia there is a tendency to recover, and that only certain cases become chronic and deteriorate. Kraepelin recognized that certain cases of catatonia recover, but he regarded the remissions as temporary.

Kirby reviewed the symptomatology of an unspecified number of cases and presented five case histories of a catatonic syndrome that seemed to him to be part of the manic-depressive category. He noted that during the catatonic episode the patients showed the same types of symptoms classically associated with catatonia. They showed complete inactivity, rigidity, mutism, insensitivity to pin prick, and waxy flexibility. He noted, however, that these catatonic attacks seemed to occur as part of a circular psychosis; i.e., they alternated with manic attacks and thus could be regarded as having replaced the usual depressive phase in the manic-depressive psychosis. Sometimes the catatonic episode seemed to be essentially an extension of a pre-existent depression. The patients showed a thought content often found in depression, such as wishes to die, belief that they were dead, or preoccupation with the concept of hell. Later, when the patients were able to report their affect, they stated that they had felt depressed.

A striking feature of these cases described by Kirby is that they showed a complete recovery. The onset was generally acute and not of the insidious type associated with schizophrenia. The premorbid personality, moreover, was not of the schizoid type usually associated with patients developing schizophrenia. He concluded that the catatonic syndrome could be broken down into two main types: (*1*) cases with an insidious onset and a poor prognosis allied to dementia praecox; and (*2*) cases with an acute onset and a good prognosis allied to manic-depressive psychosis.

BENIGN STUPOR (HOCH, 1921)

In his monograph, *Benign Stupors: A Study of a New Manic-Depressive Reaction Type,* August Hoch presented 40 cases of benign stupors. The majority of the patients were within the age range of 15–25 years. He described the following classical features in the typical cases of deep stupor.

Inactivity

There was complete cessation or marked diminution of all spontaneous or reactive movement, including such voluntary muscle reflexes as contain a psychic component. For instance, there was interference with swallowing (resulting in accumulation of saliva and drooling), interference with blinking, and even interference with the inhibitory processes involved in holding urine and feces. Often there was no reaction to pin pricks. The inactivity frequently prevented the ingestion of food, so that spoon feeding or tube feeding had to be used. The patient either kept his eyes covered or stared vacantly, his face presenting an immobile, wooden, or stolid expression. Complete mutism was the rule. When activity was not totally absent the movements were slow. The patient often had to be pushed around.

Negativism

This consisted of marked stiffening of the body, either assumed spontaneously or appearing when attempts at interference were made. There was also more active turning away or even direct warding off, sometimes with scowling, swearing, or striking.

Affect

"Complete affectlessness" was an integral part of stupor reaction. The patient seemed basically indifferent, and only certain stimuli (some cheerful remark of a relative, or a comical situation) could elicit emotional reactions.

Catalepsy

Waxy flexibility (the tendency to maintain artificial positions) was a frequent but not an essential condition of the syndrome.

Intellectual Processes

According to Hoch, the deep-stupor patients did not betray any evidence of mentation, and retrospectively spoke of their minds as being blank. Incompleteness and slowness of intellectual operations were characteristic of the partial stupors.

Ideational Content

This was elicited either while the stupor was incubating, during interruptions, or from the recollections of recovered patients. Hoch found that 35 of the 40 patients showed a preoccupation with death, which was not only a dominant topic but often an exclusive interest. After recovery, the patient frequently spoke of having felt dead, paralyzed, or drugged. Hoch stated that 25 per cent of the patients acknowledged having had the delusion of being about to die, or of being dead, or of being in heaven or hell. The delusion of death was accompanied by complete apathy. Related to this was a tendency to suicidal impulses that were ostensibly as planless and unexpected as other impulsive acts of catatonics.

The stupor reaction included the partial stupors as well as the complete stupors. Hoch made an analogy to hypomania and mania: The former is merely a dilution of the latter; both are forms of the manic reaction.

Hoch believed that the fundamental characteristic of the stupor symptoms is a change in affect that could be summed up in one word—apathy. The emotional poverty was evidenced by a lack of feeling, by a loss of energy, and by an absence of the normal urge to live. He noted that inappropriateness of affect was not observed in a true, benign stupor.

He differentiated the catatonic type of schizophrenia from benign stupors by the presence, only in the former, of peculiarities such as empty verbalizations, giggling, and fragmented speech. Furthermore, in catatonic schizophrenia the onset is characterized by the pathognomonic symptoms of schizophrenia before the actual stupor occurs.

Follow-up Studies

Rachlin (1935) attempted to chart the progress of Hoch's benign stupor cases. Unfortunately, Hoch had provided sufficient identifying data for only 19 cases. Rachlin was able to locate only 13 of the 19, some of them as long as 30 years after their initial diagnosis by Hoch. Rachlin found that 11 of the 13 had been rehospitalized, and that six, after remissions lasting an average of 10 years, had developed the typical picture of dementia praecox (chronic schizophrenia). Rachlin believed that his study indicated the basic schizophrenic nature of the so-called benign stupors. In defense of Hoch's formulation, however, is the fact that, since Rachlin's follow-up tended to locate patients who had been rehospitalized, the patients who did well were not adequately represented in his tabulation.

Rachlin later (1937) reported a follow-up of 132 cases diagnosed as benign stupor by many different psychiatrists at the Manhattan State Hospital over a 17-year period. Of these, 56 were available for further study, and 76 were not available. After reviewing the available cases, Rachlin concluded that 40 (71.4 per cent) should have their diagnoses changed from benign stupor to dementia praecox. His available follow-up sample, however, was again biased in favor of patients who had not done well, i.e., the rehospitalized group.

Although stupor was listed as a form of manic-depressive psychosis in the 1934 Classification of the American Psychiatric Association (Cheney, 1934), it has now been omitted from the official nomenclature and is rarely mentioned in the recent literature. The publication of Rachlin's work accelerated the abandonment of Hoch's concept of benign stupors. It should be emphasized, however, that although a significant proportion of cases diagnosed as benign stupor belong in the dementia praecox (or schizophrenic) category, there is a substantial proportion whose postdischarge behavior is similar to that of manic depressives.

ACUTE SCHIZO-AFFECTIVE PYSCHOSIS (KASANIN, 1933)

Kasanin described a group of nine patients he had personally studied who had aroused his curiosity because of the special clinical picture they presented. They had all been diagnosed as having dementia praecox. They were young men and women (in their twenties and thirties) in excellent physical health. Various biological tests of the urine, blood, and spinal fluid were negative. They had average or superior intelligence and they had made a satisfactory educational or occupational adjustment prior to the onset of the illness. The attacks were preceded, however, by a difficult environmental situation that served as a precipitating factor. According to Kasanin, the environmental stress was chronic in some cases and acute in others. Examples listed by the author included the loss of a job, a state of anxiety over sudden promotion, a difficult love affair, an alien environment, and hostile in-laws.

Kasanin stated that the psychosis was usually ushered in by a latent depression, and a certain amount of rumination persisted for some time until the dramatic schizophrenic picture appeared. He observed that he was able to reconstruct the psychological significance of the psychosis through reviewing the various symptoms and behavior with the patient after his recovery, and that they then became quite intelligible. He found that there was comparatively little of the bizarre, unusual, or mysterious.

In his summary, Kasanin emphasized the following clinical features:

1. The psychosis was characterized by a very sudden onset in a setting of marked emotional turmoil with distortion of the outside world and, in some cases, false sensory impressions.

2. The psychosis lasted from a few weeks to a few months and was followed by complete recovery.

3. The patients were in their twenties or thirties and usually had a history of a previous attack in late adolescence.

4. The prepsychotic personalities of the patients showed the usual variations found in any other group.

5. A good social and vocational adjustment, the presence of a definite and specific environmental stress, an interest in life, and the absence of any passivity or withdrawal were considered factors favoring recovery.

It is of some interest that Vaillant included three of these cases in his follow-up study of remitting schizophrenics (1963a); one relapsed into chronic schizophrenia after about four years, one had five recurrences after about eight years of total remission, and one died of chronic brain syndrome 10 years after remission.

Acute Remitting Schizophrenia (Vaillant, 1964a)

Vaillant (1964a) showed that since 1849 at least 16 different names have been attached to a condition characterized by (*1*) an acute picture resembling schizophrenia, (*2*) symptoms of psychotic depression, and (*3*) recovery. Proceeding from Bell's mania in 1849, these have included melancholia with stupor (1861), acute dementia (1862), mixed conditions of manic-depressive psychosis (1903), catatonic syndrome allied to manic-depressive insanity (1913), homosexual panic (1920), benign stupor (1921), hysterical twilight state (1924), schizo-affective psychosis (1933), schizophreniform state (1937), Gjessing's syndrome (1938), reactive state of adolescence (1944), acute exhaustive psychosis (1947), oneirophrenia (1950), cycloid psychosis (1960), and adolescent turmoil (1964).

In addition to the symptoms of schizophrenia and depression with recovery, most of the writers described a good premorbid adjustment, psychologically understandable symptoms, ascertainable precipitating causes, confusion, and concern with dying. These characteristics are similar to those generally associated with manic-depressive illness.

Studies of Revised Diagnoses

There is evidence that certain patients who have been initially diagnosed as manic depressive, but who show a component of schizophrenic
symptomatology, will exhibit progressively more schizophrenic symptomatology on each subsequent admission. Lewis and Hubbard (1931) studied
a group of 77 patients originally diagnosed as manic-depressive psychotics
who were followed for a number of years and finally diagnosed as schizophrenics. These writers observed that, regardless of whether the first psychosis was characterized by an elation or a depression, there was an increasingly greater tendency for the content to become schizophrenic in subsequent attacks. They stated, "These schizophrenic developments were so
pronounced that should the psychiatrist, making a diagnosis on the basis
of affect, have seen the patient in a later attack he would not have the least
hesitation in making a diagnosis of dementia praecox." The picture generally became one of schizophrenia with deterioration. The early schizophrenic signs occurred in the first observed attack but were minimized by
the diagnosing physician. These signs consisted of odd somatic feelings,
hypochondriac ideas, strange attitudes, and auditory hallucinations subjected by the patients to a mystical interpretation.

A later report by Lewis and Piotrowski (1954) was based on a study
of 5 patients who, after a first admission to the New York State Psychiatric
Institute in New York City, had received discharge diagnoses of manic-
depressive psychosis. They were rediagnosed by Lewis at least three years
and not more than 20 years after discharge. For more than 90 per cent of
the patients the follow-up interval was at least seven years long. The new
diagnosis was made on the basis of historical data and of a personal examination, except in the case of a patient hospitalized elsewhere at the time of
the study.

Of 70 patients initially discharged as manic depressives, 38 (54 per
cent) were considered to have developed a clear-cut schizophrenia. The
authors made a determination of 10 signs which appeared much more frequently in the records of patients who later developed obvious schizophrenia
than they did in the records of those who remained genuine manic-depressive psychotics (see Differential Diagnosis below). By assigning a score of
one point for each of these 10 signs, the writers found a clear-cut cleavage
between these two groups. Patients with more than two points were schizophrenics; those with less than two points were almost all manic depressives.

Hoch and Rachlin (1941) examined the records of approximately
5,800 cases of schizophrenia admitted to the Manhattan State Hospital in

New York City. From this pool they found 415 cases whose initial diagnosis of manic-depressive psychosis could not be confirmed on later admission to the hospital. In other words, 7.1 per cent of the cases of schizophrenia had been originally misclassified as manic-depressive psychosis. The authors mentioned a number of points that should be considered in making the differential diagnosis.

DIFFERENTIATION OF DEPRESSION AND SCHIZOPHRENIA

In his paper on benign stupors (1935), Rachlin points out that one rarely sees a true depressive patient throwing furtive glances or a manic patient refusing to answer questions verbally but choosing to write the reply instead; similarly, the incongruity of a patient in a state of playfulness laughing at his pranks and drooling saliva at the same time is indicative of a schizophrenic process rather than of a manic-depressive disorder. Sudden changes in behavior with impulsiveness (the refusal to eat one meal and then eating the next ravenously) are also more suggestive of schizophrenia. Finally, evasiveness and reticence upon improvement may be seen in schizophrenics but not in manic-depressive psychosis.

Hoch and Rachlin (1941) point out that, although periodicity or repeated attacks of a short duration are frequently considered a characteristic of manic-depressive psychosis, many cases of schizophrenia show complete remissions with apparent well-being between psychotic episodes. The authors suggest that in many of the so-called good recoveries a careful examination will "disclose defects in the affectivity or in the behavior."

Hoch and Rachlin also emphasize the importance of careful evaluation of the patient's ideation. Illogical remarks or incongruous statements with bizarre elaboration should arouse a suspicion of schizophrenia. Even a slight dissociation between affect and thought content is indicative of schizophrenia.

The authors point out that cases of mania with auditory hallucinations and paranoid delusions end up as schizophrenia. They emphasize particularly the importance of ideas of reference or persecution as indicative of the schizophrenic process. Also indicative of schizophrenia is the rapid changing of the delusional and hallucinatory content accompanied by fluctuating affect: A patient who rapidly alternates between laughing and crying would be more likely to be schizophrenic than manic depressive. In the pure affective disorders, the mood tends to be relatively consistent and does not show notable fluctuations over brief periods. Lewis and Piotrowski (1954) also emphasize this differential characteristic.

The ten signs listed by Lewis and Piotrowski (1954) as indicative of an underlying schizophrenic process in cases initially diagnosed manic depressive are:

Sign 1. Physical sensation with dissociation: This sign denotes delusions of perception rather than delusions of judgment. The authors cite as an example, "There is a steel plate in my forehead." "I have the skin of a monkey and I'm going to be a human being turned into an animal." "I feel as though a piece of meat is sticking out of my rectum." Also allocated to this category were electrical sensations in the body, especially in the genitals, the feeling that one is growing thinner or smaller (contrary to evidence), and the impression that the neck was crooked when it was not. These were also treated as instances of "physical sensation with dissociation."

Sign 2. Delusions regarding others: These include misidentification and misrecognition of people. One patient felt that her parents had risen from the dead and were physically present whenever she quarreled with her husband. Another believed that some of his fellow patients on the ward were his close relatives. One patient was convinced that her baby was dead even though it was alive and was being shown to her. Another patient, hearing someone cough, became convinced that this person would die, and began to cry from grief.

Sign 3. Delusions regarding physical objects: One patient felt at times that objects in her environment had become unreal. Other patients had the idea that the walls, beds, etc., were changing size or shape. Another patient spoke to objects as though they were human beings.

Sign 4. Feeling of physical isolation and personal unreality: Some patients were anxiously aware of being separated from everything else by space or air. These patients stated either that the distance was greater than it actually was or that the air or space were impenetrable. Complaints of unreality, such as are indicated by a patient's impression that he lives in a dream world, were also classified in this category.

Sign 5. Inability to concentrate: This sign was credited to patients who had complained spontaneously of inability to concentrate. It was not credited to patients who, because they were preoccupied with worries or fears, could not concentrate on a subject suggested by the examiner.

Sign 6. Feelings of having changed: The feeling of having changed applied to complaints such as: "Something slipped in my mind. Some nerve jumped." "I see myself in an institution for the rest of my life." "My mind has just disintegrated and gone down until it is nothing."

Sign 7. Speech disturbance and intellectual blocking: This sign was applied to inability to complete a sentence in the absence of physical fatigue or emotional tension, or a change in the subject matter of the patient's talk. Also classified as speech disturbance was a sudden and unintelligible mumbling, not only if it interrupted the patient's speech but also if it occurred after the patient had been silent. Other instances of speech disturbance in this category were: staring ahead in an attempt to collect the thoughts before answering questions or before making spontaneous remarks; opening the mouth to talk but remaining mute; complaining that "the thoughts are not just right," because the patient had intended to say something else.

Sign 8. Uncontrolled repeated interrupting and anxious thought: This sign included auditory and visual hallucinations. One patient complained that while he was trying to think of words his thoughts were telling him to kill people.

Sign 9. Ideas of reference and/or feeling of being controlled by inimical outside forces (paranoid ideas): This sign was credited to patients who clearly accused other persons or some external forces (magic or real) of definite attempts at harming them. This sign was particularly applicable if it implied bizarre, involved, or magical thinking.

Sign 10. Seclusiveness maintained or increased in hospital: The patient was credited with this sign if he had stayed in the hospital at least a month without becoming less seclusive, despite psychotherapy and other forms of treatment and despite participation in some organized activities on the ward. Practically all the patients who maintained or increased their seclusiveness were eventually diagnosed as schizophrenic.

The authors tabulated the frequency of each sign in schizophrenics who had originally been misdiagnosed as manic depressive and in those manic depressives who retained their diagnosis. Signs that discriminated most effectively between the two groups are 1, 6, and 10 (physical sensation with dissociation; feelings of having changed; and ideas of reference).

PRESENT STATUS OF SCHIZO-AFFECTIVE DISORDER

The concept of schizo-affective psychosis as outlined in the American Psychiatric Association nomenclature (1952) differs in at least one significant way from Kasanin's description (1933). In the present nomenclature, the condition is unequivocally classified with the schizophrenic reactions rather than in the borderland between the schizophrenic and the manic-depressive reactions. Since the glossary states that "in prolonged observation, such cases prove to be basically schizophrenic in nature," it implies that the prognosis is not better than that of schizophrenia generally.

This is at variance with the previous descriptions of a remitting schizo-affective disorder.

Vaillant (1963a), on the basis of his long-term, follow-up study of remitted schizophrenics, suggests that the term be used as defined by Kasanin. Thus, schizo-affective disorder would cover cases of good premorbid adjustment and acute onset, and manifesting affective features, confusion, and preoccupation with death.

Henderson and Gillespie (1963) are dubious about the use of the term schizo-affective psychosis and offer the opinion that it has created more diagnostic difficulties than it has solved. They assert that in the majority of cases the term has been applied incorrectly to cases which should have been diagnosed as manic depressive disorder, mixed type, in which the admixture of depressive and manic symptoms has given rise to some apparent incongruity of affect. Despite such resistance to the introduction of this new category, the International Classification of Diseases includes schizo-affective psychosis under the generic category of schizophrenic disorders (Stengel, 1959).

PROGNOSIS

A study by Clark and Mallet (1963) attempted to determine the relative frequency of readmissions for patients initially diagnosed as schizophrenic, as schizo-affective disorder, and as depressive disorder. The proportions in each group requiring readmission within three years of discharge from the hospital were: schizophrenic, 70 per cent; schizo-affective, 53 per cent; and depressive, 20 per cent. This finding was in keeping with the report of Hunt and Appel (1936) that the recovery rate for cases of psychosis "lying midway between schizophrenia and manic-depressive psychosis" was twice as good as in schizophrenia, and 50 per cent poorer than in pure, manic-depressive psychosis.

The "acute, remitting schizophrenias" described by Vaillant (1964a), characterized by acute onset of typical schizophrenic symptoms, affective components, and complete remission, would probably be classified today as schizo-affective reactions. A 50-year follow-up study of a group of 12 of those patients by Vaillant (1963a) provides valuable information about the ultimate prognosis of such cases. Eight of the 12 led independent useful lives for at least 25 years. The ultimate prognosis was not good, however; eight eventually required chronic hospitalization.

The prognosis of schizo-affective reactions may be further illuminated by examining studies of the relation of affective factors to outcome in schizophrenia. Since most of these studies were conducted before the subcategory schizo-affective type was officially adopted, the cases of schizo-phrenia with depression, "intrapunitive tendencies," self-degrading delu-sions, etc., undoubtedly correspond to the new category. The findings of these earlier studies may therefore be used as a basis for establishing the prognosis of the schizo-affective type of schizophrenia. These studies are discussed in the next section.

AFFECTIVE FACTORS AND PROGNOSIS IN SCHIZOPHRENIA

Diverse studies have indicated that in cases diagnosed as schizophrenia, the presence of depressive features in the individual or in his family history is a favorable prognostic factor. Among the examples of the relationship of depression to improved prognosis in schizophrenia have been studies of the manifest affect (Zubin *et al.*, 1961), the content of delusions (Albee, 1951; Zubin *et al.*, 1961), the content of hallucinations (Zubin *et al.*, 1961), family history of affective illness (Zubin *et al.*, 1961; Vaillant, 1963b), the specific subtypes of schizophrenia (Zubin *et al.*, 1961), and studies of the overt behavior of the patients (Albee, 1950; Feldman, Pascal, and Swenson, 1954; Phillips and Ziegler, 1964).

Manifest Affect

Zubin and his coworkers (1961) reviewed 800 studies of outcome of schizophrenia. In 159 studies the relationship of affect to prognosis was reported. In all 159 the presence of overtly expressed affect, regardless of its quality or direction, generally led to a good outcome. The types of affect mentioned were: elation, depression, anxiety, and general emotional reac-tivity. The presence of guilt, either overt or inferred, was associated with a good outcome in all 15 studies in which it was noted.

Content of Delusions

Zubin reported that in two studies in which intrapunitive delusions were distinguished from extrapunitive delusions, the presence of the former favored a good prognosis. As pointed out in Chapter 2, delusions of the intrapunitive type are characteristic of depression. Albee (1951) studied the outcome of 261 patients with schizophrenia admitted to a mental hos-pital. He distinguished self-condemnatory delusions from other types of delusion. In the former category he included: delusions of heinous crimes, horrible sins, ugliness, worthlessness, contamination, deformity, and dis-eases; also delusions that horrible odors that were offensive to other people emanated from the patient. Albee used as a criterion of outcome whether the patients were improved or recovered one year after admission to the hospital. He found that there was a relationship between recovery and self-condemnatory delulsions significant at the .01 level. Persecutory delusions, on the other hand, were found to be significantly related to poor prognosis.

Hallucinations

Zubin found that the presence of hallucinations contributed to a bad outcome in five of six studies. In one study, however, where the content of the hallucinations was of a self-accusatory nature, the prognosis was improved. As pointed out in Chapter 2, when hallucinations occur in depression, they tend to be of a self-accusatory nature.

Manic-Depressive Heredity and Outcome in Schizophrenia

Zubin noted that in six of seven studies there was a positive relationship between a family history of manic-depressive psychosis and a favorable prognosis in schizophrenia. In one study he found that there was no relationship between family history and outcome. Vaillant (1963b) also studied the relationship of manic-depressive heredity and outcome of schizophrenia. He found that among schizophrenics who recovered completely from their illness the frequency of relatives with affective psychosis was significantly higher than among those schizophrenics with an unfavorable prognosis.

Presence of Depression

Vaillant, in a prospective prediction of schizophrenic remission (1964b), found that the presence of depression was associated with full remission in 77 per cent of the cases. This was significant at the .01 level of confidence.

Patterns of Aggression in Overt Behavior

Zubin and his coworkers (1961) reported that patients with "self-directed aggression," as opposed to those with externally-directed aggression, showed a good prognosis. In eight of nine studies the prognosis was favorable for patients showing internally-directed aggression. This contrasted with eight of 13 studies that showed a bad prognosis when externally-directed aggression was present.

Albee (1950) studied 127 psychiatric patients in a mental hospital in regard to the relation of the direction of aggression to outcome of treatment. Patterns of aggression were classified as extrapunitive or intrapunitive according to whether patients involved in injuries inflicted the injuries on someone else or on themselves. He found that when the aggression was intrapunitive the improvement rate was significantly higher than when the aggression was extrapunitive. Albee analyzed the data on the 81 schizophrenics in the group to determine whether the relationship held when they were considered separately from the nonschizophrenic group. He found that more than half of the schizophrenics classified as intrapunitive improved, but only one-seventh of the extrapunitive schizophrenics improved ($p < .001$).

Feldman, Pascal, and Swenson (1954) also studied the direction of aggression as a prognostic variable in mental illness. A group of 486 hospitalized patients were categorized as improved or unimproved one year after discharge from the hospital. It was found that patients who tended to direct blame or hostility towards themselves rather than towards others had a significantly better prognosis than those who directed hostility exclusively onto the environment.

Phillips and Ziegler (1964) studied the case histories of 251 patients to investigate the relationship between the symptom clusters and two outcome measures, length of hospitalization and rehospitalization. As predicted by the authors, the patients whose symptomatology was characterized by a "turning against himself" had a shorter period of hospitalization than patients whose symptoms fell into the "avoidance of others" category.

Zubin notes that the reason for the improvement in cases with internally-directed aggression is not clear. He suggests that one should take into account the possibility that the hospital may be more willing to release patients with internally-directed aggression, since they may be more readily tolerated by the community than patients with externally directed aggression. On the other hand, many studies indicate that complete recovery, rather than simply discharge from the hospital, is associated with the presence of various characteristics of depressive illness.

Albee (1951) proposes that the self-condemnatory patient evaluates himself on the basis of social standards and therefore operates at a higher level of maturity than the patient with externally-directed aggression. Phillips and Ziegler similarly postulate that the person who assumes a "turning against the self" role has incorporated the values of society and, consequently, experiences guilt when he does not successfully meet these values. They conjecture that a pathological solution to life's demands (e.g., pronounced withdrawal) would be unacceptable to such a person; hence he would have an improved prognosis.

CONCLUSION

It is apparent from the review of the pertinent literature that the presence of affective factors significantly increases the probability of improvement in cases of schizophrenia. This finding was reported in a recent study of the schizo-affective subtype of schizophrenia, as well as in numerous studies conducted prior to the official adoption of this new subcategory. The improvement in this type of schizophrenia is greater than in the other types at all levels: In terms of the degree of improvement (mild, moderate, or marked); in terms of the proportions showing total remission; in terms of frequency of recurrence (measured by frequency of rehospitalization); and in terms of chronicity (measured by duration of hospitalization). On the other hand, the prognosis in schizo-affective disorder is not as good as in manic-depressive reaction.

These observations could be expressed graphically by viewing the cases of *functional* mental illness in terms of a spectrum: at one end are the pure manic-depressive cases with a good prognosis; and at the other are the pure schizophrenic cases with a poor prognosis. In between are varying blends of these disorders (the schizo-affective cases) with a fair prognosis. This relationship between diagnosis and prognosis may be conceptualized in terms of the operation of two variables: the schizophrenic variable linked to a poor prognosis; and the affective variable linked to a good prognosis. The cases at either end of the spectrum represent one of these variables —either the schizophrenic or the affective. The cases between the poles contain both variables, and the resultant prognosis depends on the relative strength of each.

The nature of these two diagnostic-prognostic variables has not been determined. It seems likely, however, that the determinants of schizophrenic and affective disorders include some factor (or factors) responsible for the prognosis. It could be conjectured that the schizophrenogenic determinants include a factor inhibiting recovery or promoting chronicity. The determinants of the affective disorders, on the other hand, could contain a factor promoting recovery. When the two variables are mixed, as in schizo-affective disorder, the cases also show a mixture of the recovery-inhibiting and recovery-promoting factors. The resultant prognosis is based on the balance between these two factors.

In view of the fact that the schizo-affective cases show clinical features in common with both the schizophrenic and the affective disorders, a question could be raised regarding the most appropriate classification. It might be wise to separate the schizo-affective category from the other schizophrenic subtypes, since the former show not only a different prognosis, but also a better response to antidepressant medication. Isolation of this category, moreover, might promote further investigation of its specific characteristics.

Part II.
EXPERIMENTAL ASPECTS
OF DEPRESSION

Chapter 9·
Biological Studies of Depression

The biological aspects of depression have received considerable attention in the past 60 years. Hundreds of studies have been reported in the literature; tests have been made of almost all the known constituents of the blood, the urine, and the cerebrospinal fluid; and careful pathological studies of the brain and other organs have been conducted. Yet, few "positive" findings have stood the test of time, and there is still very little basic knowledge of the biological substrate of depression.

The more recent biological studies of depression are reviewed in this chapter. As in earlier studies, the initial positive findings have often been discounted by later negative findings. One of the problems contributing to contradictory results has been the lack of adequate control of such factors as age, sex, weight, state of nutrition, and type of diet. The lack of control for age, in particular, has been responsible for many positive findings that were later disconfirmed. It has been amply demonstrated that changes in metabolism and physiological responses occur with advancing age; since depressed patients tend to fall into the older age groups, they tend to show responses different from younger control groups.

The major biological studies of depression are summarized in Table 9–1. I have attempted to assess the validity of the various findings using a scale of: certain, probable, uncertain, and doubtful. None of the findings has as yet had sufficient confirmation to justify the label "certain." To qualify for *probable* validity, a particular finding must be based on a well-designed study with both proper controls and attention to known sources of error such as diagnostic unreliability. Furthermore, the finding must be corroborated by well-designed studies by other investigators. When earlier findings based on loosely-designed studies have been contradicted by well-designed studies, or when a positive finding is more readily explained on the basis of some variable other than depression, the finding is classified as doubtful. The "uncertain" label applies to areas of conflicting results, inadequate experimental design, or lack of independent confirmation.

Table 9–1.
BIOLOGICAL STUDIES OF DEPRESSION

Area of study	Finding	Validity
Constitution	Relation to pyknic physique	Doubtful
Identical twins	Concordant for depression	Uncertain
Glucose metabolism	Decreased glucose tolerance	Uncertain
Electrolytes	Sodium retention	Uncertain
Steroids	Increased secretion	Probable*
Mecholyl test	Abnormal vascular response	Doubtful
Salivation	Decreased secretion	Doubtful
Sedation response	Decreased threshold	Doubtful
Sleep EEG	Decreased stage 4 sleep	Probable
Photoconvulsive response	Decreased threshold	Uncertain
EMG	Increased residual activity	Uncertain

* Finding not specific for depression.

Only two findings have been assigned the label probable. The increased steroid secretion seems to warrant this designation, but is not specific for depression. The EEG studies with one exception show decreased periods of deep sleep; the single contradictory finding may be explained by the administration of sedatives during the testing period.

MANIC-DEPRESSIVE DISORDER AND CONSTITUTION

The name Ernst Kretschmer has been intimately associated with the theory of the relationship between various types of psychoses and physical type. On the basis of his clinical observations, he postulated that there is a biological relationship between pyknic physique* and manic-depressive psychosis. He reported (1925) that 81 of 85 schizophrenic patients had a leptosomatic habitus; whereas 58 of 62 manic depressives had a pyknic physique.

A large number of studies have been carried out in the ensuing years. Some of these studies strongly support Kretschmer's findings, but others provide only partial support or do not support his theory. A thorough critical review of the literature has been presented by Rees (1960).

In a study of 100 manic depressives, 100 normals, and 100 schizophrenics, Clegg (1935) found only partial support for Kretschmer's theory. Burchard (1936) compared a group of 125 manic depressives and 125 schizophrenics. The patients were initially classified on the basis of a global impression of the examiner into pyknic, athletic, and asthenic types. He found an association between the pyknic type and manic-depressive psy-

* *Pyknic* type corresponds to the terms *endomorphic* or *eurymorphic* used in later reports.

choses and between the leptosomatic type and schizophrenia. He was also able to find a statistically significant relationship between the classification of the leptosomatic physique based on anthropometric indices and schizophrenia. He reported, however, that the physical type is influenced by the age of the patient; this finding, of course, casts some doubt on the significance of his results. Wittman, Sheldon, and Katz (1948) also found a significant correlation (0.51) between endomorphic (pyknic) physique and manic-depressive disorder. Age was not properly controlled, however.

Anastasi and Foley (1949) found a definite tendency towards a more pyknic body build with advancing age; this finding held for both manic depressives and schizophrenics. A similar observation was made by Farber (1938), who studied a number of physical dimensions and ratios in 18 manic depressive patients and 81 schizophrenics. He found that the pyknic physique becomes more common with increasing age. He also suggested that the greater likelihood of physical deterioration among schizophrenic patients could account for their appearing leptosomatic.

Rees (1944) compared 42 manic depressive patients with a group of normal subjects and 49 schizophrenics. Using a variety of physical measures and body-build ratios, he found a greater tendency to eurymorphic (pyknic) build in the manic depressive group. Rees concluded that this relationship could be explained only partially—not completely—on the basis of age differences, and that there was a hard-core relationship between body-build and affective disorder.

In evaluating the aforementioned studies, certain methodological problems should be taken into account: (1) The schizophrenic patients in the studies were younger than the manic depressives. Since there is a transition from leptosomatic to pyknic physique with advancing age, the differences in physique may be due to age. (2) Nutritional status may affect body-build indices. It might be expected that chronic schizophrenics would exhibit more pronounced physical effects than manic depressives as a result of longer duration of hospitalization (Bellak, 1952). Furthermore, if the reports of a relationship between high social class and manic depressive disorder are valid, the manic depressives might be expected to have had better nutrition during their developmental period. (3) The possibility of contamination or bias was present to some degree in most of the studies. An investigator making ratings of physical indices cannot be oblivious of the presence or absence of affect in the patients and may be influenced by his theoretical preconceptions. Furthermore, in making the clinical diagnosis, the investigator may be influenced by the clinical stereotype of the lean, sallow schizophrenic and the rotund cyclothymic (manic depressive). (4) As Rees (1960) has shown, there are no disparate types corresponding to pyknic and leptosomatic, but there is a continuous gradation from one extreme to the other.

SUMMARY

There has been no well-designed study to test Kretschmer's findings. With our present state of knowledge we must consider that the association of pyknic physique with depression is an artifact, resulting from intermediate variables such as age and nutritional status.

HEREDITY IN MANIC-DEPRESSIVE DISORDER

A number of writers have presented evidence in favor of the theory that some persons are *carriers* of a specific predisposition or vulnerability to manic-depressive psychosis (Kallmann, 1952; Slater, 1953). These investigators have attempted to demonstrate that the tendency to develop this disease increases in proportion to the degree of blood relationship to a patient with this disorder. The studies of manic-depressive disorder have in general yielded concordance rates consistent with the theory of transmission of the disorder via a dominant gene (Kallmann, 1952).

On the basis of his survey of 461 persons, Kallmann computed the following expectancy rates of manic-depressive psychosis among blood relatives of patients with manic-depressive psychosis. He used the *twin family* method in his studies.

> 0.4 per cent in general population
> 23.5 per cent in parents
> 16.7 per cent in half siblings
> 23.0 per cent in full siblings
> 26.3 per cent in nonidentical twins
> 100.0 per cent in identical twins

IDENTICAL TWIN STUDIES

Kallmann's Study

Kallmann (1952) isolated a group of 23 manic-depressive patients who were distinguished by their having identical (monozygotic) twin siblings. In 22 cases, the cotwin was also diagnosed as manic depressive. The essential diagnostic feature was the presence of "acute, self-limited, and unadulterated mood swings before the fifth decade of life and no progressive or residual personality disintegration before or following manic or depressive episodes."

A number of problems are raised by Kallmann's twin studies:

The problem of diagnostic unreliability. The possibility of bias by the investigator in making a diagnosis of one twin when he has full knowledge of the psychiatric status of the twin-partner must be considered. In Kallmann's study the degree of concordance is surprisingly high in view of the demonstrated low reliability of psychiatric diagnoses. It would be expected that diagnostic variability would have substantially reduced the concordance if completely independent diagnoses were rendered.

The problem of ascertainment of twins. The reliance on the patient's own report for the ascertainment of the twins is a source of error. Moreover, the selection of material from resident hospital populations introduces a sampling bias; for example, concordant cases are more likely to come to a hospital than discordant cases because it is a heavier burden for a family to take care of twin psychotics than one psychotic at home (Tienari, 1963). It is possible, furthermore, that Kallmann's attention was more likely to be called to cases in which manic-depressive disorder existed in both twin partners than to cases in which only one twin partner had the disease. This selective factory could spuriously inflate the obtained concordance.

The problem of determination of zygosity. As Gregory (1961) has pointed out, there is considerable inaccuracy in the older methods of zygosity determination (i.e., identical vs. fraternal twins) used in the psychiatric studies cited above. These inaccuracies have ranged as high as 30 per cent as compared with more refined serological typing.

Slater's Study

Slater (1953) collected a much smaller group of identical twins with affective disorders. He used more refined methods for determining zygosity than did Kallmann, and he also presented more complete data. Of the eight twin pairs, four were concordant for affective disorder. Of the discordant cotwins, three were diagnosed as normal and one as neurotic. The author points out that among the concordant twins there were many dissimilarities in the clinical picture. Although this series is too small to draw any definite conclusions, it should be noted that the degree of concordance (50 per cent) was substantially less than the 100 per cent expectancy rate presented by Kallmann.

Tienari's Study

A study that attempted to correct the methodological inadequacies and to plug the loopholes in the previous investigations of mental illness in twins has been reported by Tienari (1963). His material consisted of all live births in Finland from 1920–1929. The establishment of twinship was based on the birth register. For zygosity determination he used refined serological techniques in addition to the older methods. The investigator found 16 schizophrenic cases and one case of reactive psychosis among the identical twins (no case of affective psychosis was found). The most striking feature of the report is that in not a single instance did the cotwin of a schizophrenic patient also have schizophrenia; the degree of concordance was zero! This finding is remarkable in view of Kallmann's report of a corrected expectancy rate for schizophrenics of 86.2 per cent.

The relevance of Tienari's findings to the twin studies of depression is that Kallmann used the same techniques for twinship ascertainment, zygosity determination, and diagnostic labelling in his investigation of manic-depressive psychosis as in his investigation of schizophrenics. If the results of his studies of schizophrenia are invalid, then his findings in manic-depressive psychosis are subject to serious doubt.

IDENTICAL TWINS REARED SEPARATELY

Shields (1962) conducted an investigation into the genetic and environmental factors and variation in personality. He organized his study so that twins volunteered for the study by sending their names to the British Broadcasting Corporation. Among the volunteers were 44 monozygotic pairs separated in early life and brought up apart. Shields matched this group with 44 nonseparated monozygotic twin pairs who served as controls.

Shields found that the twins reared together were more alike on various personality ratings than the separated pairs. This difference, however, was not statistically significant. He also found that the separated as well as the nonseparated twins had considerable similarity in mannerisms, voice, temperament, and tastes. Certain extreme personality variables, such as quick temper, anxiety, emotional lability, rigidity, and cyclothymic tendencies, showed approximately the same degree of concordance in the separated group as in the nonseparated group.

On a test for extraversion, both the separated and nonseparated pairs showed significant correlations. The correlation coefficient for extraversion was higher (.61) in the separated group than in the control group (.42). Since extraversion is claimed to have some relationship to the premorbid personality of manic-depressive patients, this finding may be of some significance. The separated twins also showed a higher interclass correlation coefficient on a test for neuroticism (.53) than did the nonseparated twins (.38).

The data regarding the concordance of psychiatric disorders among the twins is inconclusive, but it is worthwhile to mention it here. One set of separated twins had psychiatric disturbances with depression and tenseness after the age of 40 and they were advised to have treatment in a mental hospital. In three cases, one of the twins had neurotic-depressive episodes. In summary, one set of twins was concordant for affective disorder and three sets were discordant for affective disorder. Obviously the sample is too small to draw any conclusions.

PEDIGREE STUDIES

Stenstedt (1952) studied 288 manic-depressive cases. He found the morbidity among the siblings, parents, and children of the patients was 11.7 per cent for the males and 11.8 per cent for the females. The patients used in this study had been admitted to psychiatric hospitals from a Swedish rural area during the years 1919–1948. Various sources of information were explored regarding the patients and their relatives. When there was a possibility of psychiatric disturbance in a relative, then the relative himself was examined. Fourteen families were excluded because of insufficient information. The period of observation ranged from 14 months to more than 20 years.

The morbidity risk for manic-depressive disorder in the investigation district was calculated to be about 1 per cent if uncertain cases were included. The morbidity risk among the relatives of the patients was as follows: parents, 7.5 per cent; siblings, 14.1 per cent; and children, 17.1 per cent.

Using data from structured interviews of 748 consecutive patients admitted to a psychiatric hospital, Winokur and Pitts (1965) attempted to determine the prevalence of affective disorders among relatives of patients diagnosed as having manic-depressive reaction, psychotic-depressive reaction, neurotic-depressive reaction, or involutional reaction. Of the initial sample, 366 patients received one of these diagnoses. Information regarding the prevalence of affective disorders among the relatives of the patients was received either from a relative accompanying the patient or from the patient himself.

The investigators found a prevalence of affective disorder in 22.9 per cent of the mothers of the patients and 13.6 per cent of the fathers of the patients. The authors determined that the prevalence of affective disorders in the siblings was much greater when one or both parents had an affective disorder than when neither parent had an affective disorder.

According to the authors, neither a single recessive gene nor a single dominant gene hypothesis is supported by the data.

Some limitations of this study are: (*1*) Information regarding the prevalence of affective disorder in the relatives was obtained either from a single relative accompanying the patient or from the patient himself. No examination was made of the relatives other than the one accompanying the patient. This leaves a wide area of uncertainty regarding the validity of diagnoses based on data that could be incomplete or biased. (*2*) The presence of a positive family history of affective disorder could have exerted some influence on the diagnosis of the patient, particularly when the clinical picture was ambiguous. (*3*) The follow-up of the members of the family did not cover a sufficient period of time to insure that all members had passed through the *risk period*. (The age of risk as proposed by Fremming (1951) ranges from 20 to 65 years.)

Summary

There is considerable variation in the reported frequency of affective disorders among relatives of patients with affective disorders. In any event, excessive frequency of a particular psychiatric disorder among relatives of a patient does not in itself prove that the disorder is hereditary. Genetic transmission is only one inference from the findings; noxious environmental influences within particular family groups could also account for the findings. The available research data does not establish conclusively whether affective disorders are genetic, environmental, both, or neither.

BIOCHEMICAL STUDIES OF DEPRESSION

Early Studies (1903–1939)

Despite the hundreds of studies of manic-depressive disorder performed during this period, there were no unequivocal findings that related this disorder to any biochemical abnormalities. Cleghorn and Curtis (1959) summarized this as follows:

> The work of the early twentieth century was performed mainly in the search for somatic pathology to account for manic-depressive psychosis as described by Kraepelin. These can be summarized quickly by saying that every accessible cell, tissue, and fluid was studied by every technique available at the time with negative results. Certain abnormalities of the glucose tolerance curve were found but in no respect did this differ significantly from that found in patients suffering from schizophrenia, anxiety, or the all-inclusive 'emotional tension.'

In 1939 McFarland and Goldstein presented an exhaustive review of the biochemical studies of manic-depressive psychosis up to that date. These authors presented in tabulated form the negative results, and in descriptive form the positive results, of 134 studies. These studies are summarized below.

Blood Glucose

The authors tabulated 19 studies in which the blood glucose was within normal limits. The largest study was by Whitehorn, and this included 520 cases; 345 were depressed, 151 were manic, and 24 were mixed. In 6 studies the blood glucose was above normal limits.

Glucose Tolerance

The glucose tolerance curve was normal in 5 studies and abnormal in 16 studies. Kooy found an elevated tolerance curve in cases of melancholia, but he also found equally elevated curves in cases of marked anxiety.

Acidity and Alkaline Reserve

Studies of the pH of the blood of manic depressives were within normal limits in 7 studies. One study by Poli of 12 depressives and 10 manics reported constant and marked lowering of the pH in excitable states and a normal or slightly lowered pH in depressive states. The alkaline reserve was markedly diminished in excitable states and almost normal in depressive states.

Serum Calcium and Phosphorous

These constituents of the blood were found to be normal in 9 studies. But 5 other studies failed to confirm these normal values in the manic depressive. Klemperer, for example, reported that calcium was diminished in agitated melancholia. Cases of melancholia with stupor also had low calcium, but cases of mania had high calcium.

Nitrogenous Substances

Ten studies indicated that the nitrogen metabolism of the manic depressive was within normal limits. Two studies, however, reported abnormal findings. Looney, for example, tested 30 cases of depression and reported a high plasma content of nitrogenous substance. He expressed the opinion that toxic amines were present in the blood of markedly depressed cases.

Lipoidal Substances

Normal cholesterol values were obtained in 4 studies, and abnormal values in 12 studies. In general, the investigations reporting abnormal values showed hypocholesteremia, and the abnormality could usually be attributed to the degree of activity of the patient.

Chlorides

The blood chlorides were reported as within normal limits in 5 studies. In one study of 11 anxious and depressive psychotics, however, the chloride values in whole blood and in plasma were increased above normal.

Critique of Studies

In analyzing the results of the biochemical studies, McFarland and Goldstein point out that the manic-depressive patients have tended to show both an intraindividual and an interindividual variability greater than that shown by normal controls. Furthermore, there seem to be indications of a slightly greater variability in the personal constants of the depressive when compared with that of the manic patient. Critical reviews and subsequent, more systematic, studies have substantially discounted the few positive findings reported above.

The abnormal glucose tolerance curve, as pointed out by Cleghorn and Curtis (1959), did not differentiate manic-depressive psychosis from other psychiatric disorders. The defective glucose tolerance was considered by Gildea, McLean and Man (1943) as an artifact, produced by delayed absorption of the test glucose from the gastrointestinal tract. When they administered glucose intravenously instead of orally, they did not obtain an abnormal glucose tolerance curve. This finding is disputed by Pryce (1958), who also used the intravenous route but found decreased tolerance among depressed patients as compared with a control group. Since glucose tolerance decreases with age, deficiency of carbohydrate in the diet, and chronic malnutrition, the finding of abnormal glucose tolerance in the depressed patients must be interpreted cautiously. The finding of hypocholesteremia has been contradicted by Whittier *et al.* (1964).

RECENT STUDIES (1940–1966)

Differences Between Manic and Depressive Phases

In 1942, Cameron presented a thoughtful review of comparisons of biochemical findings in mania and depression. He criticized the studies primarily on the basis that the so-called clinical entities in the studies had been a collection of many diverse phenomena.

The usual laboratory experimental reports simply throw together all the results obtained from patients with mood disorders, get an average and perhaps state the deviations and range of determinations and then compare such figures with similar ones obtained from unselected groups diagnosed as schizophrenic. Often no indication whatever is given as to whether individual patients included are overactive or stuporous, resentful or cooperative, fearful or secure, even though the possible effects of such differences are well known to any clinician. . . . No amount of refined statistical treatment can make data presented in such a way of any significance.

Cameron came to the following conclusions: (*1*) There is no correlation between basal metabolism and mood but there is some evidence that the basal metabolic rate in affective disorders is related to the degree of general activity, anxiety, and fear. *Manic and depressive patients do not give determinations at opposite ends of the scale.* (2) The blood pressure shows no relation to mood; variability of pressure may be marked in a given person, but the degree of lability does not correlate with lability of mood. (*3*) Blood pressure reaction to adrenaline indicates some difference between stupors and excitement but not between elation and depression. (*4*) Blood glucose level determinations after administration of ephedrine produce no significantly different results. (*5*) Glucose tolerance curves are not correlated with the direction of the mood disorder. (6) Evacuation of barium from the gastrointestinal tract shows differences; depressed patients have considerably delayed evacuation. (7) Significant differences are reported for the rate of parotid gland secretion, with the manic rates falling within the normal range and depressive rates falling well below it. (8) Elevated gastric acidity is reported for manic and agitated depressives and low values for retarded depressives.

In conclusion, Cameron emphasized the fact that the studies do not differentiate between mood disorders as such.

"The contrast most often made in the reports seemed to be associated not with mood differences but with differences in the kind and degree of action involved. Tense or agitated persons thus, may show more in common in their biological function with elated and excitable persons than they do with other depressive syndromes. *This is not compatible with the hypothesis that elation and depression are fundamentally opposed metabolical processes.*"

In the past 15 years there has been much investigation of water and electrolyte metabolism in depression although the exhaustive reviews of the literature by McFarland and Goldstein in 1939 (see above) indicated that the plasma electrolytes are within normal limits in depressed patients.

Studies of Continued Cycles

A systematic attempt to ascertain changes in metabolism in association with changes in the mental status was first made by Gjessing (1938) in cases of *periodic catatonia*. By placing his patients on a fixed intake of food and fluid over a period of many months, it was possible for him to make a detailed balance study during several cycles of the biphasic illness.

Gjessing's technique has been applied to a number of manic-depressive patients who showed rapid alternations of mood. In these cases, a period of depression and retardation of a few days' duration was followed by a normal interval of one or more days and then by a short period of elation and overactivity. These cycles continued to repeat themselves over many months or years.

The first studies in depressives were stimulated by the ancient observation that the urinary output tends to be low during the depressed phase and high during the manic phase. Despite the obvious explanation that the difference may be attributed to the fact that manic patients tend to drink more than depressed patients, investigators have sought a more important reason to account for the differences in urinary output.

Klein and Nunn (1945) studied a 67-year-old patient who had unfailing regularity of the rhythm of his manic-depressive cycles each week for 14 years. Clinical observation, continued over a period of months, had shown a period of five days of depression followed by two of mania. The writers undertook parallel clinical and biochemical investigations to correlate metabolic changes coincidental with the variations in his mental state. Various autonomic changes were associated with the changes in the mood; during the manic phases, there was a definite rise in blood pressure, pulse, and respiratory rate.

For a period of several months, this patient was given a constant balanced diet and a constant fluid intake. Urine collections were made at 12-hour intervals. He showed a cyclic metabolic fluctuation consisting of a retention of water and salt in the depressive phase and a release in the manic phase. This was accompanied by a weight gain during the depression and a corresponding weight loss during the manic phase. The sudden rise in the flow of urine started when the patient was still in his depression and was maintained at this high rate during the early stages of his manic phase. By the time he had reached the most excited state, however, the rate of urinary excretion had already decreased.

Klein described a second case in 1950. The patient was a 40-year-old male who had recurrent attacks of depression and mania, varying in duration over a period of five years. A depressive attack usually lasted about 13 days and was followed by a manic phase lasting 18 days. The manic phase was followed by about 14 days of normal mood. This patient also was studied on bed rest, with a constant diet of food and fluid. In contradistinction to the first case, there was no evidence of any fluid or electrolyte retention at any stage of the cycle.

Crammer (1959) reported a metabolic study of two chronic psychotic patients with recurring mental disturbances, who showed periodic losses and gains of body weight associated with the particular phases of the illness. Weight loss was accompanied by polyuria with increased urinary excretion of sodium chloride; weight gain by oliguria and sodium retention. In one patient, the weight loss occurred at the beginning of an attack of depression; in the other, the weight loss began just before the emergence from a depressive, semistuporous state into a hypomanic state.

Studies during Depressive Episodes

Gibbons (1960) investigated a group of 24 patients who "showed the clinical picture of so-called endogenous depression." He found that upon recovery from depression there was a decrease in exchangeable sodium. No consistent change in total exchangeable potassium was found. The author concluded that the results supported the hypothesis that depression is accompanied by retention of sodium that is excreted during recovery.

Russell (1960) investigated 15 depressed patients by the metabolic balance technique for periods of two to five weeks, during which time they received electroconvulsive treatment. He found that the patients showed a slight loss of sodium that was not statistically significant during the period of recovery.

Coppen and Shaw (1963) studied 23 patients with "severe unremitting depressions." They found that residual sodium, which includes intracellular and some bone sodium, was very significantly increased during depression. Exchangeable sodium and extracellular sodium did not change significantly. The total body water, extracellular fluid, and extracellular chloride were all greater after recovery.

Lobban *et al.* (1963) studied chloride, sodium, and potassium excretion in 20 depressed patients and compared them with 25 neurotic controls. It was found that the depressives excreted less sodium and chloride than the control groups during the day and more at night. They concluded that depressed patients showed a disturbance of the diurnal rhythm of electrolyte excretion that is not secondary to changes in behavior or diet. Of course, it could be argued that the differences between the two groups could be a sign of disturbance of the diurnal rhythm of the control group of neurotics rather than of the depressed patients.

Anderson and Dawson (1962) reported that about half of a series of 98 depressives had a high blood level of acetylmethylcarbinal. This finding was contradicted by a study by Assael and Thein (1964) which did not reveal a significant increase of this acetaldehyde metabolite in depression.

Flach (1964) investigated the calcium metabolism in 57 patients maintained on constant control diet on a metabolic unit. He found that following the administration of electroconvulsive treatment or imipramine therapy for the alleviation of depression, there was an associated significant decrease in the urinary excretion of calcium. This change was also noted in paranoid schizophrenic patients, but not in patients diagnosed as psychoneurotic. The changes, moreover, were apparent in patients who improved on therapy but were lacking among those who failed to improve clinically during the period of study.

Cade (1964) reported a significant elevation of plasma magnesium levels in schizophrenia and depressive states but not in manic patients. This finding, which persisted after clinical remission, could be the result of age differences that were not controlled in this study.

The many reports of successful treatment of manic patients with lithium ion gives further evidence that changes in electrolytes may be important in affective disorders. During the manic phase the patients have an unusually high tolerance for lithium. With the resolution of the mania this tolerance disappears and is accompanied by a massive excretion of lithium (Gershon and Yuweiler, 1960). Although the mechanisms of action of the lithium ion in the treatment of mania have no immediate explanation, these findings should provide a stimulus for further investigation.

Gibbons (1963) believes that any electrolyte changes in depression are probably *secondary effects* of the illness. Some may result from changes in the amount and composition of the diet or from the variation in motor activity. Others may be the result of the affective disturbance.

Responses of Normal Subjects to Stress

Schottstaedt, Grace, and Wolff (1956) found that depression-inducing life experiences, whether occurring in the natural course of events or artificially in the laboratory, are associated with abnormal patterns of renal excretion of water and electrolytes. The evoked reactions in the five subjects consisted of reduced physical activity, attitudes of futility or hopelessness, and feelings of depression or exhaustion. These were associated with decreased rates of excretion of water, sodium, and potassium, as compared with the excretion rates observed during neutral and tranquil periods.

Summary

It seems that in some cases of alternating mania and depression, variations of water and sodium metabolism parallel the fluctuations in mood.

But studies using the metabolic balance technique in single attacks of depressive illness have failed to reveal such variation. Some studies with radio-sodium indicate that there may be some alteration in sodium metabolism. In general, the investigations provide equivocal evidence of disturbance of water and mineral metabolism in depression. The specific findings reported above need further confirmation by independent studies. Even in the case of confirmed positive findings, it is difficult to assess the significance of changes in water and mineral metabolism because these may be secondary to abnormalities known to be associated with the depression. Among these deviations are: poor food and fluid intake; reduction in physical activity; and increased steroid secretion.

ENDOCRINE STUDIES

Steroid Metabolism

There is substantial evidence that changes in steroid metabolism accompany certain phases of depression as well as other psychiatric disorders. Some evidence suggests that an excess of adrenal hormones may produce psychiatric disturbances. Other evidence suggests that the excess adrenal hormones may be the result of, rather than the cause of, a psychiatric disturbance.

A possible association between the "humours" and mental disorder has been postulated since ancient times. Almost every newly isolated hormone has been used in an effort to treat psychiatric disorders, with inevitable failure. The development of techniques for isolating the steroids in the blood and urine, as well as the introduction of steroids into the treatment of various medical conditions has recently focused attention on the relationship between steroids and psychiatric disorders.

Michael and Gibbons (1963) have presented a comprehensive review of the relationship of steroids to psychiatric disorders. They point out that the experience of emotion by healthy subjects is associated with a rise in the plasma level of 17-hydroxycorticoids. This increase in adrenocortical activity occurs both when the emotional arousal is produced spontaneously in response to naturally-occurring environmental events and when it is induced experimentally. An increase in the plasma level of cortisol or the urinary excretion of 17-hydroxycorticoids, for instance, has been reported in the following stressful situations: in hospitalized patients just prior to major surgical procedures; in relatives accompanying severely ill or injured members of their family to the emergency room of a hospital; in students anticipating or following examinations; and in boat-race crews just prior to a race. Increases in steroid secretion have also been noted in reaction to experimentally-induced stress in the laboratory. Subjects admitted to the hospital for a sleep deprivation experiment were found to have a rise in their blood steroid levels before beginning the actual experiment. Moderate rises in the steroid level have been reported among patients subjected to stressful interviews. The level of the plasma steroids correlates more closely with the intensity of the affect (anxiety, anger, or depression) aroused than with any specific affect. Emotional arousal, in general, rather than any particular type of emotional reaction or any particular type of stress-inducing stimulus, seems to be responsible for the increased steroid levels.

Michael and Gibbons point out that notable increases in plasma steroids occur in anxious and depressed patients and in acute schizophrenic patients showing emotional turmoil. Chronic schizophrenic patients, however, displaying no appreciable disturbance of affect, have steroid levels within the normal range. Improvement of depressed patients seems to be accompanied by a decrease in the adrenal cortical activity. Adrenalectomized patients who are maintained on adequate doses of steroids experience a more serene emotional life and less fluctuation in moods than before their illness. This finding suggests to Michael and Gibbons that the changes in adrenocortical function which accompany emotion may have a role in determining the emotional experience.

Board, Wadeson, and Persky (1957) demonstrated that plasma cortisol levels were higher in depressed patients than in normal controls. The more emotional stress observed in the patient, the higher was the observed steroid level. On subsequent testing, the steroid level generally fell, although a few patients who had received electroconvulsive therapy showed increasing levels. Curtis, Cleghorn, and Sourkes (1960) investigated the relationship between urinary 17-hydroxycorticoids and various affective states. They found steroid excretion higher in the anxiety cases than in the depressed patients.

Gibbons and McHugh (1962) measured the plasma cortisol at weekly intervals in 17 depressed patients during 18 periods of stay in the hospital. The authors found elevated levels of plasma cortisol. In general, the more severe the depression the higher the cortisol level. The 18 cases' recovery from depression was accompanied by a decline in cortisol level. Kurland (1964) conducted serial studies of urinary steroid excretion in five neurotic-depressed patients and five manic-depressed patients. He found the excretion of 17-ketogenic steroids for the total group of 10 patients significantly correlated with the clinical depressive symptomatology. He also reported that the diurnal variation in the excretion of these compounds followed the usual diurnal variation recorded in the mood of depressed patients: the highest rate occurred during the early morning hours and decreased progressively throughout the day and night.

Gibbons (1964) measured the plasma cortisol in 15 depressed patients. Elevated secretion rates were found before treatment; these were higher in the more severely depressed patients. In 10 patients, relief of depression was accompanied by a substantial decrease in the secretion rate.

In a series of studies, Bunney and his coworkers demonstrated the relationship between steroid secretion and depression. In one study Bunney, Mason, *et al.* (1965) investigated the relationship between urinary steroid excretion and behavioral ratings. Seven patients were followed during periods of psychotic depressive crises. In general, they found that the onset of a depressive crisis was accompanied by a substantial increase in 17-hydroxycorticoid excretion.

In another investigation, Bunney, Hartmann, and Mason (1965) studied the behavioral and biochemical changes in a patient with 48-hour manic-depressive cycles. The 17-hydroxycorticoid excretion levels were found to alternate regularly every other day in the opposite direction from 24-hour ratings of mania. On the high manic days the 17-hydroxycorticoid levels were low, and on the immobile depressed days the levels were high.

Bunney and Fawcett (1965) also investigated the relationship between successful suicide and previous excretion of excessive 17-hydroxycorticoid levels. Three patients who committed suicide but who had previously showed relatively low ratings as suicidal behavior, revealed high mean 17-hydroxycorticoids just prior to their suicides.

Thyroid Function

There has been no consistent evidence of thyroid dysfunction in depression. Brody and Man (1950) found that the serum protein bound iodine (PBI) of depressed schizophrenics did not differ significantly from that of nondepressed schizophrenics or normals. Gibbons *et al.* (1960) found no significant differences between 17 depressives and normal controls. Most patients showed a slight decline in the PBI upon recovery from the depression.

Summary

From a large number of investigations it is apparent that increased steroid output is associated with depression, and that the greater the degree of depression the greater the steroid output. It has also been observed that the steroid levels decrease substantially following improvement or recovery.

But the increase in adrenal steroid output is by no means specific for depression. It has also been found in cases of anxiety and in disturbed schizophrenics. It seems to be related more to the intensity of the affect than to the specific kind of affect. An exception, however, is the finding that the steroid levels are low in many cases of mania.

No significant abnormalities of thyroid function have been demonstrated in depressed patients.

AUTONOMIC FUNCTION

BLOOD PRESSURE RESPONSES TO MECHOLYL

Funkenstein (1954) reported that he and his coworkers had demonstrated a relationship between blood pressure reactivity and depression. Although a number of techniques were used, the one that has continued to be employed by most subsequent investigators measures the response in blood pressure to an injection of Mecholyl. This procedure has been referred to as the *Funkenstein test*.

The test consists of the measurement of blood pressure at specific intervals before and after the intramuscular administration of Mecholyl. A positive response is defined as an excessive drop in blood pressure and a prolonged rate of return to the normal level. Funkenstein reported this effect in 32 of 36 (88.9 per cent) manic-depressive or involutional patients. He attributed this response to an excessive secretion of an epinephrine-like substance. He regarded the remaining 4 cases as showing evidence of an excessive secretion of norepinephrine. He also reported a relationship between an epinephrine-like response and a favorable outcome after electroconvulsive therapy. Another related finding was that students showing intrapunitive behavior in response to stress had an epinephrine-like pattern, whereas those showing extrapunitive responses had a norepinephrine pattern.

As has often been observed in the history of medicine, the early reports were enthusiastic and tended to support Funkenstein's findings. After several years, however, discrepant results were reported, and serious doubts were raised regarding the reliability of the test procedures and the validity of the findings. In a critical review of the literature up to 1958, Feinberg (1958) summarized the methodological inadequacies of the studies and the contradictory results. He also suggested that the relationship between the epinephrine-like pattern and depression might be a reflection of the fact that the depressed patients tended to be older than the patients in the comparison groups. Since an epinephrine-like pattern is shown in elderly normals as well as in patients in the older age groups, the relationship between depression and the particular physiological response could be spurious. Attempts have been made to improve the methodology and the design of investigations using the Funkenstein Test; these improved investigations have used more objective criteria in estimating the degree of depression and in assessing the changes in blood pressure. Hamilton (1960b) found a correlation of .42 between age and the drop in blood pressure following the injection of Mecholyl.

A critical review of the literature by Rose in 1962 failed to quell any of the doubts raised by Feinberg (1958) and Hamilton (1960b) regarding the validity of Funkenstein's findings. In a well-designed study incorporating a partial blockade of the autonomic ganglia, Rose demonstrated that the drop in blood pressure following Mecholyl administration could not be attributed to central autonomic activity, but was probably related to peripheral end-organ sensitivity. This finding tends to vitiate Funkenstein's thesis that depressed patients secrete excessive amounts of epinephrine.

Further doubt of the validity of the theory underlying use of the Funkenstein Test is raised by direct measurement of the output of adrenaline and noradrenaline. Funkenstein postulated that the vascular responses of depressed patients resemble those induced by an injection of adrenaline and are, therefore, indicative of excessive adrenaline secretion. Curtis, Cleghorn, and Sourkes (1960), however, found that the adrenaline excretion of depressed patients was *lower* than that of other psychiatric patients; in addition, contrary to Funkenstein's thesis, adrenaline excretion was higher in depression than in other psychiatric states.

Summary

The validity of the Mecholyl test and its theoretical underpinnings remain in doubt. No definite answer can be found until the parameters of the test are better defined and studies are conducted using more precise psychological and clinical measures, proper controls, and independent (blind) clinical and physiological ratings.

SALIVATION STUDIES

Complaints of dryness of the mouth have been noted by psychiatrists examining depressed patients. A number of studies have been conducted to determine whether there is any objective evidence of diminution of salivary secretion among depressed patients.

Strongin and Hinsie (1938) attempted to compare the parotid gland secretory rate in manic-depressive patients with that of deteriorated schizophrenics and normal controls. A suction cup was applied to the parotid duct, and saliva was collected. The authors concluded that the depressed patients showed decreases in salivation as compared to the nondepressed sample. In a more refined study, Peck (1959) used dental swabs to absorb the total salivary flow. Three dental rolls were placed in the mouth of each subject for a period of two minutes. Allowances were made for evaporation, and the rolls were weighed to determine the amount of salivary absorbtion. The test was applied to a heterogeneous group containing depressed and nondepressed patients. It was found that the depressed patients showed a diminished salivary secretion.

Gottlieb and Paulson (1961) applied Peck's technique to 18 hospitalized patients with the diagnosis of depressive reaction. The patients were tested again following recovery from the depression. It was found that 8 patients had increased salivary secretions and 10 patients had decreased salivary secretions after recovery; there was no significant difference between salivation rates when ill and when recovered.

Busfield and Wechsler (1961) studied 87 patients. Of the 45 judged to be significantly depressed, the diagnoses were: 20 schizo-affective and 25 neurotic or psychotic-depressive reactions. The depressive ratings were: 23 mildly depressed; 14 moderately depressed; and eight severely depressed. The depressed group was compared with 42 nondepressed patients; the diagnoses being 16 schizophrenics and 26 others. Salivary secretion was measured by using dental rolls. It was found that the depressed hospitalized patients showed significantly less salivation than did the nondepressed hospitalized patients or the normal controls. There was not, however, any significant difference among the mildly, moderately, and severely depressed patients. In another report, Busfield, Wechsler, and Barnum (1961) attempted to differentiate between reactive and endogenous depressions on the basis of the salivation. They found that the group of endogenous depressions showed a significantly lower salivation rate than did the reactive group.

Davies and Gurland (1961) found that 30 depressed patients had a slightly *higher* salivation than 11 schizophrenics. Both groups, however, secreted significantly less saliva than normal controls (age not stated). Palmai and Blackwell (1965) measured the salivary flow in 20 female patients who had a diagnosis of depressive illness. Controls were selected from the female nursing staff and, according to the authors, were "matched for age and weight." However, no statement was made as to the range of weight or the mean weight in the two groups. The investigators found that the depressed patients showed significantly diminished flow throughout the 24 hours compared to controls. There was a gradual recovery in flow on return to normal diurnal rhythm during treatment with ECT.

Critique of Salivation Studies

(*1*) Studies in which comparison groups were used did not adequately control factors such as age, sex, diet, state of oral hygiene, etc. Many of the differences shown, such as the difference between endogenous and reactive groups, may be accounted for in part or in total by the age discrepancy. It has been well-established that in the older age groups there is a notable decrease in the salivation rate of normal people (Ship and Burket, 1965). (2) The longitudinal studies (Gottlieb vs. Davies) show a definite discrepancy. In the former there was no significant change in salivation with recovery, whereas in the latter an increase in salivation was reported. (3) Age-specific values for the excretion of saliva had not been established and there is no evidence, in any event, that the degree of salivation reported was abnormally low. (4) There was no consideration given to the presence of certain oral disorders such as pyorrhea, dental caries, and stomatitis, frequently found in chronic mental disorders, especially depression; these certainly may influence the activity of the salivary glands. (5) There was no attempt to control for smoking habits. Experimenters have found that the amount of saliva in the mouths of smokers is substantially increased. (6) The nature of the food ingested prior to the salivation tests could influence the results. It is well-known that depressed patients ingest less water and food than normals.

NEUROPHYSIOLOGICAL STUDIES

SEDATION THRESHOLD

In a series of articles, Shagass reported on the use of a procedure designed to differentiate among various psychopathological groups. The procedure consists of determining the sedation threshold of the patient in terms of the amount of amobarbital sodium required to produce a specified increase in frontal EEG activity. In a study of 182 patients, Shagass, Naiman, and Mihalik (1956) found that the threshold for the psychotic depressives was low, whereas the threshold for neurotic depressives and anxiety states was high. Shagass concluded that the *sedation threshold test* could be used as an objective test to differentiate between neurotic and psychotic depressions.

A number of studies since the original reports by Shagass cast some doubt on the validity of his conclusion. Ackner and Pampiglione (1959) performed the sedation threshold test on 50 psychiatric patients. They failed to find any significant relationship between the sedation threshold and any of the diagnostic groups. Nymgaard (1959) reported that the mean sedation threshold of a group of 44 psychotic depressives was significantly lower than that of a group of 24 neurotic depressives. It is noteworthy, however, that the mean age of the psychotic depressives was 49 whereas that of the neurotic depressives was 37. Martin and Davies (1962) determined the sleep threshold by intravenous sodium amytal for 30 depressed patients and 12 normal controls. The depressed patients were categorized as endogenous, reactive, or indeterminate. The writers found no significant difference in the sedation threshold among the various groups. Martin and Davies reported another study on the sedation threshold in 1965. As in their previous report, they failed to find any difference between the neurotic and psychotic depressions in terms of the sedation threshold. Friedman and his coworkers (1965) measured the sedation threshold in a group of paranoid and depressed patients. In an initial comparison, it was found that the depressed sample had a significantly lower sedation threshold than the paranoid sample. Friedman (1966) found, however, that when the two groups were equated for age, this difference disappeared. Friedman, incidentally, found a correlation of 0.22 between age and sedation threshold score.

Summary

The work on the sedation threshold has yielded contradictory results. On the basis of the findings to date it seems there is no solid experimental support for the hypothesis that there is a significant difference in the sedation threshold of the neurotic and psychotic depressions. Whatever differences have been reported may be attributed to the age difference between the neurotic and psychotic depressives and to the fact that the sedation threshold tends to increase with age.

ELECTROMYOGRAPH (EMG) STUDIES

Whatmore and Ellis (1959) measured "residual motor activity" of depressed patients by means of the electromyograph. They found that in either an agitated or a retarded state the residual motor activity of the depressed patients was at abnormally high levels. The investigators also found, however, that the *invisible* motor activity tends to increase with age. This finding again indicates the importance of controlling for age in studies of this type.

Whatmore and Ellis (1962) presented a longitudinal study of depressed patients with severe recurrent depressions. They found that during the period of depression the EMG readings were markedly elevated. Accompanying treatment there was a temporary drop in the readings. During the period of well-being following treatment and prior to relapse the readings were markedly *elevated*.

Goldstein (1965) made basal recordings of muscle action potential during 15 minutes of rest and also in response to a noise stimulus. She found that of the various psychiatric patients the depressed patients showed the most pronounced skeletal muscular response during the noise. Autonomic activity during both rest and stimulation was also heightened in the depressed patients.

Summary

All of the studies of muscle potential in depression must be regarded as preliminary. The finding that retarded and mute patients show increased muscular activity is intriguing. Larger samples and the establishment of age-specific norms are necessary, however, before any definite conclusion may be reached.

ELECTROENCEPHALOGRAM (EEG) SLEEP STUDIES OF DEPRESSED PATIENTS

Diaz-Guerrero, Gottlieb, and Knott (1946) performed continuous sleep recordings of the entire night's sleep of six patients diagnosed as having manic-depressive psychosis, depressive type, and compared the data with those obtained from normal subjects. The investigators found considerable variability among the patients in terms of the percentage of time that each type of electroencephalographic (EEG) tracing appeared during the entire night's recording. This variability became less when the waking records were excluded and only the tracings that occurred during sleep were considered.

The authors found that the patients had almost twice as much low voltage activity as the normal controls and approximately one-half as much spindle plus random activity as the normal controls. In a comparison of the minute-by-minute fluctuations from one EEG pattern or level to another, they found that the fluctuations for the patients were more frequent than those for the controls. The percentage of the minutes that contained two or more of the EEG sleep levels during the night's sleep was nearly twice as great for the patients as for the normal controls.

The authors concluded that the disturbed sleep of patients with manic depressive psychosis is characterized not only by difficulty in falling asleep and by early or frequent awakening, but also by a greater proportion of light sleep. In addition, the patients showed more frequent oscillation from one level of sleep to another than did the normal controls.

Oswald *et al.* (1963) conducted a study of the sleeping patterns of depressive patients compared to those of matched normals. Continuous nocturnal recordings of EEG, eye-movement, and bed movement were carried out on six normal controls. The six psychiatric patients, ranging in age from 33–67 years, had in common a depressive component to their illness, although they differed considerably in terms of the rest of the psychiatric picture. Each patient was matched with a corresponding paid control of the same sex. Four women and two men were in each group, and the age differences between patient and control ranged from three to eight years.

According to the authors, all patients were suffering from an autonomous melancholia. In an expanded definition of this condition, the authors state that the patient had "an illness of a kind which we believe may sometimes develop in the absence of severe environmental stress, while in others it may be clearly provoked by circumstances. But the illness as it develops may take on a form which becomes largely independent of the environmental circumstances, and may continue even when the provoking factors are past. It has become an *autonomous melancholia*. It will be apparent that by autonomous melancholia we mean an illness shown by clinical experience to respond especially well to electroplexy."

The experiment was carried out over a period of five nights. On the first night, intended for adaptation to the laboratory setting, electrodes were attached, but no recording was made. On the following four nights recordings were made. The investigators were not only interested in natural sleep, but also in the effects of barbiturates on sleep patterns. Consequently, the patients and the control group received either heptabarbitone or dummy tablets. A total of 48 records were obtained. "Blind interpretation" of the EEG was carried out by the senior author. The following significant findings were made: (1) The patients spent significantly more minutes awake than did the controls; (2) percentage of time spent by the patients in paradoxical sleep (REM sleep) and frequency of shifts in the depths of sleep were not significantly different from those of the controls; and (3) when the patients did sleep, they spent a significantly larger percentage of time in the *deeper* stage of sleep (Stage E) than did the controls. Heptobarbitone greatly decreased the duration of rapid eye movement (REM) periods and also the frequency of eye movements within these periods. The drug decreased the duration of time awake, especially in patients in the early hours of the morning, and decreased the frequency of body movement.

In addition to substantiating clinical observations that depressed patients sleep less than do normals, the study was notable in that it showed that when the patients did sleep, they showed a higher percentage of sleep in the deeper stages than do the normals (contrary to findings of Diaz-Guerrero and his coworkers.) The authors explained this particular finding as a kind of compensation for the sleep deprivation. Among the limitations of this study are: (1) the small number of patients included; (2) the broad criteria for inclusion of patients in the psychiatric group; (3) the use of a normal control group rather than nondepressed psychiatric controls (consequently, it is difficult to know whether the findings are specific for depressed patients or characteristic of psychiatric patients generally.); and (4) since all the patients had electroconvulsive therapy at some time during their illness, there is a question as to whether these treatments might have in some way influenced the EEG recordings.

Another study of the effect of depressive disorders on sleep EEG responses was conducted by Zung, Wilson, and Dodson (1964). The sample consisted of 11 hospitalized men ranging in age from 37 to 69 years. The characteristics of the normal control subjects are not specified. In one part of the study the patients served as their own controls. The diagnostic criteria were more rigorous than those in Oswald's study. "The diagnosis of the depressive disorder was made clinically, based upon the presence of a pervasive depressed affect and its physiological and psychological concomitants." The specific criteria utilized are specified, and include 20 indices of depression; no reliability studies are cited, however. In addition, the patients quantitated the severity of their own symptoms by means of a self-rating depression scale.

Observations and analyses were made of continuous EEG records obtained from an entire night's undisturbed sleep. On the second consecutive night, pretaped sounds of approximately equal intensity were played at various stages of sleep. For six of the patients these studies were repeated after remission of the symptoms.

Results: (1) Mean time from retiring to sleep state, 20 minutes (range 7.5–63 minutes); mean duration of sleep, seven hours; and the number of fluctuations between Stage E (the deepest stage) to Stage A (the lightest stage), 11 per patient. (2) The distribution of the sleep recorded in A, B, C, D, and E were 26.6 per cent, 20.2 per cent, 20.5 per cent, 23.1 per cent, and 9.0 per cent respectively. These findings are consistent with those of Diaz-Guerrero, but not with those of Oswald *et al.*, quoted above. The present study, unlike the Oswald study, showed a smaller percentage of time in the deepest levels of sleep.

Responses to auditory stimulation by the depressed patient group indicate that the patients before treatment responded in the B, C, D, and E Stages of sleep 79.2 per cent, 77.1 per cent, 61.8 per cent, and 54.4 per cent, respectively. A comparison with the results obtained from normal control subjects indicates that the depressed patient group showed a significantly higher degree of response at all stages of sleep. This was interpreted by the authors as indicating a *heightened arousal response*. After treatment, the responses to auditory stimulation in the B, C, D, and E Stages of sleep were 62.5 per cent, 34.8 per cent, 31.8 per cent, and 25.0 per cent, respectively. A comparison of the post-treatment responses with those obtained from normal control subjects indicates that they did not differ significantly.

The findings of these authors indicate that the patients' duration of sleep was similar to that recorded in a normal population. The patients, however, spent more time in the lighter stages of sleep. The responses to auditory stimulation are consistent with the suggestion that the depressed patients have a greater responsivity during sleep than do normals.

Other possible interpretations of the data are possible. It is conceivable, for instance, that the increased responsivity of the depressed patients to auditory stimuli may be due to a lower degree of physical fatigue because of lessened activity during the day that is not due to the depressive illness itself, but related more to the low activity level of depressed patients. The normalization of the records after ECT and drug treatment should be considered in terms of the effect of these treatments on the electrical rhythm of the brain, quite apart from whether the patient was in the depressed or nondepressed state. When a control group was used, age and sex were not adequately controlled. In addition, since psychiatric controls were not used, there is no indication that the findings are specific for depressive illness.

Gresham, Agnew, and Williams (1965) conducted a more refined study than any previously reported. Instead of relying on clinical impressions alone to determine the depressed group, they used a variety of clinical and psychometric measures. Eight depressed psychiatric inpatients were selected on the basis of six tests and were compared with closely matched controls for four consecutive nights in a laboratory controlled for noise, temperature, and lighting, with continuous all-night EEG and eye movement recording.

The first night's records were not used for analyses. The duration of the stages of sleep over three nights were estimated by observers other than the experimenter. The investigators found that the patients showed more wakefulness, less Stage 4 sleep, and a slightly longer sleep latent state than the controls. Four patients were available for re-examination after their depressions were substantially reduced by therapy. On re-examination they showed a change in the direction of the values obtained by the controls.

Mendels, Hawkins, and Scott (1966) also reported a deficiency in Stage 4 sleep. This correlated with the severity of the depression.

Summary

The consensus of the studies of the sleep EEG's of depressed patients is that depressed patients tend to have excessive periods of light or restless sleep and a shorter period of total sleep. In addition, they tend to be more sensitive to noises when they are asleep. The studies reported to date are hampered by the small number of patients in each study, the use of normal controls instead of nondepressed psychiatric patients, and the lack of age-specific values for the various EEG patterns. Some studies, moreover, have not excluded the possible influence of sedation on the EEG tracings.

ELECTROENCEPHALOGRAM (EEG) AROUSAL RESPONSE

Paulson and Gottlieb (1961) made a longitudinal study of the electro-encephalographic arousal response in 11 depressed patients. The rationale behind their study was that the depressed patient seems in general to be self-absorbed and preoccupied, and has a corresponding impairment in his alertness to environmental stimulation. The presence of an apparent deficit in attention provided the basis for the following hypotheses: (1) If the patients' thresholds for responding to environmental stimulation are excessively high during depression, then the EEG arousal response to environmental stimulation should occur less frequently during depression than upon recovery. (2) If the peripheral rate of responsiveness is retarded during depression, then the latency of the arousal response should be longer during depression than upon recovery; (3) If the central responsiveness and integrative activities are retarded during depression, then the duration of the arousal response should be longer during depression than upon recovery.

The investigators found that eight of the 11 patients showed more frequent arousal upon recovery, but the latency was unchanged. The average duration of the arousal response was shortened. The writers interpreted these results as being consistent with the assumption that the attentional threshold is higher than usual during depression and the central integrative processes are slower.

Shagass and Schwartz (1962) investigated the cerebral cortical reactivity in psychotic depressives. The mean cortical reactivity cycles were determined for 21 psychotic-depressive patients and 13 nonpatient control subjects. The nonpatient subjects showed an early phase of response recovery, whereas early recovery was much less in the psychotic depressives before treatment. As the depressed patients improved, however, they showed progressively more early response recovery.

Wilson and Wilson (1961) investigated the duration of photically elicited arousal responses in psychotic depressed patients. They found that the mean arousal response duration for 16 patients was significantly increased when compared with the control group of normal subjects.

Some contradictory evidence is presented in a study by Driver and Eilenberg (1960). The investigators measured the photoconvulsive threshold in 27 patients with a severe depressive illness. The findings are not different from those reported elsewhere for other nosological syndromes and also for normal subjects. The authors concluded that the threshold had no clinical differentiating value. The estimation was repeated in 18 patients after they had received a course of ECT. No change was found in the photoconvulsive threshold. The investigators concluded that it was unwise to assume that any aspect of diencephalic function was assessed by an estimate of the photoconvulsive thresholds.

Summary

The results of the studies of reactivity of the central nervous system are contradictory. Many of the studies have serious methodological shortcomings. The most frequent finding (contradicted by one study) has been an increased threshold for external stimulation during depression and a reduction in the threshold upon recovery. Also, the duration of the arousal response was increased during depression but decreased after recovery. Further confirmatory work is necessary.

CONCLUSIONS

Despite the hundreds of studies in this area, there is little, if any, solid knowledge of the specific biological substrate of depression. With almost monotonous regularity initial positive results have failed to be confirmed by later investigations. Many of the widely accepted findings such as the genetic and constitutional factors in manic-depressive disorders are clouded with doubt because of methodological inadequacies in the original studies. Other promising findings such as an excessive physiological reaction to drugs such as methylcholine or amobarbital have been contradicted by later studies that have controlled for age.

Among the positive findings that have been consistently associated with depression have been excessive levels of steroids, sodium retention, and changes in sleep EEG patterns. Excessive steroid secretion is not a specific characteristic of depression and appears to be associated with many states of emotional arousal. Sodium retention has so far been demonstrated in only a few studies. Several EEG studies have indicated a deficit in the deeper levels of sleep.

Numerous sources of error have been present in the biological studies. These include inadequate, heterogeneous samples; diagnostic methods of dubious reliability and validity; and inadequate control for variables such as age, sex, diet, state of nutrition, and activity level. The lack of control for age may be singled out as one of the most frequent factors responsible for initial positive findings that were discomfirmed by later better controlled studies. These discrepant results may be attributed to the practice of using schizophrenics or neurotic depressives as comparison groups; both of these diagnostic groups tend to be substantially younger than psychotic depressives or manic depressives.

With the tightening of the experimental methods it may be expected that much of the uncertainty surrounding the biological aspects of depression will be dissipated.

Chapter 10.
Psychological and Psychodynamic Studies

PSYCHOMOTOR PERFORMANCE

Most clinical descriptions of depression have emphasized psychomotor retardation and have assumed that the patients' complaints of being slowed down in their thinking are an indication of inhibition of thought processes. Objective evidence to substantiate the proposition of an inhibition of psychomotor functions, however, has been lacking.

Rapaport (1945), comparing a depressed group with a schizophrenic group, reported a significant lowering of digit-symbol scores within the depressed group. He concluded that performance on this test is sensitive to the retardation assumed to be associated with depression. A further analysis of Rapaport's data, however, indicated that his depressed group was significantly older than his schizophrenic group and that the difference in age might account for the inferior performances by the depressed patients. To clarify the relationship between depression and performance on tests such as the Digit-Symbol test, we conducted a study with statistical controls for age and intelligence (Beck, Feshbach, and Legg, 1962). The Digit-Symbol test and the vocabulary test were administered to a sample of 178 psychiatric patients. The results indicated that the digit-symbol scores decreased in a step-wise fashion with increasing age, and increased in the same fashion with increasing vocabulary scores. When the variables of age and intelligence were controlled, it was found that there was no relationship between digit-symbol scores and depression. The depressed patients performed as well as did the nondepressed patients.

Granick (1963) performed a comparative analysis of the performances on the Wechsler Adult Intelligence Scale Information and Similarities tests and on the Thorndike-Gallup Vocabulary test of 50 psychotic depressives and 50 normals matched for age, sex, race, education, religion, and nativity. The investigator failed to find any significant difference in performance between the psychotically depressed group and the normal group.

Friedman (1964) administered 33 cognitive, perceptual, and psychomotor tests to 55 depressives and 65 normals matched for age, sex, education, vocabulary score, and nativity. In all, 82 test scores were derived from the various tests administered. The depressives ranked lower than did the normal group in only 4 per cent of the test scores, a finding that could be due to chance. The author concluded that actual ability and performance during severe depression is not consistent with the depressed patient's unrealistically low image of himself.

In one of our studies (Loeb *et al.*, 1966), 20 depressed and 20 matched nondepressed male patients were given two card sorting tasks. Although the depressed patients tended to underestimate their performance, their actual performance was as good as that of the nondepressed patients.

Another study that indicates that depressed patients do not have significant impairment of psychomotor ability was conducted by Shapiro *et al.* (1958). They found that depressed patients following recovery (produced by ECT) did not show any significant change in their performance on a battery of psychomotor tests when compared to a control group.

Tucker and Spielberg (1958) compared the Bender-Gestalt scores of 17 depressed outpatients with those of 19 nondepressed psychiatric outpatients. In general, the various Bender-Gestalt scores did not discriminate between the two groups. Of 20 items, only two, tremor and design distortion, were significant at the 5 per cent level in discriminating between the depressed and the nondepressed group. No test items were significantly different at the 1 per cent level. The finding of only two discriminating items out of 20 could be due to chance. Comparisons were also made of average initial reaction and average response time to each test card. Contrary to expectations, the depressed patients showed a *faster* mean reaction time than the nondepressed group. This finding was short of statistical significance.

In summary, although the depressed patients tend to complain of cognitive inefficiencies, they perform as well in test situations as do nondepressed patients.

CONCEPTUAL PERFORMANCE

Payne and Hirst (1957) investigated conceptual thinking in depressed patients. In a previous study, Payne had found that schizophrenic patients showed a tendency toward "overinclusion" when administered the Epstein Overinclusion test; this finding was consonant with Norman Cameron's formulation that the schizophrenic is unable to preserve his conceptual boundaries so that irrelevant ideas become incorporated into his concepts, making his thinking more abstract and less lucid.

The authors administered the Epstein Overinclusion test to 11 depressed patients and 14 normal controls matched for age, sex, and vocabulary level. Their findings indicated that depressives show a significantly greater tendency towards overinclusion than the normals. They found, in fact, that depressed patients seem to be more extreme with respect to overinclusion of thinking than are schizophrenics. This is inconsistent with Cameron's theory, since he regarded this type of thought disorder as specific to schizophrenics. The authors suggest that the overinclusion tendency may be related to psychosis generally, rather than to any specific psychosis such as schizophrenia or depression.

PERCEPTUAL THRESHOLD

Hemphill, Hall, and Crookes (1952) attempted to measure the pain and fatigue tolerance of depressed patients as compared with other psychiatric patients. The depressed patients showed a significantly higher threshold for both pain and fatigue than the other groups. It should be noted, however, that the mean age of the depressed patients was substantially higher than that of the other groups, which could account for the differences in thresholds for perception of fatigue and pain. It is also worth noting that the depressed patients were more persevering in a fatiguing task than were the nondepressed patients. Wadsworth, Wells, and Scott (1962) found no difference in fatigability or work performance between a group of depressives and a group of schizophrenics.

In an attempt to relate perceptual regulation to mental disorders, Dixon and Lear (1962) measured the visual threshold for one eye while presenting neutral and emotive material below the awareness threshold to the other eye. The five depressive patients showed a consistent raising of threshold ("perceptual defense") as compared to the six schizophrenics who showed a lowering of threshold ("perceptual vigilance"). Caution is necessary in interpreting these results because of the small samples and because all the patients were on drug therapy.

DISTORTION OF TIME JUDGMENT

Many writers have described a distortion of the time sense in affective disorders. The existential writers in particular have commented on the relevance of time distortion to the existential experience of the patient

(Chapter 16). Although it seems fairly well established from the clinical description that depressed patients feel that time is passing more slowly than normal, there is no objective evidence that actual judgment of time is impaired.

Mezey and Cohen (1961) investigated the subjective experience of time and the judgment of time of 21 depressed patients. The study included introspective statements about time experience as well as objective tests involving projection-reprojection and verbal estimation of time intervals ranging from one second to 30 minutes. The authors found that about three-fourths of the patients felt that time was passing more slowly than normal; this feeling tended to disappear on recovery. The objective tests, on the other hand, indicated that the verbal estimation of time under experimental conditions was as accurate during the depressed phase as during the recovery phase.

DISTORTION OF SPATIAL JUDGMENT

A number of articles have suggested that psychiatric patients experience some changes in spatial perception. Neurotics and schizophrenic patients have been reported to have distortions in the perceived distance between themselves and others. Other phenomena reported to occur in psychiatric patients have been the assignment of different qualities to the right and left aspects of space, and fading of the third-dimensional aspect of objects (Fisher, 1964). There is also some experimental evidence that the individual's mood state influences his spatial perception. Distortion in locating the nearness or distance of objects has been reported to be related to personal insecurity.

Depression has been shown to be related to up-down perception in several studies. Rosenblatt (1956) found that in contrast to manic patients, depressed patients have a tendency to focus on the downward rather than the upward aspect of a spatial situation. Wapner, Werner, and Krus (1957), in a parallel study of college students, related the experience of academic failure to a consequent downward effect on the subjective judgment of eye level ("apparent horizon"). Fisher (1964) tested the specific hypothesis that the degree of downward bias of perception is positively related to the level of sadness or depression. Fifty-two subjects were evaluated. The measure of sad affect was made in terms of the number of sad terms used in describing a series of faces. Upward vs. downward directionality of perception was estimated by means of the autokinetic phenomenon and by judgments requiring the adjustment of a luminous rod to the horizontal. The results supported the proposition that subjects with a sad affect showed a downward bias in perception, whereas subjects with a neutral affect showed an upward bias.

FACTOR ANALYTIC STUDIES

Hamilton (1960a) administered a 17-item rating scale to 49 depressed male patients. The product-moment correlations were computed for the 17 variables and the correlation matrix was factored and then transformed to orthogonal simple structure. Four factors were extracted. The first factor was defined by suicidal thoughts, loss of libido, retardation, depressed mood, and loss of insight. The second factor consisted of gastrointestinal complaints, sleep difficulty, loss of interest, body preoccupation, and loss of weight. The third factor consisted of anxiety items. The fourth factor was equivocal.

Grinker *et al.* (1961) conducted an extensive study to determine the prominent trait-dimensions of depression. In a pilot study, a group of 21 patients diagnosed as depressed by experienced psychiatrists were studied intensively to define the major trait factors. The raw data from the study were translated into a list of "Feelings and Concerns" and a list of "Current Behaviors." The Feelings and Concerns list dealt with the verbalized experiences of the patient such as envy of others, sense of failure, and fear of death or dying. The Current Behavior list dealt with the visible actions of the patient or with traits that require only a low level of inference on the part of the rater. The reliability of the Feelings and Concerns list was high. Factor analysis of the data uncovered three factors. The reliability of ratings on the Current Behavior list was too low to justify factor analysis.

In the large scale study, 96 patients diagnosed as depressive by various psychiatrists were investigated. Ten nondepressed patients were used as a control group. Analysis of the data from this study revealed five factors in the Feelings and Concerns list. The factors made sense psychologically and were described as follows: (1) depression; (2) projective defense; (3) restitution; (4) free anxiety; and (5) attempt to manipulate the environment.

An analysis of the Current Behavior list revealed ten factors. These were characterized roughly as follows: (1) isolation, withdrawal, and apathy; (2) retardation of thought processes and speech; (3) general retardation in behavior and gait; (4) angry, provocative behavior; (5) somatic complaints; (6) organic syndrome; (7) agitation, tremulousness, and restlessness; (8) rigidity; (9) somatic symptoms such as dry skin and hair; and (10) ingratiating behavior.

Certain traits that were expected to be important in depression did not appear in any of the factors. These included loss of interest in oral satisfaction, suicidal ideas, fatigue, wishes to cry, loss of esteem by others, relief after hospitalization, and ambivalence towards important personal issues. In the pilot study, an investigation of precipitating factors suggested that there was rarely a single clear-cut precipitating event or experience. Almost invariably, a series of events led up to the clinical illness.

The factors derived from the Feelings and Concerns list did not correlate with the factors for current behavior. The subjective symptom *anxiety*, for instance, did not correlate with the behavioral factor *agitation*. This finding suggests a lack of correspondence between the self-reports of the patients and the clinicians' inferences based on their overt behavior.

This study by Grinker and his associates is an important pioneering effort to demarcate the important dimensions of depression. The absence of an adequate control group, however, raises questions to to whether the factors are characteristic of depression, or whether they are applicable to psychiatric patients generally.

A number of studies of psychotics by Overall and his group (1961, 1962, 1964) have attempted to isolate the basic dimensions of psychiatric disorders. Overall and Gorham (1961) studied 120 chronic schizophrenics in an effort to identify the primary dimensions of change in their symptomatology. Six independent processes were identified. These were labelled as mental disorganization, distortion of thought processes, guilt-conversion, retardation, depression in mood, and anxiety. The depression factor was defined by feelings of inadequacy, depression, and suicidal impulses.

Friedman *et al.* (1963) obtained factors similar to those previously reported by Grinker. One-hundred-seventy psychotic-depressed patients were rated independently by two psychiatrists on a rating scale of symptoms, traits, and themes. Two experienced psychiatric interviewers rated each patient on the 60 item PPH Depression Rating scale.

Five factors were extracted. Factor A contained the items relevant to the affective component of depression; this included loss of self-esteem, guilt feelings, degree of depression, and loss of satisfaction. Factor B was defined by retardation and apathy, loss of energy, withdrawal and isolation. Factor C was characterized by the vegetative signs of depression such as loss of appetite, sleep disturbance, constipation, and work inhibition. Factor D was defined by items relevant to irritability, preoccupation, complaining and agitation. The fifth factor was equivocal.

McNair and Lorr (1964) attempted to determine the basic mood factors in a neurotic population. A mood scale was administered to a series of psychiatric samples. Five moods were identified: tension; anger; depression; vigor; and fatigue. The depression was defined by a series of adjectives such as worthless, helpless, unhappy, discouraged, and blue.

Pichot and Lempérière (1964) factor analyzed the Depression Inventory. (See Chapter 12 for a more complete account of their findings.) The following orthogonal factors were extracted: (*A*) vital depression; (*B*) self-debasement; (*C*) pessimism-suicide; and (*D*) indecision-inhibition.

Critique

Any comparison of the factors obtained by the various investigators cited above is hampered by each investigator's using different measures. It is possible, however, to find certain regularities among the studies. The vegetative signs of depression, for example, appear as a factor in several studies. Another obstacle to interpreting the findings is that most studies did not include nondepressed psychiatric patients. It is, therefore, not possible to ascertain whether the factors are characteristic of depression, of psychiatric disorders in general, or of the general population. There has not been any independent replication of any of the studies so the findings must be regarded as tentative.

EXPERIMENTAL STUDIES

An intriguing study concerned with the effect of serum from manic-depressed patients on the behavior of dogs has been reported in the Russian literature. Polyakova (1961) reported that the time taken for five dogs to negotiate a labyrinth increased from a mean of 6.37 seconds to 19 seconds when the dogs received serum from depressed patients. The time decreased to a mean of 5.8 when the blood came from patients in the manic phase. The profound implications of this study certainly warrant independent replication.

In the first of several studies in which depressed patients were exposed to varying experimental conditions, we randomly assigned a group of 20 depressed and 22 nondepressed patients to an experimentally induced superior and inferior performance condition (Loeb *et al.*, 1964). Prior to and immediately following the experimental task, the patients rated their own mood. Indices of self-confidence were also obtained. The depressed patients tended to be more affected by task performance than the nondepressed patients when estimating how they would do in a future task. The groups did not differ, however, in performance effect on self-ratings.

In a later study, we measured the effects of success and failure on mood, motivation, and performance (Loeb *et al.*, 1966). Twenty depressed and 20 nondepressed male patients were selected on the basis of their having, respectively, high or low scores on the Depression Inventory *and* high or low ratings of depression made independently during a psychiatric interview. In an experiment designed as part of the psychiatric outpatient evaluation procedure, the depressed patients were significantly more pessimistic about their likelihood of succeeding and tended to underrate the quality of their performances, although their actual output was the same as that of nondepressed patients. On a second task the previous experience of success and failure had contrasting effects on the actual performances of the two groups. Success improved the performance of the depressed patients, and failure improved the performance of the nondepressed patients.

Harsch and Zimmer (1965) selected 62 male and 34 female college students on the basis of their performance on the Zimmer Sentence Completion test. Forty-eight students were considered to exhibit a predominantly extrapunitive behavior pattern, and 48 students were considered to exhibit a predominantly intrapunitive behavior pattern. Since the intrapunitive behavior pattern was considered characteristic of depression, this experiment has relevance to the understanding of depression. The experiment endeavored to produce abandonment of the characteristic behavior pattern and adoption of a different behavior pattern. This was attempted by rewarding subjects for statements contrary to the basic behavior pattern or punishing the subjects for statements conforming to the behavior pattern. As a result of the experimental manipulation, both groups showed significant shifts in behavior pattern as measured by the Zimmer test. The experimentally induced changes in a direction opposite from the starting points persisted over an eight-day follow-up period.

FAMILY BACKGROUND AND PERSONALITY

Wilson (1951) investigated the role of family pressures in the socialization of manic depressives. On the basis of his review of case records and the intensive study of 12 patients and their families, he concluded that during childhood the manic depressives felt excessive pressure to conform to the attitudes of their parents and had less freedom than did the control group.

In 1954, Cohen *et al.* reported the results of an intensive psychoanalytic investigation of 12 cases of manic-depressive psychosis. A consistent findings in all 12 patients was that during the patient's childhood his family felt set apart by some factor that singled it out as "different." Among these factors were membership in a minority group, serious economic reversals, or mental illness in the family. In each case, the patient's family felt the social distinction keenly and reacted to it by trying to improve its acceptability in the community. The family placed a high premium on conformity and made a great effort to improve its social status by raising its economic level or by achieving other symbols of prestige. In order to reach his goal, the children were expected to conform to a high standard of behavior, based primarily on the parents' concepts of what the neighbors expected. The patient's role was experienced by him as being in the service of the family's social striving.

The responsibility for winning prestige was generally delegated by the mother to the child who was later to develop a manic-depressive psychosis. The reason a particular child was selected was either because he was exceptional in terms of intelligence or other gifts or because he was the oldest, the youngest, or the only child. The emphasis on achievement and competition usually caused the child to have serious problems with envy.

Gibson (1957) used a more refined technique to test the findings of Cohen's study. He studied a group of 27 manic-depressive patients and 17 schizophrenic patients from St. Elizabeth's Hospital in Washington, D.C., to determine whether Cohen's description of the early life history and family background could differentiate manic-depressive from schizophrenic patients. Hospital records and interviews with the families by specially trained social workers provided the basic data. The data were evaluated according to a questionnaire specifically designed to measure the degree to which a patient's history conformed to the concepts formulated by Cohen and her group. The 12 patients of the original Cohen study were also evaluated according to the questionnaire.

The two manic-depressive groups were differentiated from the schizophrenic groups on three of the five scales of the questionnaire. The manic depressives were statistically different from the schizophrenics in terms of the following characteristics: (1) The manic depressive comes from a family in which there is marked striving for prestige and the patient is the instrument of his parents' prestige needs; (2) The manic-depressive patient has a background in which there has been intense envy and competitiveness; and (3) The parents of the manic-depressive patients show a high degree of concern about social approval.

Certain methodological inadequacies are apparent in this study. Among these are the possibility of contamination in the social workers' evaluations of their data and the lack of control for age.

Becker and his associates, in a series of systematic studies, attempted to test the hypotheses derived from Cohen's study and the systematic investigation by Gibson. According to their reformulations of Cohen's findings, persons who develop manic-depressive reaction in adulthood have experienced excessive parental expectations for conformity and achievement as children. They react to these demands by adopting the prevailing values of their parents and other authority figures in order to placate them and win approval. The authors attempted to investigate the extent to which chronic dependence on others for guidance and approval is manifested in the opinions and attitudes of the manic-depressive patient. In an initial study, Becker (1960) compared 24 remitted manic depressives with 30 nonpsychiatric controls who were matched for age, education, and literacy level. The manic depressives scored significantly higher than the controls on measures of value achievement, authoritarian trends, and conventional attitudes. The manic depressives did not differ from the nonpsychiatric controls in direct self-rating of achievement motivation or on performance output.

In another study, Spielberger, Parker, and Becker (1963) essayed a broader investigation of the formulations derived from the studies of Cohen, Gibson, and Wilson. The subjects of this investigation consisted of 30 remitted manic depressives and 30 nonpsychiatric controls. Four objective psychological scales or tests were administered. These consisted of the California Fascism Scale, the traditional family ideology scale, the value achievement scale, and the need achievement scale. The manic depressives obtained significantly higher scores than the controls on all these experimental measures except need achievement. The authors interpreted their findings as indicating that the adult personality structure of manic depressives is characterized by conventional authoritarian attitudes, traditional opinions, and stereotyped achievement values, but not by internalized achievement motives.

Some doubt of the specificity of these findings is raised by another study by Becker, Spielberger, and Parker (1963). In this study, the scores of manic depressives on various attitude measures were compared with the scores of neurotic depressives, schizophrenics, and normal controls. No significant difference in value achievement or authoritarian attitudes was found between the psychiatric groups, although they differed significantly from the normal controls. The investigators found, however, that age and social class significantly affected the scores; this indicates the need for empirical or statistical control of these variables in personality studies of this kind.

SELF-CONCEPT

We developed a self-concept test, consisting of traits and characteristics such as appearance, intelligence, sex appeal, selfishness, and cruelty (Beck and Stein, 1960). Each patient rated himself on each of these traits using a five point scale. He also made ratings of how he felt about having each of these traits (the self-acceptance score). We found a significant correlation (–.66)) between self-concept scores and Depression Inventory scores; the correlation between self-acceptance scores and DI scores was also significant (–.42). This study indicated that depressed patients tended to give themselves low ratings on socially desirable traits and high ratings on undesirable traits. We concluded that the self-concept is low in depressed as compared with nondepressed patients.

Laxer (1964) used the semantic differential test to investigate changes in the self-concept of neurotic depressive and other psychiatric patients. The depressives showed a low self-concept on admission to a hospital but moved to a higher self-concept at the time of discharge. The paranoids, on the other hand, began with a relatively high self-rating and did not change appreciably at the time of discharge.

SUMMARY

There has been a dearth of systematic psychological and psychodynamic studies of depression as compared with the biological studies reviewed in the preceding chapter. In addition to presenting the usual methodological problems such as inadequate attention to diagnosis and the control of extraneous variables such as age, investigations of the psychological and psychodynamic aspects of depression have not been followed by replication studies by other independent investigators. Any conclusions must, therefore, be regarded as tentative.

One interesting group of findings demonstrates that in test situations the depressed patient is able to perform as effectively as matched controls. Experimental studies indicate that the experience of success significantly improves the performance of depressed patients. These findings suggest that the inertia in depression may be related more to factors such as loss of motivation than to physiological inhibition. The studies also indicate that the depressed patients greatly underestimate their capacity and actual performance.

The finding of a high threshold for fatigue also suggests that in actual work situations the depressed patient does not become as fatigued as is generally believed. No objective evidence was obtained to substantiate the notion of a disturbance of judgments of time. Some studies, however, suggest that the depressed patient tends to have a downward bias in spatial perception.

The factor analytic studies have opened a new era for exploration. The differences in clinical and psychometric measures used in the various investigations, however, preclude any definite conclusions about the basic dimensions of depression at this time.

The studies of the personality and of the family backgrounds of depressed patients have not fulfilled early expectations. Efforts to test the hypothesis generated by the clinical studies of M. B. Cohen and her group provided some initial support. Investigations using a tighter design, however, suggest that the obtained differences between depressed and nondepressed patients may be due to extraneous factors such as age, social class, and educational level. Studies of the self-concept indicate that depressed patients rate themselves much lower than nondepressed patients, but return to average ratings upon recovery from the depression.

Part III.
A SYSTEMATIC INVESTIGATION OF DEPRESSION

Chapter 11.
Résumé of the Research

AN OVERVIEW

The psychodynamic factors in depression have engaged the interest of psychiatric writers since Abraham's first exploration of this subject in 1911. The psychiatric literature contains a wide variety of theories of depression including increased orality (Abraham, 1911), retroflected hostility (Freud, 1917), and needs to manipulate the significant persons in the environment (Rado, 1928).

In view of the numerous clinical papers on depression (Mendelson, 1960), the paucity of controlled studies testing the various hypotheses is surprising. A major factor is the number of highly complicated conceptual and methodological problems confronted in subjecting these hypotheses to systematic test. One problem is that of specificity: The same psychodynamic formulations that have been provided to explain the phenomena of depression have also been applied to conditions quite different from depression. The concept of oral fixation, for instance, has been applied not only to depression, but also to a diversity of conditions including schizophrenia, alcoholism, and peptic ulcer. Another problem is that many of the theories, such as Freud's formulation of depression in *Mourning and Melancholia* (1917), are so complex and remote from observables in the clinical material that they are not readily reduced to operational terms for systematic study.

In undertaking a study of the psychodynamic factors of depression, I felt that it would be necessary to satisfy two prerequisites. First, it should be possible to isolate a particular psychodynamic constellation or construct that has a meaningful relationship to depression but not to other syndromes. Second, it should be possible to develop methods for identifying the referents of this construct in the clinical material.

The evolution of the present investigation may be of interest. In an

The research described in Part III was supported in part by Grant #3358, from the National Institute of Mental Health, Bethesda, Maryland.

earlier study, I had collected data from five soldiers who became psychotically depressed after having accidentally killed a comrade (Beck and Valin, 1953). (See Chapter 5 for illustrative cases.) A detailed examination of the ideational productions of these patients (hallucinations, fantasies, dreams, and obsessive ruminations) revealed direct evidence of self-punitive tendencies. In a typical case, for example, the patient had a visual hallucination of the dead buddy in which the buddy told him to kill himself. All the patients expressed a desire to be punished for their deeds and all but one had made suicidal attempts.

The next event in this evolution was the observation that the dreams of neurotically depressed patients in intensive psychotherapy or analysis showed a particularly high frequency of themes of being disappointed, thwarted, injured, punished, incompetent, or ugly. These themes occurred occasionally in the dreams of nondepressed patients, but much less frequently*

This observation of the dreams of depressed patients suggested the possibility that there might be a particular psychodynamic variable or constellation that was characteristic of depression but not of other psychiatric conditions. The common denominator of these dream themes was that the dreamer experienced some unpleasantness or suffering in the manifest dream. Proceeding on Freud's theory that dream content represents wish fulfillment, I speculated that these dreams represented a wish to suffer.

When this observation of the dreams of depressed patients was aligned with the previous observation of the punishment themes in the ideational productions of the psychotically depressed soldiers, there appeared to be one feature common to both, namely, self-imposed suffering. I conjectured that the unpleasant dream themes might reflect the same psychological variables as the self-punitive hallucinations and verbal statements of the psychotically depressed soldiers. This formulation led to the formal hypothesis that a central feature in depression is the need to suffer. The term "masochism" was employed to designate this particular variable.† To confirm this hypothesis experimentally, it was necessary to demonstrate that depressed patients show a significantly higher degree of "masochism" than nondepressed patients.

To develop a method for measuring "masochism," it was first necessary to obtain a kind of data that could be readily defined, collected, and

---

* I received the stimulation to review the dreams of depressed patients as the result of attending weekly seminars on "Quantitative Studies of Dreams" conducted by Leon J. Saul. Dr. Saul's clinical and experimental approaches to dreams provided the starting point for my studies in this area.

† The word "masochism" is used here in the general sense of a tendency toward self-suffering rather than with the more restricted meaning of gaining sexual gratification through physical pain.

analyzed. Dreams seemed to fit these requirements. The reported dream is a discrete entity, in contrast to other types of clinical material (such as discursive responses to questions, free associations, or nonverbal behavior). In addition, it is relatively easy to subject dreams to content-scoring systems that have a high degree of interjudge reliability (Saul and Sheppard, 1956).

In attempting to provide a theoretical framework to explain the "masochistic" tendencies in depressed patients, I considered two alternative conceptualizations: (1) "Masochism" could be regarded as a manifestation of inverted hostility. In accordance with Freud's thesis in *Mourning and Melancholia* (1917), the patient is primarily angry at somebody else (the lost love-object), but turns this anger against himself. The insults and rebukes initially intended for the lost love-object are focused on himself. (2) The need to suffer could be viewed as a direct expression of self-punishment tendencies. (This thesis is different from the first in that it does not presuppose the presence of hostility). According to the second formulation, the patient has either done something contrary to his primitive moral code (superego), or he has some unacceptable wish. This deed or wish arouses guilt in the patient, and the guilt then leads to the wish to punish himself.

Several objections were immediately apparent. The first formulation was concerned with inverted hostility. The presence of hostility could not be demonstrated in the manifest content of the dream of the depressed patient or in the feeling experienced during the dream. The second formulation assumed the presence of guilt over some unacceptable wishes or deeds. Neither guilt nor the unacceptable wishes or deeds could be directly identified in the manifest content of the dreams. Since these elements could not be demonstrated directly in the clinical material, the formulations could not be subjected to direct test.

Another problem to be confronted was that Freud's theory of dreams is based upon the assumption that the dream represents a wish fulfillment of some kind, i.e., the content of the dream represents a particular wish or set of wishes. If this assumption is invalid, then the whole formulation of the need to suffer collapses.

As the research developed, I attempted to circumvent these problems by adopting a different approach. It seemed more satisfactory to stay at the level of the patients' experiences than to infer some underlying process. If the patient has a dream in which he perceives other people as frustrating him, it would be more economical to simply consider this a conception of people as being frustrating rather than to read into the dream an underlying "masochistic" wish. This revised conception also fitted in with some later observations of the thematic content of the verbalized statements of patients (see Chapter 15). The focusing on the material in terms of the patient's perception of himself and of external reality gradually shifted the emphasis from a motivational model to a cognitive model.

The first stage in the systematic investigation of depression was a content analysis of the dreams of patients in psychotherapy. The hypothesis that depressed patients show a greater frequency of "masochistic" dreams than do a control group of nondepressed patients was confirmed (Chapter 13).

This initial finding seemed to warrant a more complete investigation, using a much larger patient sample and more refined techniques.

In order to provide a more solid empirical basis for the large-scale investigation, a number of preliminary studies were carried out. The first stage consisted of a series of studies evaluating current methods of clinical diagnosis. On the basis of these studies, a decision was made to use psychiatrists' ratings and various psychometric techniques to isolate the depressed group. The second stage was the development of an inventory for measuring depression, and a refinement of the clinical rating scale.

In the third stage, the studies were oriented to testing the hypothesis that depressed patients are characterized by a number of distinctive patterns that lead to suffering disproportionate or inappropriate to the reality situation. Two major approaches were used to demonstrate these self-suffering (or "masochistic") patterns: Ideational material (dreams, responses to structured projective tests, and free associations) was analyzed to determine whether depressed patients show a greater frequency of "masochistic" themes in these productions than nondepressed patients; and controlled experimental stress-situations were set up, to determine whether the reactions of depressed patients were more self-debasing than the reactions of nondepressed patients.

In a collateral study to determine whether there were any significant differences in the backgrounds of depressed and nondepressed patients, a computation of the relative incidence of parental loss during childhood was made. In addition, the verbal productions of depressed patients in psychotherapy were studied to determine whether there were any patterns that were characteristic of depression.

Part III of this volume is designed to integrate the findings of our research, much of which has been published in separate articles in various journals. A general review of the procedures and findings will be presented in the remainder of this chapter. In the following four chapters, the major studies will be presented in detail. The theoretical formulations based on these studies will be presented in Part IV.

THE MEASUREMENT OF DEPRESSION

DIAGNOSIS OF DEPRESSION

The first problem in determining the psychodynamic correlates of depression was that of establishing a reliable and valid measure of depression. There has been considerable skepticism among psychiatric researchers regarding the traditional nosology as embodied in the accepted Standard Nomenclature. Some investigators question the value of the entire diagnostic system, particularly in view of the reports of relatively low inter-psychiatrist reliability. Others, focusing on the broad category of depression, doubt the utility of the subtypes (manic-depressive, psychoneurotic-depressive reactions, etc.). Since the previous studies of the reliability of psychiatric diagnoses showed methodological defects, we decided to conduct a reliability study ourselves. In designing our reliability study, we attempted to remedy those defects, and to reduce the influence of extraneous factors that might artificially raise or lower the degree of agreement.

As the first step in ascertaining the usefulness of formal diagnostic categories for identifying the experimental groups, a study was made of the degree of agreement between psychiatrists diagnosing psychiatric patients in an outpatient clinic (Beck, Ward *et al.*, 1962). To determine the degree of agreement, 154 cases were diagnosed by a group of four board-certified psychiatrists, randomly paired so that each patient was interviewed separately by two of the psychiatrists, and the diagnoses were rendered completely independently.

A comparison of the diagnoses of the paired diagnosticians indicated overall agreement on the narrow nosological categories (neurotic-depressive reaction, schizophrenic reaction, etc.) in 56 per cent of the cases. The agreement on the category of neurotic-depressive reaction was 63 per cent. The agreement on the broad divisions (neurosis, psychosis, personality disorder) was 70 per cent.

The expected agreement that might be expected by chance alone, i.e., if each diagnostician diagnosed the cases according to his own system of diagnostic preferences, was computed. In order to arrive at this figure, the "base rates" for each diagnostician were calculated on the basis of the frequency of his selection of each diagnostic category. The obtained agreement was significantly higher than might have been expected on the basis of chance. This rate of agreement on the refined categories was higher than that obtained in other comparable studies reported in the literature.

In 31 cases in which both diagnosticians indicated that they were certain of the diagnoses, the agreement rate was 81 per cent, which was significantly higher than the agreement (49 per cent) in the remaining 123 cases, in which at least one of the diagnosticians was not completely certain of his diagnosis.

When the diagnosticians presented both a preferred diagnosis and an alternative diagnosis (differential diagnosis), it was found that there was at least one matching pair of diagnoses in 82 per cent of the cases. This suggested that the diagnosticians may have been closer in their appraisals than was indicated by the scoring of only the preferred diagnoses. The possible influence of clinical experience on the rate of agreement was suggested by the fact that the diagnostician in the group of four who had substantially less experience than the other three had a significantly lower rate of agreement than the others.

Reasons for Diagnostic Disagreement

On the basis of this study, we felt that the current system of diagnosis did not yield sufficiently high concordance rates to justify its use for our investigation. Nonetheless, we were reluctant to abandon the traditional nosological system completely. In the first place, the Standard Nomenclature is part of the common language of psychiatrists, and communication of our findings in terms of the familiar categories would be much more useful and meaningful than operational definitions in terms of rating systems or inventories. Second, since there is a multiplicity of rating scales and inventories being used by various investigators, it is difficult to compare results based on dfferent instruments. Third, there is no evidence that diagnostic variability is the result of irremediable defects in the nomenclature; in fact, the variability might be more closely related to psychiatrist inadequacies such as lack of uniformity in obtaining the basic psychiatric information and in selecting the appropriate diagnostic label. In view of these considerations, we decided to make a more thorough study of the process of diagnosis, with the ultimate goal of determining whether the system employing the standard nosology could be sufficiently improved to meet research standards.

One step in this direction was a systematic study by the diagnosticians of the reasons for disagreements (Ward *et al.*, 1962). Each patient was seen by at least two psychiatrists. In each case in which there was disagreement, the diagnosticians conferred and tried to determine the reasons for disagreement. The causes of disagreement in 97 cases were grouped into three major categories: cases of disagreement attributed to fluctuations in the clinical state of the patient, 5 per cent; cases of disagreement attributed to inconsistencies by one of the psychiatrists, 37 per cent; cases of disagreement attributed to inadequacies in the present nosological system, 58 per cent.

On the basis of the joint experience in rendering formal diagnoses, the diagnosticians attempted to construct a system to standardize and revise some of the processes of arriving at a diagnosis. The new procedure, for example, provided a method for determining which major diagnostic category should be listed first when two were present in the same patient. For example, in cases of psychoneurotic reactions in patients with personality disorders, it was decided that the psychoneurotic disorder would be listed first. Some improvement in the degree of agreement was obtained using the new system, but it still fell short of the minimum requirements of our research plan.

RATINGS OF DEPRESSION

An alternative approach to identifying the criterion group consisted of clinical ratings on the dimension of *depth of depression*. Prior to making these ratings, the diagnosticians discussed the criteria to be used in assessing the depth of depression and agreed on 22 signs and symptoms which would be used as indices of depression. Each diagnostician rated the intensity of each sign and symptom on a 4-point scale (none, mild, moderate, or severe). His final rating of the overall intensity of the depression took into account his quantitative estimate of the severity of each of the 22 signs and symptoms (see Chapter 12 for list of indices), as well as a global judgment of the severity of the depression. There was complete agreement on the depth of depression in 57 per cent of the cases, and the diagnosticians were one interval apart in 42 per cent of the cases; hence, in 99 per cent of the cases, the diagnosticians showed no more than one scale unit difference in their ratings. The product-moment correlations of the ratings of the paired diagnosticians ranged from .78 to .92.

Clinical vs. Psychometric Ratings

The question then arose as to whether we should rely solely on the clinical ratings of depression or should use a more *objective* measure such as the Depression Inventory, which was developed concurrently with the clinical diagnostic study.

We recognized that the use of clinical judgments has the advantage of being based on careful appraisals by judges who are specialists in identifying the clinical phenomena. In contrast to testers applying purely verbal measures, the diagnostician can evaluate the nonverbal as well as the verbal behavior of the patient. With the application of his specialized skills, the psychiatrist can isolate and weigh the various signs and symptoms of a specific patient, can deal with distorting factors such as evasiveness or exaggeration, and can make a global judgment which takes into account the total behavior of the patient as well as the individual signs and symptoms.

On the other hand, the diagnosticians' appraisals presented certain problems. The individual diagnostician was frequently inconsistent in applying his diagnostic techniques and in making judgments. A more serious problem was that while the diagnosticians were able to achieve a reasonable degree of uniformity through a painstaking process of discussing their differences, there was no assurance that other diagnosticians at different psychiatric centers would show any appreciable agreement with their ratings; diagnostic differences between various institutions have been demonstrated many times. It seemed likely that, unless specifically trained to conform to the specified techniques and indices employed by our diagnosticians, other psychiatrists assessing a complicated phenomenon such as depression would be prone to diverge according to their individual predilections. This would impede generalizing our findings to patients diagnosed by other psychiatrists and would pose problems if we should change diagnosticians during our investigations. Because of these problems, it was necessary to consider the alternative method, namely the Depression Inventory, for isolating the experimental group.

INVENTORY FOR MEASURING DEPRESSION

Since a psychometric technique such as our Depression Inventory consists of a standard set of items presented in a uniform way, it is not subject to the inconsistencies and biases originating with the interviewer that may occur in the psychiatric evaluation. Because of this, the inventory could be used as a criterion measure by other investigators and, thus, facilitate replication of our studies. Furthermore, the precision afforded by the relatively wide range of scores on the inventory provides finer discriminations between patients and allows for comparisons with other types of quantitative data. Finally, the inventory is readily adaptable to continual refinement as additional data regarding its reliability and validity is accumulated.

Reliance on the inventory, on the other hand, posed a number of special problems. First, the accuracy with which patients can discriminate between alternative statements in each item is variable. Second, inventory responses are especially susceptible to distorting tendencies on the part of the patient. There is considerable evidence, for instance, that part of the variance of self-report instruments is due to response sets. Third, some of the basic assumptions underlying the interpretation of the scores on such measures may not be tenable. There is a reasonable question, for example, regarding the validity of the assumption that the cumulative score over a large number of items on a personality scale reflects the intensity of the variable being measured. It also could be argued that *fractionating* a form of disturbed behavior into a number of separate scorable units (the items on the inventory) actually produces a distorted measure of this behavior, which can be appropriately evaluated only by a holistic approach.

Our approach in coping with these problems was to use the clinical ratings of the depth of depression as the initial criterion against which to judge the validity of the Depression Inventory. In several of our studies, moreover, we used both the Depression Inventory and the diagnosticians' ratings to define the clinical groups. In this way, we hoped to maximize the advantages of both approaches.

After we had determined that there was a reasonably high correlation between scores on the inventory and clinical ratings, we assessed the ability of the inventory to predict behaviors assumed to be associated with depression. Since the results of these studies supported the construct validity of the inventory, it was then feasible to refine it on the basis of an analysis of its properties and its correlations with the other test and nontest behavior.

It is apparent that we have by no means reached the ultimate in measures of depression. A good deal of basic research must be done to elucidate the various determinants of patients' interview behavior and test responses and of clinicians' judgments to provide a solid empirical basis for our diagnostic and psychometric techniques.

BEHAVIORAL TESTS OF DEPRESSION

One approach to circumvent the difficulties posed by the use of clinical judgments or psychometric techniques is to use behavioral tests that are not dependent on the self-evaluations of the patients. A behavioral test would attempt to measure an individual's performance directly rather than to rely on his subjective appraisal of himself. Some of the supposed characteristics of depressives which we attempted to assess in this way were: psychomotor retardation, constriction of handwriting, distortion of judgment of time and distance, loss of mirth response, and indecisiveness.* We found, however, that only the loss of mirth response showed a significant relationship to depression.

* We found initially a positive relationship between the performance on these behavioral tests and depression. When the age was controlled, however, the relationship disappeared.

TESTING THE HYPOTHESIS

Once we had established reasonably reliable measures of depression, we were ready to proceed with determining whether the self-defeating patterns ("masochism") could be identified in the dreams and other ideational productions (early memories and story-telling), responses to verbal tests, and reactions to experimentally induced stresses. The major hypothesis to be tested was: There is a significant association between "masochism" (as defined below) and depression.

DEFINITION OF "MASOCHISM"

We defined "masochism" in terms of a cluster of related behaviors. Some typical repetitive behavior patterns observed in individuals considered "masochistic" but not necessarily depressed are: the tendency to interpret the lack of complete success as failure; to have self-doubts even when successful; to magnify the importance of personal defects; to react to criticism with self-debasement; and to expect rejection. This type of behavior pattern was conceptualized as (*a*) a manifestation of *a need to suffer* or as (*b*) a manifestation of an enduring cognitive distortion which negatively biases the individual's evaluation of his own worth, adequacy, social acceptability, or achievements. Which of these formulations is the more applicable still remains to be demonstrated empirically. In either case, the individual tends to structure his experiences in such a way that he reacts to life situations with inappropriate or excessive suffering. The type of dysphoria experienced includes feelings of humiliation, deprivation, frustration, and social isolation.

Previous clinical experience, and a systematic study based on this experience (Beck and Hurvich, 1959), indicated that dreams in which the dreamer is deserted, frustrated, deprived, or injured are characteristic of depression-prone or "masochistic" people. As a broad test of this finding, we attempted to determine whether the self-representation of the depressed patients as degraded, impotent, or deprived may be found consistently in various types of ideational material. Since there is no definitive criterion of "masochism," it was necessary to make a series of predictions based on the underlying concept of "masochism" and to design tests and experiments to confirm or disconfirm these predictions. As a first step, it was predicted *a priori* that the scores on various tests that were designed to facilitate a certain type of response ("masochistic") would correlate significantly with measures of depression. Since these tests dealt with various forms and levels of behavior including dreams, memories, story-telling, and self-reports, on an inventory and on a self-concept test, a fairly broad area of verbal behavior was tapped. That scores on each of these measures showed a significant relationship to measures of depression offers supporting evidence for the hypothesis.

DREAM STUDY

In our preliminary study, a scoring system had been devised for identifying "masochistic" dreams. In our large-scale study, this system was applied to the dreams of 219 patients. The depressed group was found to have a significantly higher number of "masochistic" dreams than the non-depressed group (see Chapter 13).

Assumptions and Interpretations

A major problem in using the test of dreams, memories, and story-telling responses to projective tests is concerned with whether the basic assumptions regarding the identification and measurement of constructs in this material are justified. Dreams, for instance, have been postulated to be an expression of a wide variety of personality processes. Some of the specific assumptions regarding dream content that are most relevant to our research and that have been considered by us in interpreting our findings are that dream content is: (*a*) an expression of motivations, such as hostility, dependency, the need to suffer, etc.; or (*b*) a representation of the individual's concept of himself and/or of his concept of personal and impersonal forces in the environment; or (*c*) an expression of characteristic patterns of behavior; or (*d*) a translation of affects, such as sadness, into pictorial imagery; or (*e*) a manifestation of an attempt at problem-solving; or (*f*) a condensation of random waking impressions, thoughts, worries, and memories.

Two more general assumptions interwoven with those listed above are that dream imagery may be regarded as (*g*) a symbolic, indirect, or disguised representation of a psychological process, or (*h*) a direct, un-camouflaged representation that can be appraised at its face value, i.e., relatively little inference is required to categorize it. The various assumptions are not necessarily mutually exclusive.

As mentioned previously, our utilization of dreams in the project originally rested on at least two of the above assumptions. The first (assumption *a*), was that the construct, "masochism," would be expressed in dreams because of its motivational properties: Thus, the "masochistic" dream of being subjected to a painful experience was regarded as the expression of a motivation, viz., the need to suffer. The second (assumption *b*), was that the dream can be usefully categorized on the basis of its superficial content and the specific themes may be taken literally (irrespective of any possible symbolic or disguised meaning). These two assumptions (which also appear to underlie research with the TAT in which Murray's "need system" is used) were made in our work with the projective tests.

After we had determined that there was a significant relationship between our measures of depression and the incidence of "masochistic" dreams, the question of how to interpret these findings arose. Since any interpretation is dependent on the underlying assumptions, these were re-examined. Our assumption that the dream is an expression of a motivation, led to the interpretation of the "masochistic" dream as the representation of a need to suffer. However, an equally plausible (or more plausible) explanation of "masochistic" behavior in general had to be considered. This was that the typical "masochistic" behaviors, characterized by suffering disproportionate to the reality situation, are the result of the specific way the "masochistic" individual structures his experiences. As a result of his particular conceptual systems, he might introduce a systematic bias (against himself) in evaluating specific experiences; he would, for example, be prone to interpret any difficulties or disappointments as manifestations of his own inadequacies. In accordance with this formulation, the "masochistic" dream would be regarded as a manifestation of the individual's distorted self-concept, negative interpretation of experience, and unpleasant expectations.

Our other initial assumption was that the dramatic action and imagery in the dream can be analyzed in a relatively literal way on the basis of the superficial themes. Thus, the "masochistic" dream of being betrayed by a spouse would be assigned to the category of *rejection*. A corollary of this is the assumption that the themes in the dreams have observable counterparts in the waking behavior or conscious mental activity of the individual. Thus, the individual who dreams of himself as ugly would be expected to show unusual concern about his appearance as manifested by, say, frequently looking into the mirror or worrying about his physical attractiveness.

Dreams and Overt Behavior

Since we were relying on the assumption that dream themes reflect specific behavior patterns, it was considered important to determine whether this assumption is tenable. One approach to the problem was to ascertain whether the thematic content of dreams bears any relevance to overt behavior. An initial line of inquiry has been to select individuals whose actions have been unusual or extreme in some regard, and to attempt to predict this behavior on the basis of their dreams. For this reason, we conducted a study of the dreams of various types of convicts (sexual offenders, murderers, and burglars) to determine whether their manifest dreams are significantly related to the type of offense for which they were imprisoned.

Ten consecutive dreams were collected from each of eight prisoners convicted of sexual offenses against children and from a matched control group of eight prisoners with no history of sexual offenses (Goldhirsh, 1961). A scoring system for identifying undisguised sexual elements and *criminal sexual activity* in the manifest content of dreams was constructed. Agreement between two judges as to whether or not a dream contained a sexual element or a theme relating to sexual offenses was 99 per cent on 200 dreams that were scored. It was found that there was a significantly higher frequency of dreams with both uncamouflaged sexual elements and *criminal* sexual activity in the sexual offender group than in the control group ($p < .01$, Wilcoxon Matched-Pairs Signed-Ranks test). These findings were regarded as consistent with the assumption that dream themes are relevant to observable patterns of behavior.

EARLY MEMORIES

Each patient in our studies was routinely asked to report his three earliest memories, and in about 80 per cent of the cases it was possible to obtain at least three early memories. A scoring manual to identify "masochistic" themes in the early memories was drawn up. It was found that the same categories used in scoring the dreams could be adapted for scoring the memories. Agreement between independent ratings of two judges was 95 per cent. The verbal reports of 25 patients who reported their three earliest memories were analyzed blindly for the presence of "masochistic" themes. It was found that the frequency of "masochistic" early memories reported by patients in the depressed group was significantly higher than for patients in the nondepressed group. The association between the scores on the Depression Inventory and the frequency of "masochistic" early memories was evaluated statistically by the Mann-Whitney U test and was found to be significant at the 0.05 level (Beck, 1961).

FOCUSED FANTASY TEST

This test consists of a set of four picture cards. Each card has four frames that portray a continuous sequence of events. The action in the sequence centers essentially around two figures, who are sufficiently similar to make it equivocal which figures in one frame correspond to the figures in the subsequent frames. One of the two figures is subjected to an unpleasant experience, and the other figure avoids the unpleasant experience or has a pleasant experience.

The subject is presented one of the pictures and then is asked to tell a story about the sequence. After listening to the story, the examiner determines which of the two characters in the story recounted by the subject is the main character or hero. The hero, by definition, is the character who is present in all four frames in the story, i.e., he is identified as the solitary figure in the first frame. The outcome is label "masochistic" or "nonmasochistic" depending upon whether the hero or the secondary character is identified with the figure hurt in the final frame.

This test was administered to 87 patients. Since four cards were used, the score for each patient ranged from 0–4. The patients were divided according to their Depression Inventory scores into depressed and nondepressed groups and ranked according to the scores on the Focused-Fantasy test. It was found that the scores were significantly higher (p.$<$0.0003, Mann-Whitney U test) among the depressed than among the nondepressed patients (Beck, 1961).

"Masochism" Inventory

This inventory consists of 46 items relevant to the following behaviors: "masochism" (20 items), hostility (20 items), and submission (6 items). The items were primarily clinically derived. The "masochism" items were based on clinically observed behaviors considered consistent with the definition of "masochism" and observed in patients who were not clinically depressed. Each item in the inventory consists of a statement that is read aloud to the patient, who is then asked to select one of five alternative phrases to complete the statement. The alternatives are scaled on a frequency dimension as follows: never (0), sometimes (1), often (2), usually (3), always (4).

This test was administered to 109 patients. The scores on the "masochism" items were then compared with the scores on the Depression Inventory. It was found that there was a Spearman rank correlation of 0.51 between these two tests (p$<$0.001). The correlation between scores on the Depression Inventory and on the hostility items was substantially lower, the coefficient being 0.24 (Beck, 1961).

Self-Concept Test

Another interviewer-administered schedule has been developed to index the negative self-concept considered to be characteristic of "masochistic" patients. It was observed clinically that "masochistic" and depressed patients tend to downgrade themselves in regard to certain attributes that are of special importance to them; it was also observed clinically that other types of attributes, such as the conventional virtues (kindness, goodness, generosity), were often selected by the depressed patients as characteristics in which they were superior to others. The inventory consists of 25 personal attributes such as personal appearance, conversational ability, sense of humor, and success. The patient compares himself with other people on a 5-point scale ranging from "worse than anybody I know" (1) to "better than anybody I know" (5). He similarly indicates "how I feel about being this way." The items are keyed so that a low total score indicates a low self-regard.

This test was administered to a sample of 49 psychiatric inpatients and outpatients. The product-moment correlation between scores on this self-concept test and the scores on the Depression Inventory was $-.66$ (p.$<$.01). A similar negative correlation ($-.42$) was found between self-acceptance scores on the Self-Concept test and the scores on the Depression Inventory. The results support the hypotheses that the depressed patient has a negative view of himself and rejects himself for his presumed failings.

Experimental Studies

Another approach used to investigate the relationship of specific psychodynamic constructs to depression, and to develop measures of the constructs, was through the manipulation of the specific variables in a controlled experiment. In two of the experiments described below, predictions were made regarding the expected response of depressed patients when the experimental situation was designed to elicit "masochistic behavior."

Effects of Inferior Performance on Depressed Patients

One of the characteristic behaviors assumed to be typical of "masochistic" individuals is the tendency to be disproportionately affected by inferior performance. To test this assumption empirically, an experiment was designed to determine the differential effects of superior and inferior performance on the reported mood of depressed and nondepressed patients (Loeb *et al.*, 1964). The Depression Inventory was individually administered to 32 male patients on the intensive treatment ward of a Veterans Administration neuropsychiatric hospital. On the basis of their inventory scores, patients were divided into three groups: high-depressed, moderate-depressed, and low-depressed. On the same day that they were given the Depression Inventory, subjects were scheduled in groups of three for the experiment. Patients rated their present mood on an 11 point scale (with "extremely sad" and "extremely happy" as the anchor points) both before and after the experimental manipulation of success and failure. In addition, a post measure on the level of expectation (in regard to the estimated number of words they could write in three minutes) was obtained from all subjects.

During the experiment, the patients worked on a series of four word-completion tasks that they believed were identical, but that in reality varied in difficulty. Consequently, in each group of three, one of the subjects consistently scored high (superior), one medium (neutral), and one low (inferior). The moderate-depressed were always assigned to the neutral position and are not considered in the results. Half of the high-depressed were assigned to the inferior performance group and half to the superior performance group; the low-depressed were treated in the same way. After each word-completion task, scores were posted on a blackboard to dramatize the relative performance of the subjects. After the final posting of scores, the patients rated their mood for the second time.

The results indicated that the high-depressed patients showed a greater drop in mood level (as indicated by self-ratings) following failure, and a greater increase after success, than did the low-depressed patients. This difference was short of statistical significance (p = .10). The high-depressed had a significantly higher level of expectation (number of words they estimated they could write in three minutes) following superior performance, than each of the other three groups; following inferior performance, the high-depressed had a lower level of expectation than the other groups.

Effects of Success and Failure on Expectancy and Performance

A study was designed to determine the effects of success and failure on the probability-of-success estimate, the level of aspiration, and the actual performance of depressed and nondepressed patients. Twenty depressed and 20 nondepressed patients were individually given two card sorting tasks. The experimenter deliberately interrupted the second task so that all the subjects "failed".

It was found that the depressed patients were more sensitive to failure than the nondepressed patients. They reacted with significantly greater pessimism (as measured by probability-of-success estimates) and a lower level of aspiration. Despite consistently greater pessimism than the non-depressed patients, the depressed patients' actual performance was consistently as good as that of the nondepressed patients (Loeb *et al.*, 1966).

COLLATERAL STUDIES

COGNITIVE PATTERNS IN VERBAL MATERIAL

While the systematic studies of newly-admitted patients to our psychiatric outpatient clinics or hospitals was being conducted, I began to review the case records of depressed and nondepressed patients in psychotherapy to determine whether any consistent differences could be detected in the verbal (i.e., non-dream) material. As described in Chapter 15, I found that the depressed patients tended to distort their experiences in an idiosyncratic way: They misinterpreted specific events in terms of failure, deprivation, or rejection. They also tended to make negative predictions of the future. I was not able to find any tangible evidence of a need to suffer. Such a need, if it exists, could not be identified directly in the clinical material nor in any of the systematic studies.

Since the studies could not demonstrate (nor rule out) that the depressed patient is motivated by a need to suffer, I considered alternative explanations for the findings in the dream studies and the studies of the verbal materials. In both the dreams and in the reports of waking experiences, the patients frequently pictured themselves as thwarted, deprived, defective, etc. This led to the conclusion that certain cognitive patterns could be responsible for the patients' tendency to make negatively-biased judgments of themselves, their environment, and their future. These cognitive patterns, although less prominent in the nondepressed period, became activated during the depression. The theoretical elaboration of this formulation is contained in Chapters 17 and 18.

LONGITUDINAL STUDIES

In another approach to understanding depression, past-history information was obtained to determine whether the depressed patients had been exposed to any particular types of developmental stresses that might account for their sense of deprivation and hopelessness. It was anticipated that the death of a parent in childhood, because of the intensity and finality of the loss, might be expected to sensitize the child to react to future life situations in terms of deprivation and hopelessness. It was found that in a group of 100 severely depressed adult patients, 27 per cent had lost one or both parents through death before the age of 16; whereas in a control group of nondepressed psychiatric patients, only 12 per cent had been orphaned before 16 (Chapter 14). It appeared that these results were consistent with the concept that depressed patients may develop through traumatic life experiences certain cognitive-affective patterns which, when activated, produce inappropriate or disproportionate reactions of deprivation and despair.

Chapter 12.
Measurement of Depression: the Depression Inventory

The difficulties inherent in obtaining consistent and adequate diagnoses for the purposes of research and therapy have been pointed out in Chapter 11. Pasamanick, Dintz, and Lefton (1959) viewed the low interclinician agreement on diagnosis as an indictment of the present state of psychiatry, and called for "the development of objective, measurable and verifiable criteria of classification based not on personal or parochial considerations, but on behavioral and objectively measurable manifestations."

In 1954 Lorr summarized the rating scales and check lists for the evaluation of psychopathology that had been used up until the time of the preparation of his review article. Since then a number of rating scales have been reported. These include rating scales by Hamilton (1960a), Cutler and Kurland (1961), Kanter (1961), Friedman et al. (1963), Wechsler, Grosser, and Busfield (1963), and Zung (1965).

This chapter will be concerned with self-rating instruments rather than with psychiatrists' rating scales.

PSYCHOMETRIC TESTS OF DEPRESSION

In 1930 Jasper devised the Depression-Elation test. This was derived from a study of normal college students, and his report does not refer to any studies with a psychiatric population. So far as I can determine, this test is no longer in use.

The Depression Scale (D-Scale) of the Minnesota Multiphasic Personality Inventory (MMPI) has been widely used for the measurement of depression for clinical and research purposes. Despite the tremendous amount of work that has been done using the MMPI (Hathaway and McKinley, 1942), we found that it had certain disadvantages that made us question its usefulness for our purposes. Factor analytic studies revealed that the depression scale contains a number of heterogeneous factors, only one of which is consistent with the clinical concept of depression (Comrey,

1957). O'Connor, Stefic, and Gresock (1957) isolated five separate parameters identified as hypochondriasis, cycloid tendency, hostility, inferiority, and depression. Since only one of these clusters was relevant to the clinical definition of depression, the authors questioned the practice of attributing unitary significance to the D-Scale. A wide variety of studies, furthermore, have suggested that the MMPI is peculiarly sensitive to response sets such as the acquiescence response set and the social desirability response set (Messick, 1960).

In recent years, a number of tests consisting of adjective check lists have been developed for the measurement of depression and other affects. (Clyde, 1961; Zuckerman and Lubin, 1965). These check lists include adjectives frequently used by depressed patients to describe their subjective states. Unfortunately, the subjective feeling tone is only one aspect of the entire depressive syndrome, and there is evidence that the failure to tap the other dimensions of depression impairs the usefulness of this kind of test. It was observed in our studies that not all patients diagnosed by clinicians as depressed acknowledge that they have any depressed feelings. Of the mildly depressed patients in our series, for instance, only 50 per cent acknowledged feelings of depression or unhappiness, and of the moderately depressed, 75 per cent acknowledged having these feelings. Pichot and Lempérière (1964) found that the reported affect had a substantially lower correlation with the general factor of depression than did several other depressive phenomena. Furthermore, there is considerable doubt that depression should be conceived of simply as a mood disorder rather than as a complex disorder involving affective, cognitive, motivational, and behavioral components.

RATIONALE FOR THE INVENTORY

In planning our research, we decided that it would be useful to develop an inventory for measuring the depth of depression. We felt that it could be used in combination with clinical ratings of the depth of depression (Chapter 11) for some studies and as the sole measure of depression for other studies. We concluded that if we could develop an inventory that approximated clinical judgments of the intensity of depression it would offer a number of advantages for research purposes. First, it would meet the problem of the variability of clinical diagnoses and would provide a standardized, consistent measure that would not be sensitive to the theoretical orientation, the idiosyncracies, or the inconsistencies of the individual administering it. It would ask each patient the same questions in exactly the same way. Second, since the inventory could be administered by an easily trained interviewer, it would be far more economical than a clinical psychiatric interview. Third, since the inventory would provide a numerical score, it would facilitate comparison with other quantitative data, and would also lend itself to various types of statistical manipulation. Finally, because of the wide range of scores, the inventory might be a more sensitive indicator of changes of the depth of depression than would clinical judgments based on a psychiatric interview.

When faced with the problem of assessing some diagnostically relevant behaviors as, for example, are presented by states of depression, the clinician is disposed to rely upon clinical observation and tends to mistrust personality inventories. This objection to so-called objective instruments is formally expressed by Horn (1950), who, in commenting on the "relative sterility" of personality inventories in predicting behavior, challenges the assumption that the items in an inventory convey the same or similar meaning to everyone who takes the test. He argues that "a personality self-rating questionnaire is in the nature of a projective test: each item serves as an ambiguous stimulus whose interpretation is affected by the subject's needs, wishes, fears, etc." This approach, in his opinion, removes from consideration the efficacy of a self-rating inventory as an accurate self-evaluation. However, the adequacy of any test as an accurate index of what it is supposed to measure is essentially an empirical question and can only be settled through systematic investigation.

The objective in applying the Depression Inventory to a given sample of psychiatric patients was to identify as many of the depressed patients as possible and to exclude as many of the nondepressed patients as possible. In constructing the instrument, we sought to maximize the differences between the depressed and the nondepressed patients. The form of the instrument was related to two observations. (1) With increasing severity of depression, the number of symptoms increases and there is a steplike progression in the frequency of depression symptoms from nondepressed, to mildly depressed, to moderately depressed, to severely depressed patients (Chapter 2). (2) The more depressed a patient is, the more intense a particular symptom is likely to be.

The inventory, consequently, was designed to include all symptoms integral to the depressive constellation and at the same time to provide for grading the intensity of each. Each symptom category was constructed to include a series of statements reflecting varying degrees of severity. The scoring system took into account the number of symptoms reported by the patient by assigning a numerical score for each symptom. The intensity of each symptom was registered by assigning graduated numerical values to each statement within a category. The patient's total score, therefore, represented a combination of the *number* of symptom categories he endorsed and the *severity* of the particular symptoms.

METHOD

CONSTRUCTION OF THE INVENTORY

The items in this inventory were primarily clinically derived. In the course of the psychotherapy of depressed patients, I made systematic observations and records of their characteristic attitudes and symptoms. I selected a group of these attitudes and symptoms that appeared to be specific for these depressed patients, and which were consistent with descriptions of depression contained in the psychiatric literature. On the basis of this selection, I constructed an inventory composed of 21 categories of symptoms and attitudes. Each category describes a specific behavioral manifestation of depression and consists of a graded series of four to five self-evaluative statements. The statements are ranked to reflect the range of severity of the symptom, from neutral to maximal severity. Numerical values from 0–3 are assigned each statement to indicate the degree of severity. In many categories, two alternative statements are presented at a given level and are assigned the same weight; these equivalent statements are labeled *a* and *b* (e.g. 2*a*, 2*b*) to indicate that they are at the same level. The items were chosen on the basis of their relationship to the overt behavioral manifestations of depression and do not reflect any theory regarding the etiology or the underlying psychological processes in depression.*

The symptom-attitude categories were:

1. Mood	12. Social withdrawal
2. Pessimism	13. Indecisiveness
3. Sense of failure	14. Distortion of body image
4. Lack of satisfaction	15. Work inhibition
5. Guilty feeling	16. Sleep disturbance
6. Sense of punishment	17. Fatigability
7. Self-dislike	18. Loss of appetite
8. Self accusations	19. Weight loss
9. Suicidal wishes	20. Somatic preoccupation
10. Crying spells	21. Loss of libido
11. Irritability	

* An amended version of the Depression Inventory and instructions for administering it are presented in the Appendix.

Administration of the Inventory

The inventory was administered by a trained interviewer (a clinical psychologist or a sociologist) who read aloud each statement in the category and asked the patient to select the statement that seemed to fit him best at present. In order that the instrument reflect the current status of the patient, the items were presented so as to elicit the patient's attitude at the time of the interview. The patient also had a copy of the inventory so that he could read each statement to himself as the interviewer read it aloud. On the basis of the patient's response, the interviewer circled the number adjacent to the appropriate statement.

The total score was obtained by summing the scores of the individual symptom categories.

Description of Patient Population.

The patients were drawn from routine admissions to the psychiatric outpatient department of a university hospital (Hospital of the University of Pennsylvania) and to the psychiatric outpatient department and psychiatric inpatient service of a metropolitan hospital (Philadelphia General Hospital). The outpatients were seen either on the day of their first visit to the outpatient department, or an appointment was made for them to come back a few days later for the complete work-up. Hospitalized patients were all seen the day following their admission to the hospital, i.e., during the first full day in the hospital. The demographic features of the population are listed in Table 12–1. It will be noted that there are two patient samples: one, the original group of 226 patients; the other, the replication group of 183 patients.* The original sample (Study I) was taken over a seven-month period starting in June, 1959 and the second (Study II) over a five-month period starting in February, 1960. The completion of the first study coincided with the introduction of some new projective tests not relevant to this report.

Salient aspects of this table are the predominance of white patients over Negro patients, the age concentration between 15 and 44, and the high frequency of patients in the lower socioeconomic groups (IV and V). The social position was derived from Hollingshead's Two-Factor Index of Social Position, which uses the factors of education and occupation in class level determination.

The distribution of diagnoses was similar for Studies I and II. Patients

* In later studies, the inventory was administered to an additional 557 patients. See Table 2–2 for characteristics of total sample of 966 patients.

Table 12–1.

PERCENTAGE DISTRIBUTION OF DEMOGRAPHIC CHARACTERISTICS
OF PATIENT SAMPLE

	N	Male	Female	White	Negro
Study I	226	40.7	59.3	67.6	32.4
Study II	183	37.2	62.8	61.2	38.8
Combined	409	39.1	60.9	64.7	35.3

			Age		
	15–24	*25–34*	*35–44*	*45–54*	*55 +*
Study I	24.5	33.3	25.8	11.1	5.3
Study II	21.3	31.2	23.5	16.9	7.1
Combined	23.0	32.4	24.8	13.7	6.1

	Social index				
	I–III	*IV*	*V*	*Inpatient*	*Outpatient*
Study I	13.7	40.6	45.7	33.6	66.4
Study II	17.4	34.8	47.8	34.4	65.6
Combined	15.3	38.1	46.6	34.0	66.0

with organic brain damage and mental deficiency were automatically excluded. The proportions among the major diagnostic categories were: psychotic disorder 41 per cent, psychoneurotic disorder 43 per cent, personality
disorder 16 per cent. The distributions among the subgroups were, in order
of frequency, as follows:

	Per cent
Schizophrenic reaction	28.2
Psychoneurotic-depressive reaction	25.3
Anxiety reaction	15.5
Involutional reaction	5.5
Psychotic-depressive reaction	4.7
Personality trait disturbance	4.5
Sociopathic personality	4.5
Psychophysiological disorder	3.4
Manic-depressive, depressed	1.8
Personality pattern disturbance	1.8
All other diagnoses	4.8
	100.0

External Criterion

The patient was seen, either directly before or directly after the administration of the Depression Inventory, by an experienced psychiatrist who interviewed him and rated him on a four-point scale for the depth of depression. The psychiatrist also rendered a psychiatric diagnosis and filled out a comprehensive form designed for the study. In approximately half the cases, the psychiatrist saw the patient first; in the remainder, the Depression Inventory was administered first.

Four experienced psychiatrists participated in the diagnostic study. They may be characterized as: having approximately 12 years' experience in psychiatry, holding responsible teaching and training positions, being certified by the American Board of Psychiatry, and being interested in research.

The psychiatrists had several preliminary meetings during which they reached a consensus regarding the criteria for each of the nosological entities and focused special attention on the various types of depression. In every case, the *Diagnostic and Statistical Manual of Mental Disorders* of the American Psychiatric Association (1952) was used, but it was found that considerable amplification of the diagnostic descriptions was necessary. After they reached complete agreement on the criteria to be used in making their clinical judgments, the psychiatrists composed a detailed instruction manual to serve as a guide in their diagnostic evaluations.

The psychiatrists then participated in a series of interviews, during which two of them jointly interviewed a patient while the other two observed through a one-way screen. This served as a practical testing ground for the application of the agreed-upon instructions and principles and allowed further discussion of interview techniques, the logic of diagnosis, and the pinpointing of specific diagnoses.

Since the main focus of the research was to be on depression, the diagnosticians also established specific indices to be used in making a clinical estimation of the depth of depression. These indices represented the pooled experience of the four clinicians and were arrived at independent of the Depression Inventory. For each specified sign and symptom the psychiatrists made a rating on a four-point scale of none, mild, moderate, and severe. The purpose of specifying these indices was to facilitate uniformity among the psychiatrists. In making the over-all rating of the depth of depression, however, they made a global judgment and were not bound by the ratings in each index. They also concentrated on the intensity of depression at the time of the interview; hence, the past history was not as important as the mental status examination.

The indices of depression devised and used by the psychiatrists were as follows:

I. *Appearance*
  Facies
  Gait
  Posture
  Crying
  Speech
    Volume
    Key
    Speed
    Amount

II. *Thought content*
  Reported mood
  Helplessness
  Pessimism
  Feelings of inadequacy and inferiority
  Somatic preoccuation
  Conscious guilt
  Suicidal content

III. *Vegetative signs*
  Sleep
  Appetite
  Constipation

IV. *Psychosocial*
  Performance
  Indecisiveness
  Loss of drive
  Loss of interest
  Fatigability

The diagnosticians also rated the patient on the degree of agitation and overt anxiety, and filled out a check list to indicate the presence of other specific psychiatric and psychosomatic symptoms and disturbances in concentration, memory, recall, judgment, and reality testing. They also made a rating of the severity of the present illness on a four-point scale.

To establish the degree of agreement, the psychiatrists interviewed 100 patients and made independent judgments of the diagnosis and the depth of depression. All four diagnosticians participated in the double assessment and were randomly paired with one another so that each patient was seen by two diagnosticians. First one psychiatrist interviewed the patient and then, after a resting period of a few minutes, the other psychiatrist interviewed the same patient. After the second interview, the clinicians usually met and discussed the cases seen concurrently to ascertain the reasons for any disagreement.

RESULTS

RELIABILITY

Reliability of Psychiatrists' Ratings

The agreement among the psychiatrists regarding the major diagnostic categories of psychotic disorder, psychoneurotic disorder, and personality disorder was 70 per cent in the 154 patients seen by two psychiatrists. For the finer categories of schizophrenia, anxiety reaction, neurotic-depressive reaction, etc., the agreement was 56 per cent. The agreement on neurotic-depressive reaction was 63 per cent. This level of agreement, although higher than that reported in many investigations, was considered too low for the purposes of our study.

The degree of agreement, however, in the rating of depth of depression was much higher. Using the four-point scale (none, mild, moderate, severe) to designate the intensity of depression, the diagnosticians showed the following degree of agreement:

Complete agreement	56 per cent
One degree of disparity	41 per cent
Two degrees of disparity	2 per cent
Three degrees of disparity	1 per cent

This indicates that there was agreement within one degree on the four-point scale in 97 per cent of the cases.

Reliability of Depression Inventory

Two methods for evaluating the internal consistency of the instrument were used. First, the protocols of 200 consecutive cases were analyzed. The score for each of the 21 categories was compared with the total score on the Depression Inventory for each individual. With the use of the Kruskal-Wallis Non-Parametric Analysis of Variance by Ranks, it was found that all categories showed a significant relationship to the total score for the inventory.* Significance was beyond the .001 level for all categories except category 19 (Weight-loss category), which was significant at the .01 level. A later item analysis of 606 cases showed that the categories correlated positively with the total DI score (range .31–.68). These correlations were all significant at the .001 level (see Table 12–6).

The second evaluation of internal consistency was the determination of the split-half reliability. Ninety-seven cases in the first sample were selected for this analysis. The Pearson r between the odd and even categories was computed and yielded a reliability coefficient of .86; with a Spearman-Brown correction, this coefficient rose to .93.

Certain traditional methods of assessing the stability and consistency of inventories and questionnaires, such as the test-retest method and the

* This procedure is designed to assess whether variation in response to a particular category is associated with variation in total score on the inventory. For each category, the distribution of total inventory scores for individuals selecting a particular alternative response was determined. The Kruskal-Wallis test was then used to assess whether the ranks of the distribution of total scores increased significantly as a function of the differences in severity of depression indicated by these alternative responses.

inter-rater reliability method, were not appropriate for appraisal of the Depression Inventory for the following reasons: If the inventory were readministered after a short period of time, the correlation between the two sets of scores could be spuriously inflated because of a memory factor. If a long interval were provided, the consistency would be lowered because of fluctuations in the intensity of depression occurring in psychiatric patients. The same factors precluded the successive administration of the test by different interviewers.

Two indirect methods of estimating the stability of the instrument were available. The first was a variation of the test-retest method. The inventory was administered to a group of 38 patients at two different times. Each time, a clinical estimate of the depth of depression was made by one of the psychiatrists. The interval between the two tests varied from 2–6 weeks. It was found that changes in the score on the inventory tended to parallel changes in the clinical rating of the depth of depression, indicating a consistent relationship of the instrument to the patient's clinical state (see Table 12–5).

An indirect measure of inter-rater reliability was achieved as follows. Each of the scores obtained by each of the three interviewers was plotted against the clinical ratings. A very high degree of consistency among the interviewers was observed for the mean scores respectively obtained at each level of depression. Curves of the distribution of the Depression Inventory scores plotted against the depth of depression were notably similar, again indicating a high degree of correspondence among those who administered the inventory.

VALIDITY

The evaluation of the validity of personality tests involves many complex problems. In trying to assess how well a given test measures a particular personality variable, the investigator is generally hampered by the absence of any established external criterion that defines the variable in question. Of the four types of validity described in the manual, *Technical Recommendations for Psychological Tests and Diagnostic Techniques* by the American Psychological Association (1954), concurrent validity and construct validity are relevant in evaluating personality tests.

CONCURRENT VALIDITY

Concurrent validity is evaluated by demonstrating how well the test scores correspond to other measures of depression, such as clinical evaluation and scores on other psychometric tests of depression.

Table 12–2.

DISTRIBUTION OF MEANS AND STANDARD DEVIATIONS OF DI SCORES ACCORDING TO DEPTH OF DEPRESSION

		Depth of depression											
		None			Mild			Moderate			Severe		
Total N		N	Mean	S.D.	N	Mean	S.D.	N	Mean	S.D.	N	Mean	S.D.
Present study 409*		115	10.9	8.1	127	18.7	10.2	134	25.4	9.6	33	30.0	10.4
British study 120†		32	5.4	5.8	44	14.3	8.3	24	24.2	10.8	20	29.5	6.5

* N = No. of patients.
† N = No. of ratings

Relation to Clinical Ratings

The means and standard deviations of DI scores for each of the depth-of-depression categories are presented in Table 12–2. It can be seen from inspection that the differences among the means are as expected; that is, with each increment in the magnitude of depression, there is a progressively higher mean score. The Kruskal-Wallis One-way Analysis of Variance by Ranks was used to evaluate the statistical significance of these differences; for both the original group (Study I) and the replication group (Study II), the p-value of these differences is < 0.001.

For purposes of comparison, the means and standard of deviations of a similar study in England by Metcalfe and Goldman (1965) are included in Table 12–2. It is worthy of note that their results closely paralleled ours, particularly in the moderately and severely depressed groups. Their lower score in the nondepressed group may be explained by the fact that their entire sample consisted of depressives who were psychiatrically well when they recovered. Our nondepressed group, however, consisted of patients diagnosed as having schizophrenia, anxiety reaction, etc.; hence, it could be expected that even in the absence of depression, a certain amount of their pathology could be reflected in their scores on the inventory.

Correlation with Clinical Ratings

A Pearson biserial r was computed to determine the degree of correlation between the scores on the Depression Inventory and the clinical judgment of depth of depression. To perform this correlation, the criterion ratings were reduced from four to two (none and mild, moderate and severe). The obtained biserial coefficients were .65 in Study I and .67 in Study II (Table 12–3).

In Metcalfe's study, using British patients, Kendall's rank correlation coefficient was calculated to determine the degree of association between

CLINICIANS' RATINGS OF DEPTH OF DEPRESSION*

Table 12–3.

CORRELATIONS BETWEEN DEPRESSION INVENTORY SCORES AND

	N	Correlation coefficient	Standard error	q
Study I	226	.65	.068	$<.01$
Study II	183	.67	.059	$<.01$

* Pearson biserial r.

psychiatrists' ratings and the DI score. The correlation coefficient was .61 (p < .001).

A drug study by Nussbaum, Wittig, *et al.* (1963), in which clinical ratings of depression, the Depression Inventory, and the D Scale of the MMPI were used as criterion measures, provides further data on the concurrent validity of the DI. As shown in Table 12–4 the DI showed a prod-

Table 12–4.
CORRELATION OF DI SCORE WITH CLINICAL RATING,
LUBIN CHECK LIST, AND MMPI D-SCALE

	N	DI	MMPI
Pretreatment rating	19	.66	.50
Posttreatment rating	19	.73	.37*
Change of score	19	.67	.22*
Lubin check list (F)	73	.66	.31
MMPI D-scale	19	.75	

* Not significant.

uct moment coefficient of .66 with the clinical ratings before treatment, and .73 after treatment; the correlation of the change of scores in these two measures was .67. All these correlations were significant. The correlation of the MMPI with the clinical ratings were lower, and two of the three were not significant.

The relationship between the Depression Inventory and the Hamilton Rating Scale has been evaluated by Schwab, Bialow, and Holzer (1967). Using a sample of 153 medical inpatients, these investigators obtained a Spearman Rank Correlation Coefficient of .75 between these two measures.

Prediction of Clinical Change

A pertinent test of the inventory's power to assess the intensity of depression is its ability to reflect changes after a time interval. A group of 38 hospital patients who had received the complete work-up including diagnostic evaluation, on the first full day in the hospital, were examined a second time by the same psychiatrist and received the same battery of tests. The time interval between the two tests ranged from 2–5 weeks. In five cases, the psychiatrist found that the changes were not sufficient to warrant changing the patient from one depth-of-depression category to another; he was aware, however, of finer changes in the severity of depression in these cases. In 33 cases, there was enough gross change in the clinical picture to warrant a change from one depth-of-depression category to another. The Depression Inventory scores changed in all cases; this was consistent with the expectation that the Depression Inventory would reflect minor changes, since its range is much greater than the clinical rating scale.

Table 12–5 shows the results of the determination of the number of

Table 12–5.

RELATIONSHIP OF CHANGES IN DEPRESSION
INVENTORY SCORE TO CHANGES IN DEPTH
OF DEPRESSION RATING

Depression inventory score	*Depth of depression*	
	Decreased	*Increased*
Decreased	26	2
Increased	3	2

cases in which a change in the depth of depression was predicted by a change in the Depression Inventory score; in 28 of the 33 cases (85 per cent), the change in the clinical depth of depression was correctly predicted. Similar correlations between DI scores and clinical assessment of change have been reported by Nussbaum, Wittig, *et al.* (Table 12–4) and by Pichot (1966).

Other self-rating instruments have been less useful in detecting changes in the level of depression. Several studies, for example, have reported that the Clyde Mood Scale is relatively insensitive to improvement in the depth of depression (Snow and Rickels, 1964).

Correlation with Other Tests

Lubin (1965) developed a set of Depression Adjective Check Lists (DACL) with which to measure transient depressive mood. These were administered to samples of males and females; normals and patients. The correlations of the individual list scores with the DI score in the patient group ranged from .40 to .66. The correlations in the female patient group were generally higher (.58 – .66) than in the other groups. Those results are contained in Table 12–4. Correlations of the DI Score with the MMPI D-Scale score obtained in Nussbaum's study are also presented in Table 12–4. The highest correlation was that between the DI score and MMPI. This may be attributed to similarity in the type of measure and to some similarities in item content. Also, both instruments might be affected in a similar way by extraneous factors such as response set. Since the DI score also correlated fairly highly with clinical ratings, however, it does not seem likely that its validity was substantially reduced by response set.

Discrimination between Anxiety and Depression

Since anxiety and depression are often associated in a given patient, it is important to have a test that discriminates between these two variables. In a study of 606 patients we found that the DI scores correlated .59 (Pearson r) with clinical ratings of depression and .14 with clinical ratings of anxiety. A positive association between anxiety and depression should be expected, since the clinicians found a correlation of .16 in their ratings of these variables. The individual items of the DI also correlate more highly with the clinical ratings of depression than with clinical ratings of anxiety (with the exception of item "Irritability"). The correlations of the DI items with the DI score and the clinical ratings are shown in Table 12–6.

Table 12–6.

PRODUCT-MOMENT CORRELATIONS OF DEPRESSION INVENTORY ITEMS WITH
TOTAL DI SCORE AND WITH CLINICAL RATINGS ($n = 606$)

	DI score	*Clinical ratings**		
		Depression	Severity	Anxiety
1. Sadness	.68	.44	.26	.07
2. Pessimism	.68	.45	.19	.11
3. Failure	.62	.37	.12	.11
4. Dissatisfaction	.68	.43	.19	.09
5. Guilt	.61	.36	.21	.12
6. Punishment	.50	.29	.14	.06
7. Self-dislike	.57	.39	.12	.10
8. Self-accusations	.51	.30	.07	.11
9. Suicidal	.60	.40	.23	.02
10. Crying	.51	.25	.16	.04
11. Irritability	.31	.08	.07	.10
12. Withdrawal	.60	.34	.18	.10
13. Indecisive	.63	.37	.22	.09
14. Self-image	.51	.33	.20	.07
15. Work inhibition	.54	.42	.16	.15
16. Insomnia	.50	.30	.17	.05
17. Fatigue	.54	.31	.11	.12
18. Anorexia	.54	.35	.21	.02
19. Weight loss	.32	.12	.10	.01
20. Hypochondria	.38	.18	.09	.14
21. Libido loss	.51	.27	.13	.23

* Clinical ratings made by psychiatrists on four-point scale, independently of administration of DI. *Severity* refers to severity of the specific illness (e.g. anxiety reaction, schizophrenic reaction of psychotic depressive reaction). Correlations of .12+ are significant at .01 level.

The inventory is evidently more effective in distinguishing depression from anxiety than are the various adjective check lists. Zuckerman and Lubin (1965), e.g., found that the Anxiety scale of their Multiple Affective Adjective Check List correlated .68 and .72 with clinical ratings of anxiety and depression, respectively. Their Depression scale correlated .34 with anxiety and .41 with depression but these correlations were not significant. They also found that the MMPI D-Scale did not distinguish between anxiety and depression (correlations .64 and .67, respectively). The Taylor Manifest Anxiety scale, surprisingly, correlated more highly with depression than with anxiety.

In summary, the concurrent validity of the DI has been supported by a number of studies employing clinical ratings and/or other psychometric measures. In separate studies at three different research centers, employing different samples and different types of psychiatric procedures, the separate DI correlations with the psychiatric ratings were very close (.61, .65, .66, and .67). The change in DI score over a period of time also correlated at this level with changes in the psychiatric evaluation of patients. The DI also showed significant correlations with other tests of depression. It correlated more highly with the MMPI D-scale and with the Lubin check list than the latter tests correlated with each other. Unlike some other tests (MAACL and MMPI D-Scale), the DI was also able to discriminate between anxiety and depression.

CONSTRUCT VALIDITY

Cronbach and Meehl (1955) have asserted that when there is no generally accepted criterion for a variable, a complicated logical and empirical attack is required. In studies of construct validity, the investigator is validating not only the test, but the theory or construct underlying the test. Two steps are involved in the validation procedure. First, the investigator inquires: What predictions can be made, using this theory, regarding the variation of scores from person to person or from occasion to occasion? Second, he gathers data to confirm these predictions (American Psychological Association, 1954).

The problem of validation of the construct is presented in more technical language by Cronbach and Meehl (1955): "A necessary condition for a construct to be scientifically admissible is that it occur in a nomological net, at least some of whose laws involve observables (p. 290). . . . unless the network makes contact with observations, and exhibits explicit, public steps of inference, construct validation cannot be claimed (p. 291.)"

In attempting to measure the construct *depression*, we defined it as follows, "Depression is conceived of as an abnormal state of the organism manifested by signs and symptoms such as low subjective mood, pessimistic and nihilistic attitudes, loss of spontaneity and specific vegetative signs." This variable may be construed in terms of a continuum, extending in a series of fine gradations from the neutral point (no depression) to an end point (maximal depression). This particular variable may occur together with any combination of other psychopathological variables such as anxiety, obsessions, phobias, and hallucinations.

The concept of depression as a psychopathological variable or constellation should be distinguished from the use of the term to designate specific nosological categories such as neurotic depressive reaction or psychotic depressive reaction. These nosological categories are generally believed to have a specific onset, course, prognosis, and etiology (Chapter 3). In our use of the term, depression might occur in pure form, such as neurotic-depressive reaction or psychotic-depressive reaction, or it might occur in association with another psychopathological state such as schizophrenia or anxiety reaction. The construct, depression, might be identifiable in many diverse types of patients. By grouping patients together on the basis of their having scored high on a test of intensity of depression we would have a population that would be congruent so far as this particular variable was concerned, but that might be vastly different in terms of other characteristics, such as degree of conceptual disorganization, presence of anxiety, prognosis, etc.

The theory being tested contained certain implications about the nature of the depressive constellation. In brief, the theory is that patients scoring high on the depression inventory have had life experiences during the developmental period that predispose them to react to stress later by the appearance of, or exacerbation of, depressive symptomatology. It was postulated further that, because of these early life experiences, these individuals have a negative view of themselves and of the world that is manifested in their dreams, in their responses to certain projective tests, and in their conscious self-concept. (For a further elaboration of this theory see Chapters 17 and 18.)

The major predictions were: The most depressed patients were likely (1) to have a certain type of dream characterized by a "masochistic" content (themes of deprivation, thwarting, and other unpleasantness); (2) to have a negative self-concept; (3) to identify with the "loser" on projective tests dealing with success and failure; (4) to have had a childhood history of deprivation that sensitized them to depression later in life; and (5) to respond to experimentally induced failure with a disproportionate drop in self-esteem and increase in hopelessness.

Using the Depression Inventory as the criterion measure (either alone or in combination with clinical ratings of the degree of depression), we found these hypotheses largely supported. We found a significant relationship between depression and "masochistic" dreams (Beck and Ward, 1961); the scores on a self-concept test, the high scores indicating a negative concept (Beck and Stein, 1960); the tendency to identify himself with the "loser" or underdog in responses to a series of pictorial stimuli (Beck, (1961); childhood bereavement (Beck, Sethi, and Tuthill, 1963); the tendency to make excessively pessimistic predictions after inferior task performance (Loeb *et al.*, 1964); and the tendency to underestimate actual performance (Loeb *et al.*, 1966).

The use of the Depression Inventory by other investigators provides further evidence of its construct validity. Gottschalk, Gleser, and Springer (1963) found a significant correlation (.47) between scores on the DI and scores on a *hostility-inward* scale, designed to measure the direction of hostility in samples of free associations of patients; as expected, there was a negative correlation with the *hostility-out* scale. Nussbaum and Michaux (1963) found a significant negative association between scores on a sense of humor test and scores on the DI. In both studies the results confirmed the hypotheses.

The prediction of response of patients to antidepressant drugs is another index of the construct validity of a measure of depression. Patients scoring in the depressive range on the DI* showed a significant decrease in their scores following the administration of imipramine. The change in the DI scores, furthermore, paralleled the clinical improvement (Pichot, 1966).

FACTOR ANALYTIC STUDIES

Delay *et al.* (1963) administered a French translation of the Depression Inventory to 79 depressed patients. Although a factor analysis was not performed because of the small sample, the writers found that the individual items of the DI correlated positively with the total DI scores; the authors concluded that this indicated the presence of a "general factor" of depression. The positive correlations were further evidence of the homogeneity of the inventory.

In a subsequent study, Pichot and Lempérière (1964) collected 56 additional cases of depression and added these to the initial sample, making

* On the basis of our experience with the DI, we established the cut-off point between depressed and nondepressed patients at 13 or 14. Since psychopathology other than depression could result in scores as high as 13 or 14, our cutting score was higher than it would have been if the nondepressed group consisted of normals or of medically ill patients with psychopathology. In a study of medically ill patients, for example, Schwab *et al.* (1967) used 10 as the cut-off point.

a total of 135 cases of depression tested with the Depression Inventory. The data was factor analyzed and four centroid factors were extracted. One of these was a general factor, all of the items having a positive and significant loading on this factor. The items with the heaviest loadings were: pessimism, indecision, suicidal wishes, and work inhibition. Since the other factors were not interpretable, the authors subjected the data to an orthogonal rotation in order to achieve simple structure. The following factors were extracted:

A. Vital Depression
Fatigability	.601
Loss of appetite	.592
Somatic preoccupation	.424
Weight loss	.348
Difficulty sleeping	.325
Loss of libido	.323

B. Self-Debasement
Self-dislike	.590
Sense of failure	.564
Expectation of punishment	.563
Guilty feeling	.452

C. Pessimism-Suicide
Pessimism	.397
Suicidal wishes	.344

D. Indecision-Inhibition
Indecision	.399
Work inhibition	.338

These factors appear to have significance. Factor *A* consists of the physiological signs of depression. It has been noted many times that these symptoms are often absent in depression. When they are present, some psychiatrists apply the diagnostic label, "vital depression."

Factor *B* contains items relevant to the sense of unworthiness and self-derogation. The themes of self-dislike, view of self as failure, desiring or expecting punishment, and feelings of guilt appear to be congruent with this over-all concept.

Factor *C* revolves around the items of hopelessness and suicide. This provides some empirical support to the notion that, in depressed patients, hopelessness is a fundamental precursor to suicidal wishes; the patient seeks suicide as an escape from problems he considers insoluble.

Factor *D* is concerned with two motivational symptoms. The work-inhibition category is closely related to motivation (e.g., "I have to push myself very hard to get started at doing something"). Similarly, the indecision category is related to loss of *constructive* motivation and to avoidance wishes ("I am less sure of myself and try to put off making decisions").

In a more recent study of the effects of imipramine on depressed patients, Pichot (1966) extracted 10 factors all of which were interpretable. The general factor score correlated .74 with the improvement as judged by clinical ratings. Some of the other factors had a relatively high correlation with improvement and others had a nil correlation.

In our own study of 606 patients we have computed the intercorrelations of the DI items but have not as yet performed a factor analysis. The intercorrelation matrix may be found in the appendix.

INFLUENCE OF EXTRANEOUS VARIABLES

We analyzed the records of 606 of the patients included in our study of 975 psychiatric patients. The characteristics of this sample approximated those described in Table 12–1. The correlations between the total DI score and the background variables were computed. Product moment correlations were obtained for the continuous variables, and point biserial r's for the dichotomous variables. The results are summarized in Table 12–7. For

Table 12–7.
CORRELATIONS OF BACKGROUND VARIABLES WITH
DEPRESSION INVENTORY SCORES AND DEPTH OF
DEPRESSION RATINGS (D of D) ($n = 606$)

Background variables*	DI score	D of D rating
Female	.189†	.217†
White	—.023	.055
Age	.025	.050
Education	—.163†	—.026
Vocabulary	.083	.027

* Pearson point-biserial correlations obtained for sex and race; product-moment correlations obtained for age, education and vocabulary.
† Significant at .01 level.

purposes of comparison, correlation coefficients between each of the variables and the 4-point depth-of-depression ratings were also computed.

Sex: There was a significant positive correlation between the females and the DI score (point biserial $r = .189$). The presence of a similar positive correlation with the psychiatrists' depth-of-depression ratings (point biserial $r = .217$) indicates that this was not an artifact. There is no immediate explanation for the tendency of the women to be more depressed than the men. It is important, however, to take this factor into consideration in selection of cases for the study of depression.

Race: The point biserial correlation between race and DI score and depth-of-depression ratings were negligible.

Age: The product moment correlations with age were negligible. This is contradictory to the frequently expressed idea that older patients tend to be more depressed.

Educational Level: The educational level was used as an index of social class. After considerable exploration of current methods for evaluating socioeconomic status, including the Hollingshead Scale, we decided that the number of grades completed in school provided the most reliable index for our particular population. As shown in Table 12–7, there was a significant negative correlation between educational level and DI score ($p < .01$). In other words, patients with lower educational attainment tended to have higher DI scores than those with a higher education.

This relationship was *not* found in the correlation with the depth-of-depression ratings. The reasons for this discrepancy are not apparent; it is possible that it is the result of a response set in the less-educated patients. The major contribution to the correlation is made by the white males. The correlation cannot be explained on the basis of lower vocabulary skills in the lower educational group, since the correlation between vocabulary scores and DI scores was minimal.

Vocabulary Score: The score on the vocabulary test showed only slight correlation with the DI score and the depth-of-depression ratings. The vocabulary score was used an an index of intelligence (Thorndike, 1942).

RESPONSE SET

In evaluating the validity of the Depression Inventory, we attempted to determine how much of the variance could be attributed to response set (or style). Since the individual items were of the multiple-choice type, the measures of acquiescence set designed for true-false items were not applicable. To obtain some idea of the effect of the social-desirability response set, we designated an inventory whose form was similar to the DI, but whose content did not deal with symptoms.

In administering this *social-desirability* inventory to depressed patients, we found that they selected those alternatives that reflected unfavorably upon themselves. It was noted, for instance, that in rating themselves on the dimensions of intelligence, ability, or appearance, the depressed patients consistently down-graded themselves. We were faced with the fact, therefore, that since depressed patients view themselves as undesirable, they attribute unfavorable characteristics to themselves. If a response set is operating, it is likely that it is a social undesirability set which in itself might be diagnostic of depression.

The basic question in considering response sets may be reduced to: Is the validity of the Depression Inventory materially reduced by the presence of a response set? This question may be answered by referring to the results of the various studies described above. We found, for instance, that the DI yielded approximately the same results as the psychiatrists' ratings when used as a criterion measure in testing various hypotheses about depression. It was noted, furthermore, that the correlations between the DI scores and the clinicians' ratings were consistently in the moderately high range wherever it has been used (United States, Great Britain, and France). If the validity of the DI was substantially reduced by response sets, we would expect much greater inconsistency when the DI scores were correlated with clinicians' ratings in such different settings.

As compared to other psychometric instruments, the Depression Inventory was found to be highly effective in discriminating between depression and anxiety. Again, if response sets were undercutting the effectiveness of the DI, we would expect more blurring in the differentiation between these two states.

In view of the above considerations, we concluded that response sets do not materially detract from the validity of the DI.

Chapter 13.
Patterns in Dreams of Depressed Patients

PRELIMINARY STUDY

Statistical techniques have been used in the content analysis of dreams for several decades. In 1935, Alexander and Wilson applied quantitative techniques to the manifest dreams of patients for the purpose of quantifying psychoanalytic material. Saul and Sheppard (1956) devised a rating scale for measuring hostility in the manifest dream. In a later paper (Sheppard and Saul, 1958), they outlined a comprehensive rating system for estimating ego functions in dreams. These studies provided a stimulus for the investigations reported in this chapter.

In the course of the psychotherapy of outpatients, I noted that the manifest content of the dreams of neurotically-depressed patients contained a relatively high frequency of unpleasant themes; these unpleasant themes were observed much less frequently in other types of neurotic patients. The striking characteristic of the unpleasant dream was the presence of a particular kind of thematic content: that the dreamer was the recipient of a painful experience such as being rejected, thwarted, deprived, or punished in the dream action. The affect, when reported, was consistent with the dream theme and was described as a feeling of sadness, of loneliness, or of frustration.

On the basis of the associations to the dream, as well as the other clinical material, I concluded that the unpleasant dreams were the outcome of certain personality processes in the depressed patient that produced suffering disproportionate to his reality situation. The dreams were regarded as analogous to the kind of suffering the depressed patient experienced in his waking life. Because of the salience of suffering in these dream themes, I selected the term "masochistic" to designate this type of dream. Although this label is unsatisfactory in several respects, it seems to be the best term available for this class of dreams.

In order to determine whether this clinical observation was valid, I started a systematic study of the dreams of depressed patients in my practice. The data for the subsequent investigation were limited to the manifest content of the dream; the free associations to the dream and other clinical material were excluded from consideration for methodological reasons.

The hypothesis for this study was: Consecutive dreams of neurotic depressed patients in psychotherapy show a greater incidence of manifest dreams with "masochistic" content than a series of dreams in a matched group of nondepressed patients.

METHOD

In order to test this hypothesis, I designed a systematic study in collaboration with Dr. Marvin S. Hurvich. Relying primarily on clinical observations, we developed a provisional scoring manual. We then reviewed several hundred dreams of patients diagnosed as depressed and nondepressed. Examples of unpleasant themes that were found frequently in the dreams of the depressed patients but that were found infrequently in the dreams of the nondepressed patients provided the basis for expanding and refining scoring categories.*

The typical theme consists of something unpleasant happening to the patient. The unpleasantness may be *static*: the patient appears deformed; or *dynamic*: in the course of the dream he is thwarted or subjected to direct or indirect psychic or physical trauma. The scoring categories are listed below:

1. Deprived, disappointed, or mistreated
2. Thwarted
3. Excluded, superseded, or displaced
4. Rejected or deserted
5. Blamed, criticized, or ridiculed
6. Legal punishment
7. Physical discomfort or injury
8. Distorted appearance
9. Being lost
10. Losing something of value

No score was given for dreams with "threat" or "shame" content unless there was a specific "masochistic" element or theme as indicated above. The complete scoring manual is found in the Appendix.

After the scoring system was developed and we had attained a high

---

* It should be noted that the dreams of the 12 patients who were the subject of this investigation were not included in the construction and refinement of the scoring manual.

degree of agreement in scoring dreams, the system was applied to our experimental and control groups. The records of six female patients with the diagnosis of neurotic depression and those of six nondepressed female patients were selected from my files. The two groups were matched patient-for-patient as closely as possible on the basis of age, marital status, and an estimate of the severity of the illness. The characteristics of all the patients are listed in Table 13–1.

Table 13–1.

IDENTIFYING DATA ON DEPRESSED AND NONDEPRESSED PATIENTS

	Age		Marital status		Diagnosis of nondep.
Pair	Dep.	Nondep.	Dep.	Nondep.	
A	23	20	S	M	Anxiety reaction
B	28	28	M	M	Character neurosis
C	31	29	M	M	Spastic colitis
D	31	33	M	M	Cardiac neurosis
E	36	36	M	M	Character neurosis

I abstracted the first twenty dreams in treatment from each case record. These were typed on individual sheets of paper. The total sample was 240 dreams (20 per patient for 12 patients), arranged in random order. These were then presented to Dr. Hurvich, who rated each dream according to the "masochistic" theme scale. He had no knowledge of any of the patients; this insured an unbiased blind scoring procedure. These blind ratings were subjected to the statistical valuation reported below. In order to obtain an estimate of the reliability of the ratings, I also rated the dreams, and the percentage agreement between our ratings was calculated.

The criteria for establishing the diagnosis of neurotic-depressive reaction in these patients were as follows: depressed mood, feelings of discouragement, unwarranted self-criticism and self-reproaches, inertia or apathy, sleep disturbance, anorexia, and suicidal wishes. The following signs were also considered in the diagnosis: psychomotor retardation, weight loss, and melancholic facies associated with weeping and crying. Each patient showed at least 11 of the 13 diagnostic signs and symptoms. The absence of any evidence of conceptual disorganization, inappropriate affect, or bizarre behavior ruled out a psychotic process.

The estimate of severity of illness was based on the intensity of the symptoms and the degree of impairment of social adjustment. An estimate of socioeconomic standing indicated that all subjects would probably be labelled upper-middle class or lower-upper class. A rough clinical estimate of intelligence suggested that all patients in both groups were of at least bright average intelligence. The range of social class and intelligence was thus somewhat restricted; there were no systematic differences between the two groups on either continuum.

RESULTS

For the 240 dreams, the raters agreed regarding the presence or absence of a "masochistic" element on 229 of the dreams, which is slightly in excess of 95 per cent agreement. This indicates that the scoring procedure is highly reliable. The results of the comparison between the two groups are listed in Table 13–2.

Table 13–2.
FREQUENCY OF "MASOCHISTIC" DREAMS OF
MATCHED DEPRESSED AND NONDEPRESSED PATIENTS

| Pair | Number of dreams out of 20 scoring "masochistic" | |
	Depressed	Nondepressed
A	13	1
B	9	3
C	14	3
D	13	3
E	7	3
F	9	2

p < .025 (one-tailed test).

It will be seen that there is no overlap between the groups. More than one-half (54 per cent) of the dreams of the depressed patients contained one or more "masochistic elements," whereas in the nondepressed group, one-eighth (12.5 per cent) of the dreams contained one or more of these elements.

Statistical evaluation of the frequency differences between groups with the Wilcoxon Matched-Pairs Signed-Ranks test results in a probability figure of .025 (one-tailed test).

DISCUSSION

The obtained differences between the depressed group and the control group were statistically significant and clear-cut. On the basis of these results, the hypothesis that the depressed patients show a greater incidence of dreams with "masochistic" content than the nondepressed patients appeared to be clearly confirmed.

Several qualifications of the scope of these results should be stressed, however. The smallness of the sample, the use of the dreams of females only, and the restricted socioeconomic and IQ ranges represented by these private patients all limited the possible generalizability of the findings. Further, although the present dream sample was not explicitly used as a basis for construction of the rating scale, it is probable that some aspects of the rating scale were at least partly based on the dreams of patients in the present sample, since the dreams were known to me when the scoring manual was developed.

PRINCIPAL STUDY

In view of the obvious limitations in the initial study, we considered it desirable to test the findings on a substantially larger patient sample and to employ more refined procedures as well as a tighter experimental design. The larger study was designed to eliminate the possibility of suggestion by the data collector, as well as the possibility of biased reporting of the dreams; these possibilities of contamination had not been excluded in the first study. In addition, by using a substantially larger sample we were able to test the generalizability of the findings to patients of different nosological, socioeconomic, age, and intelligence categories from those represented by private patients in psychotherapy. Moreover, we could determine whether the findings applied to males as well as to females, who were the sole subjects in the first study. Finally, by using a standardized inventory for measuring depression, in addition to clinical ratings, we were able to circumvent a number of the complex problems associated with the low reliability of psychiatric diagnoses.

A precise replication of the original study was not feasible. Although we had planned to collect dreams at weekly intervals from the patients in the sample, this was not possible because of a number of insuperable problems. We had to limit our collection of dreams, consequently, to the first dream reported by the patient on admission to the outpatient clinic or the hospital.

The likelihood of the introduction of any systematic bias by the data collector was minimized by using a group of interviewers who were not aware of the hypothesis under investigation. A blind scoring procedure by two judges was used to classify the dreams.

METHOD

Identification of the Depressed Groups

In order to determine the reliability of the conventional clinical methods of classifying patients according to nosological categories, a group of four experienced psychiatrists interviewed a series of patients and rendered independent diagnoses according to the APA *Diagnostic and Statistical Manual*. Degree of agreement obtained on the primary diagnosis of depression, as well as on diagnoses of the other nosological categories, was considered to be too low for the purposes of this study. Consequently, psychiatrists' ratings of the depth of depression were used, since they had a higher degree of reliability (Chapter 11). Also the Depression Inventory (DI) was used as another index of the degree of depression.

Sample

The 287 patients in the initial sample were drawn from random admissions to the psychiatric outpatient department of the Hospital of the University of Pennsylvania and the psychiatric outpatient and psychiatric inpatient service of the Philadelphia General Hospital. The outpatients were interviewed during the period of evaluation prior to starting treatment; the hospitalized patients were interviewed during their first full day in the hospital. Sixty-one per cent of the sample were females and 39 per cent males; 65 per cent were white and 35 per cent Negro. The age range was from 15 to 60, with a median age of 38. Determination of the social index, as derived from the Two-Factor Index of Social Position (Hollingshead, 1957), indicated that the patients were, for the most part, of the lower socioeconomic groups (15 per cent in groups I, II, and III; 38 per cent in group IV; and 47 per cent in group V). Sixty-six per cent were outpatients; 34 per cent were inpatients. Cases of mental deficiency were automatically excluded from the series. Two-hundred eighty-seven patients received a complete workup.

The distribution of the patients among the major diagnostic categories was: psychotic disorders 41 per cent; psychoneurotic disorders 43 per cent; personality disorders 16 per cent. The diagnoses were: schizophrenic reaction, 28 per cent; neurotic-depressive reaction, 25 per cent; anxiety reaction, 16 per cent; psychotic-depressive reaction, 10 per cent; personality disorder, 10 per cent; and miscellaneous, 11 per cent.

Collection of the Data

The Depression Inventory was administered by a trained interviewer (a clinical psychologist or a sociologist), who read each statement in each category aloud to the patient, who was then instructed to select the statement that seemed to fit him best. The patient also had a copy of the inventory, so that he could read each statement to himself while the interviewer read the statement aloud.

After administering the Depression Inventory, the interviewer asked the patient to tell his most recent dream. This was reported orally and recorded. Only the first dream reported by a patient was used in this study. Following this procedure, the interviewer administered a short intelligence test and several other short projective and questionnaire-type tests.

Either immediately before or immediately after the above procedure, one of the four psychiatrists in our research group saw the patient, conducted a thorough psychiatric evaluation, and made a psychiatric diagnosis and a rating of the depth of depression.

Measurement of "Masochistic" Themes in Dreams

The scoring manual used in this study is described in detail in the Appendix. The reliability was shown to be high; the agreement between the two raters in the earlier study was approximately 95 per cent. A further check by Dr. Clyde Ward and me on the scoring of the present data revealed a similarly high degree of agreement (96 per cent).

The most recent dreams collected from the patients were typed on individual sheets identified only by the patients' file numbers. We scored the dreams independently, and differences were resolved by the conference method. A dream was considered scorable so long as there was a subject and a verb in the dream text. An example of a short, scorable dream is "My mother was sick." On the other hand, the following would not be scorable: "It was about my cousin. That's all I can remember."

RESULTS

Two-hundred eighty-seven patients received the complete clinical and experimental evaluation. Dreams were obtained from 228 of these patients. Ten dreams were not scorable because of brevity or unintelligibility; thus, 218 patients reported scorable dreams. The cases were ranked according to the scores on the Depression Inventory and divided into three groups of approximately equal size. A comparison of the incidence of "masochistic" dreams in each of these groups is presented in Table 13–3. It was found that significantly more "masochistic" dreams occurred in the high depressed group than in the nondepressed group ($p < 0.01$). An analysis of the overall association between the degree of depression and the incidence of "masochistic" dreams indicated a relationship which was significant at the 0.01 level.

Table 13–3.
COMPARISON OF INCIDENCE OF "MASOCHISTIC" DREAMS WITH
SCORES OF DEPRESSION INVENTORY (DI)

Range of DI scores	N	Patients reporting "masochistic" dreams	Patients reporting "nonmasochistic" dreams
26–45	73	22 (30%)	51 (70%)
15–25	73	21 (29%)	52 (71%)
0–14	72	8 (11%)	64 (89%)

Total distribution: $\chi^2 = 9.08$, p $= 0.01$.
Upper $\frac{1}{3}$ vs. lower $\frac{1}{3}$: $\chi^2 = 8.00$, p < 0.01.

When both psychometric and clinical measures were used to demarcate the extreme groups, the incidence of "masochistic" dreams in the depressed groups was again found to be significantly greater than in the nondepressed groups. With the more stringent criterion, the proportion of "masochistic" dreams in each group remained approximately the same as in the previous analysis, although there was some decrease of significance (p < 0.02) due to the smaller number of cases. The results of this analysis are shown in Table 13–4.

Table 13–4.
INCIDENCE OF "MASOCHISTIC" DREAMS USING TWO MEASURES OF
DEPRESSION AS CRITERION: CLINICAL RATINGS OF DEPTH OF
DEPRESSION (D OF D) AND SCORES ON DEPRESSION INVENTORY (DI)

Rating of D of D and range of DI scores	N	Patients reporting "masochistic" dreams	Patients reporting "nonmasochistic" dreams
D of D: moderate or severe DI: 26–45	51	16 (31%)	35 (69%)
D of D: none DI: 0–14	38	4 (11%)	34 (89%)

$\chi^2 = 5.43$, p < 0.02.

Another approach to analyzing the data was utilized by dividing all the cases into a group reporting "masochistic" dreams and a group reporting "nonmasochistic" dreams. When the data was organized in this way, it was found that 84 per cent of the "masochistic" dreams were obtained from patients whose scores placed them in the mildly to severely-depressed range. The differences in the ranks of the DI scores of the cases in the "masochistic"-dream group and of those in the "nonmasochistic"-dream group were evaluated with the use of the Mann-Whitney U test, and a highly significant difference between the two groups was obtained ($p < .003$).

Specific analyses were performed to determine whether there were any significant differences in the distribution of "masochistic" dreams attributable to age, sex, race, IQ, or socioeconomic position. None were obtained.

The initial study evaluated a series of 20 consecutive dreams collected from each of six depressed patients and from a matching group of six non-depressed patients (total number of dreams, 240). It was found that while all of the patients reported "masochistic" and "nonmasochistic" dreams, the proportion of "masochistic" dreams was significantly higher for the depressed patients. In contrast to the previous study, the data of the present investigation consisted of only one dream per patient from a much larger patient sample (218). On the basis of the previous findings, it was expected that the probability of any single dream's being "masochistic" would be greater if the patient were depressed than if he were not depressed. This was borne out by the finding of a significantly higher percentage of depressed patients than nondepressed patients who reported "masochistic" dreams.

Almost as many mildly- or moderately-depressed as severely-depressed patients reported "masochistic" dreams. This suggests that the "masochistic" dream is associated with the presence of depression, regardless of its intensity. On the other hand, this finding may be due to the fact that, since the dream scoring procedure permitted only a dichotomy of dream content into "masochistic" and "nonmasochistic," quantitative differences in the degree of "masochism" could have been obscured.

A consideration of the general significance of the "masochistic" dream raises certain important issues. Since many individuals who have never had a clinical depression or other psychiatric illness state that they occasionally have dreams of this nature, the dream itself is not necessarily a sign of illness. Moreover, many patients with recurrent depressions continue to report the "masochistic" dreams with the same degree of frequency during the symptom-free intervals. Furthermore, some patients recall having had repetitive dreams of this nature long before having been depressed. Consequently, the "masochistic" dream cannot be construed as being associated only with the state of depression. It seems more likely to be a correlate of certain personality characteristics of individuals who are prone to develop depressions.

The dynamic relationship of the "masochistic" dream to depression may be further explored by comparing the typical dream themes with other behaviors observable in the depressed patient. For example, the dreams of failing, of being rejected, or of losing something of value may be compared with the depressive's waking feelings of inadequacy, of undesirability, and of deprivation. Another characteristic dream is that of trying to attain some goal and of being consistently thwarted by circumstances. This type of dream is suggestive of the depressive's constantly seeing barriers against any goal-directed activity, a kind of behavior which conveys a general attitude of indecisiveness or of hopelessness.

SUMMARY

In the course of the psychotherapy of patients with neurotic-depressive reactions, it was noted that there was a high incidence of dreams with unpleasant content. This unpleasant content was of a particular kind: the patient was the recipient of rejection, of disappointment, of humiliation, or of similar unpleasant experiences in the dream content.

A rating scale was constructed for the objective identification of these unpleasant themes, which were labelled "masochistic." This rating scale was applied to the first 20 dreams in treatment of (*a*) six patients who were diagnosed as neurotic depressives, and of (*b*) six matched but nondepressed patients. The depressed patients showed a significantly higher number of dreams with "masochistic" content than did the nondepressed patients.

Because of the findings of this preliminary study, a large-scale investigation was carried out to test these findings in a more carefully designed study. The dreams of 218 patients were rated independently by two judges for the presence or absence of "masochistic" themes. There was 96 per cent agreement between the judges. Patients were divided into three groups according to their scores on the Depression Inventory: nondepressed, moderately depressed, and severely depressed. The moderately and severely-depressed groups reported significantly more "masochistic" dreams than the nondepressed group. Analysis of background factors such as age, sex, race, intelligence, and socioeconomic position indicated that these variables were not responsible for the attained results.

Chapter 14.
Childhood Bereavement
and Adult Depression

The association of early parental deprivation with the subsequent development of psychopathology has been reported by many authors. Up to the present time, more than fifty papers in this area have been published. The systematic studies published before 1958 have been well-summarized in a critical review by Gregory (1961), who focused particularly on their sources of error.

Brown (1961) reported a significant relationship between parental loss in childhood and adult depression. He found that 41 per cent of 216 depressed adult patients had lost a parent through death before the age of 15; this incidence was found to be significantly greater than the incidence of orphanhood in the general population in England (12 per cent) and in a comparison group of 267 medical patients (19.6 per cent).

Most studies of orphanhood and psychopathology had certain methodological defects that pose difficulties in evaluating the obtained relationships. First, when the isolation of the criterion group depends on the conventional system of diagnosis, many complex problems related to the variability of psychiatric diagnoses are introduced and restrict the generalization of the findings. In Brown's study, the basis for diagnosing depression was "the presence of an unpleasant affect, not transitory, and without schizophrenia or brain disease." Such a broad definition could make clinical identification of the depressed patients particularly vulnerable to inconsistency and over-inclusiveness. A second problem encountered in this type of investigation is the comparison of a specific nosological group with a normal control group. In Brown's study, for example, the use of nonpsychiatric medical patients as the control group raises a question as to whether the high incidence of orphanhood was a specific characteristic of his depressed group or was associated with psychiatric disorders in general. A third difficulty is presented by the fact that there is considerable discrepancy in the base rates of parental death for the various demographic classes in the general population from which samples of patients are drawn. These variations need to be taken into account in any epidemiological studies.

The present study presents further findings regarding the relationship of the development of depression in late adolescence and adulthood to the death of a parent in childhood. To circumvent the difficulties posed by the variability of psychiatric classifications, the Depression Inventory (DI) was used as the major criterion measure. As an additional measure of depression, clinical ratings of the depth of depression, irrespective of the specific diagnostic category, were also obtained. Nondepressed psychiatric patients were used as the comparison group, and provision was made to determine the influence of background variables such as age, race, and sex.

METHOD

Two-hundred ninety-seven patients were selected from routine admissions to the psychiatric outpatient clinic of the University of Pennsylvania and the psychiatric outpatient clinic and psychiatric wards of the Philadelphia General Hospital. The demographic characteristics and the distribution of the patients among the standard nosological categories are tabulated in the section on "Results" (Tables 14–3 and 14–5). Cases diagnosed as having brain damage were excluded from the study.

Each patient was studied by the research team during his initial period of evaluation at the outpatient clinic or on the day following admission to the psychiatric ward. The research study included a thorough psychiatric evaluation by one of four psychiatrists who made both a diagnosis according to the 1952 edition of the Standard Nomenclature of the American Psychiatric Association and also a rating on a four-point scale of the depth of depression irrespective of the nosological category. The indices used in making the judgment of the depth of depression and the interrater reliability of these ratings are described in Chapter 12.

The Depression Inventory was administered to each patient by a trained interviewer. Each patient was specifically questioned about whether his parents were living and, in the case of the death of a parent, the interviewer attempted to determine the patient's age at the time of the death.

RESULTS

The patient sample was divided into three groups of approximately equal size according to the scores on the Depression Inventory. The results for all three groups are included in the tables. In the formulation of the research design, however, it was decided that the comparison would be made only between the extreme groups, since previous experience with the inventory indicated that there was a considerable overlap of clinically depressed and nondepressed patients in the middle group.

The incidence of parental loss in each group is presented in Table 14–1. It was found that in the high-depressed group (DI score 25 +), 27

Table 14–1.
COMPARISON OF INCIDENCE OF DEATH OF PARENT BEFORE AGE 16
WITH DEPRESSION INVENTORY SCORES

| Depression Inventory score | N | Death of parent(s) | | | | |
		Mother only	Father only	Both	Total	%
25+, High-depressed	100	6	17	4	27*	27.0
14–24, Medium-depressed	97	3	9	3	15	15.5
0–13, Nondepressed	100	3	7	2	12*	12.0
TOTAL	297	12	33	9	54	

* Significance of difference between extreme groups: $\chi^2 = 7.17$, p $<$ 0.01.
N = Total no. of cases in each category of depression.

per cent of the patients reported the loss of a parent before the age of 16 as compared with 12 per cent in the nondepressed group (DI score 0–13). The difference in incidence between these two groups was found to be highly significant (p $<$ 0.01).

Table 14–2.
COMPARISON OF INCIDENCE OF DEATH OF PARENT BEFORE AGE 16
WITH CLINICAL RATINGS OF DEPTH OF DEPRESSION

| Clinical rating of depression | N | Death of parent(s) | | | | |
		Mother only	Father only	Both	Total	%
Severe	33	4	5	3	12*	36.4
Moderate	114	3	13	2	18	15.8
Mild	84	2	9	3	14	16.7
None	66	3	6	1	10*	15.2
TOTAL	297	12	33	9	54	

* Significance of difference between extreme groups: $\chi^2 = 5.73$, p $<$ 0.02.

A similar analysis was performed to determine the incidence of parental loss when clinical judgments of the depth of depression were used as the criterion measure (Table 14–2). When the extreme groups were compared, it was again found that the severely depressed groups showed a significantly higher proportion of parental death (36.4 per cent) than the nondepressed group (15.2 per cent). There was no significant difference in incidence among the groups judged clinically to be moderately depressed, mildly depressed, or nondepressed.

A comparison of the sex of the patient with the sex of the dead parent showed that for both males and females a loss of the father occurred appreciably more frequently than a loss of the mother. The greater frequency of paternal loss held for both sexes across all levels of depression. Furthermore, when the extreme groups are compared, loss of father was over-represented in the high-depressed group for both males and females.

The incidence of cases of orphanhood when the sample was subdivided according to inpatient vs. outpatient status, race, sex, and age is shown in Table 14–3. It should be noted that the over-all incidence of orphanhood is significantly higher in the Negro than in the white group and in the older (31–60) than in the younger (16–30) group.

Inspection of the distribution shows that within each demographic class the incidence of orphanhood is consistently higher for the high-depressed than for the nondepressed patients. A χ^2 analysis indicated that these differences between extreme groups were significant in the following categories: inpatients ($p < 0.02$); Negroes ($p < 0.02$); females ($p < 0.02$); and younger age group ($p < 0.05$). The differences between the extreme groups in the remaining categories were in the predicted direction, the p-value in each case being < 0.20.

Further inspection of Table 14–3 indicates an association of age with depression as well as with orphanhood. There is also a suggestion of a relationship between sex and depression, since females are over-represented in the high-depressed group.

In order to evaluate statistically the significance of the relationship among orphanhood, age, and depression, the data were reorganized with the Depression Inventory scores as the dependent variable. An appropriate number of cases were randomly eliminated from each of the age categories in the nonorphan group in order to make the cells proportional for the analysis of variance. The total number thus was reduced from 297 to 162 for this analysis.

The results of the analysis of variance are presented in Table 14–4. The F of 3.81 for the comparison of depression with orphanhood falls just short

Table 14–3.
INCIDENCE OF DEATH OF PARENT BEFORE AGE 16 IN DEPRESSED GROUPS ARRANGED ACCORDING TO HOSPITAL STATUS, RACE, SEX, AND AGE

Depression Inventory score	Inpatient	Outpatient	White	Negro	Sex M	Sex F	Age groups 16–30	Age groups 31–60
25+, High-depressed	35 / 31.4%	65 / 24.6%	55 / 18.2%	45 / 37.8%	29 / 31.0%	71 / 25.4%	46 / 21.7%	54 / 31.5%
14-24, Medium-depressed	33 / 21.2%	64 / 12.5%	57 / 12.3%	40 / 20.0%	36 / 8.3%	61 / 19.7%	50 / 10.0%	47 / 21.3%
0-13, Nondepressed	34 / 8.8%	66 / 13.6%	54 / 9.3%	46 / 15.2%	51 / 15.7%	49 / 8.2%	56 / 7.1%	44 / 18.2%
Over-all %	102 / 20.6%	195 / 16.9%	166 / 13.3%	131 / 24.4%	116 / 17.2%	181 / 18.8%	154 / 12.3%	143 / 24.5%

Numeral in upper right-hand corner of each cell is the total number for that cell. Percentage refers to proportion of patients in cell who lost one or both parents.

Significance of differences between high-depressed vs nondepressed within demographic groups:

	x^2	P		x^2	P
Inpatient	5.45	<0.02	Male	2.60	<0.20
Outpatient	2.56	<0.20	Female	5.72	<0.02
White	1.83	<0.20	Age: 16-30	4.54	<0.05
Negro	5.96	<0.02	Age: 31-60	2.26	<0.20

Significant differences obtained in comparing overall incidence of parental loss for specific demographic groups:

	x^2	P
White vs Negro	6.14	<0.02
Age: 16-30 vs 31-60	7.34	<0.01

Table 14–4.

SUMMARY OF ANALYSIS OF VARIANCE FOR DEPRESSION INVENTORY SCORES
AS A FUNCTION OF ORPHANHOOD AND AGE

Source of variance	SS	df	MS	F
Age	608.52	4	152.13	1.16
Orphanhood	498.78	1	498.78	3.81*
Age × Orphanhood	441.85	4	110.46	0.84
Error	19,905.13	152	130.95	
TOTAL	21,454.28	161		

* p < 0.06.

of the 0.05 level of significance (when $F = 3.84$, $p < 0.05$). This analysis indicates that the major portion of the variance in the Depression Inventory scores is attributable to the association between these scores and orphanhood. The interaction between age and orphanhood is not significant.

To explore the possibility that the obtained differences between the high-depressed and nondepressed patients might be related to the specific nosological classes, the patients were grouped according to their specific formal diagnoses as well as according to their scores on the Depression Inventory. The comparison of the incidence of orphanhood in these groups is presented in Table 14–5. (Only those diagnostic categories that contained at least 12 cases were included; the remaining 53 cases were distributed among various diagnostic categories, predominantly those in the generic class of "personality disorders," in the *Standard Nomenclature.*)

Inspection of Table 14–5 reveals that within each nosological category the group scoring highest on the Depression Inventory consistently shows a greater incidence of orphanhood than the low-scoring group. This consistent difference across all categories was evaluated by the Sign test and was found to be significant at the 0.03 level.

Although the over-all incidence of orphanhood in the psychotic-depressed group was higher than in any other nosological category, the difference was not significant when this group was compared with the schizophrenic group. The over-all incidence of orphanhood in the neurotic-depressive group approximated that in the schizophrenic group.

To determine whether any of the late-adolescent depressions occurred during the mourning period following bereavement, the cases who lost their parents just before age 16 were reviewed. Of the four who lost a parent at the age of 14 or 15, three reported symptom-free intervals of 15, 29, and 30 years, respectively, between the time of bereavement and the onset of the depression. The remaining patient was 19-years-old at the

Table 14–5.

INCIDENCE OF PARENTAL DEATH BEFORE AGE 16 IN SPECIFIC DIAGNOSTIC GROUPS

Nosological category, reaction	Depression Inventory scores			
	25+	14–24	0–13	Over-all
Neurotic depressive	32 31.3%	30 10.0%	20 10.0%	82 18.3%
Schizophrenic	28 28.6%	23 21.7%	24 8.3%	75 20.0%
Anxiety	14 7.1%	22 13.6%	17 5.9%	53 9.4%
Psychotic depressive	13 30.8%	6 33.3%	3 0%	22 27.3%
Psychophysiological	3 66.7%	4 0%	5 20.0%	12 25.0%

Numeral in upper right-hand corner of each cell is the total number for that cell. Percentage refers to proportion of patients in cell who lost one or both parents.

The 53 cases not included in this table were distributed primarily among the various subgroups of personality disorders.

time of admission to the hospital. At that time he reported a symptom-free interval between the loss of the parent and the onset of depression, and dated the onset of the depression to one year following the death of his parent (at age 15).

COMMENT

The finding of a significantly greater incidence of loss of a parent during childhood in the high depressed as compared with the nondepressed patients is consistent with the results reported by Brown. Some of the methodological problems presented by his study were dealt with by using a comparison group of nondepressed psychiatric patients and employing a standardized instrument to identify the depressed group rather than relying on clinical diagnoses of uncertain reliability. In addition, in analyzing the data, an attempt was made to control certain relevant background variables. Although the incidence of orphans and of depressed patients was increased in the older age groups, it was found that the factor of age did not account for the obtained relationship between orphanhood and depression.

The finding of significant differences in the incidence of orphanhood between various demographic groups (e.g., whites vs. Negroes) underscores the necessity for introducing methods in the design of such studies for controlling the background characteristics. Overlooked in many previous studies, for instance, is that during the past 50 years there has been a gradual decline in the incidence of orphanhood in the general population. Gregory's abstract of the census data for the Province of Ontario (1961) shows an appreciable drop in the frequency of death of a parent before age 16 when individuals born in 1921 are compared with those born a decade later. This decrease is reflected in our comparisons of the relative incidence of orphanhood in the older and younger groups.

The use of an inventory as the principal measure of depression naturally presents problems. In view of the demonstrated vulnerability of some inventories to noncontent variables such as response styles, reservations must be made in interpreting the scores on the instruments that consist of self-descriptive items. On the other hand, the obtained differences between the extreme groups were confirmed when a different measure of depression, viz., the psychiatrists' ratings of the depth of depression, was used. The Depression Inventory was selected as the preferred criterion measure because it has the major advantage over clinical ratings of being easily applied by different investigators, a characteristic that facilitates replication of the study.

Another feature that may justify further elaboration is the conceptual basis for defining the criterion group. The concept of depression as a psychopathological state that may exist to varying degrees irrespective of the formal diagnosis is more congruent with the "polydimensional model" described by Lorr (1961) than with the model on which the Standard Nomenclature is based. It seemed *a priori* that for the purposes of this investigation the former model was more appropriate than the latter. In fact, when the patients were grouped according to the conventional nosological system, no significant relationships were found between specific diagnostic categories and the incidence of orphanhood; however, within each diagnostic category there was a consistent tendency for high scorers on the Depression Inventory to show a greater incidence of orphanhood than low scorers.

The relevance of the findings to the understanding of the pathogenesis of depression can be established only by further research. The present findings (if confirmed by other studies) suggest that a drastic experience such as the loss of a parent in childhood may be determinant in the later development of severe depression.

Since this study was completed, two relevant controlled studies have been published by other investigators. These do not show a significant relationship between parental loss and the clinical diagnosis of depression. In this respect, their findings are similar to ours in that we did not find any association between orphanhood and the *nosological category* of depression. Although neither of these studies employed the same approach or methods as did our study, the findings raise doubts about the relationship of orphanhood to depression.

Pitts *et al.* (1965) did not find a significant association between childhood bereavement and any diagnostic category in their adult patients. However, their control group consisted of medical inpatients. Several studies have shown that depressive symptomatology is widely distributed among medical inpatients (Schwab, *et al.*, 1965; 1967). Hence, it is necessary to control for the presence of depression even when nonpsychiatric patients are used as the comparison group. Gregory (1966) made systematic comparisons of parental loss and psychiatric diagnoses. Using clinical diagnoses and MMPI high points as his criterion measures, he was unable to establish a significant association between parental loss and any of the diagnostic groups.

Since our study used clinical ratings of the depth of depression and DI scores as the criterion measure, it may be valuable to replicate this study before discarding the hypothesis of a relationship between parental loss and depression.

SUMMARY

A group of 297 inpatients and outpatients were studied during their initial period of evaluation on a psychiatric ward or at a psychiatric clinic to determine the relationship of orphanhood to depression. The state of depression was investigated as a psychopathological dimension, irrespective of specific diagnoses, by the use of the Depression Inventory and by clinical ratings by experienced psychiatrists.

The 100 patients who received high-depressed scores on the Depression Inventory showed a significantly higher incidence of orphanhood before age 16 (27 per cent) than did the 100 low scorers (12 per cent). A similar difference between the extreme groups was obtained when psychiatrists' ratings of the intensity of depression were used as the criterion measure.

The obtained difference in the incidence of orphanhood between the high-depressed and nondepressed groups provides evidence that the death of a parent in childhood may be a factor in the later development of a severe depression in a significant proportion of psychiatric patients. The precise nature of this relationship cannot be determined without further research.

Chapter 15.
Cognitive Distortions in Depression

Clinical and theoretical papers dealing with the psychological correlates of depression have generally utilized a motivational-affective model for categorizing and interpreting the verbal behavior of patients. The cognitive processes as such have received little attention except insofar as they are related to variables such as hostility, orality, or guilt (Mendelson, 1960).

This lack of emphasis on the thought processes in depression may be a reflection of—or possibly a contributing factor to—the widely held opinion that depression is an affective disorder and that any impairment of thinking is the result of the affective disturbance (American Psychiatric Association, 1952). This opinion has been buttressed by the failure to demonstrate any consistent evidence of abnormalities in the formal thought processes in the responses to the standard battery of psychological tests (Schafer, 1948). Furthermore, the few experimental studies of thinking in depression have revealed no consistent deviations other than a retardation in the responses to speed tests (Payne and Hewlett, 1961) and a lowered responsiveness to a Gestalt completion test (Cohen, Senf, and Huston, 1956).

In his book on depression, Kraines (1957) described, on the basis of clinical observations, several characteristics of a thought disorder in depression. The objective of the present study has been to ascertain the nature of the thought processes of depressed patients. An important corollary of this objective has been the specification of the differences from, and the similarities to, the thinking of nondepressed psychiatric patients. This chapter will focus on the following areas: (1) the verbalized thought content indicating distorted or unrealistic conceptualizations; (2) the processes involved in the deviations from logical or realistic thinking; (3) the formal characteristics of the ideation showing such deviations; and (4) the relation between the cognitive distortions and the affects characteristic of depression.

CLINICAL MATERIAL

The data for this study were accumulated from interviews with 50 psychiatric patients seen in psychotherapy or formal psychoanalysis. Of these patients, four were hospitalized for varying periods during treatment. The rest were seen on an ambulatory basis.

The frequency of interviews varied from one to six a week, with the median number three a week. The total length of time in psychotherapy ranged from six months to six years; the median was two years. In no case did a single episode of depression last longer than a year. Many patients continued in psychotherapy for a substantial time after the remission of their initial depressive episode. Thirteen either had recurrent depressions while in psychotherapy or returned to psychotherapy because of a recurrence. In this recurrent depression group, six had completely asymptomatic intervals btween the recurrences, and seven had some degree of hypomanic elevation. It was, therefore, possible to obtain data from these patients during each phase of the cycle.

Of the 50 patients in the sample, 16 were men and 34 were women. The age range was from 18 to 48, with a median of 34. An estimate of their intelligence suggested that all were of at least bright average intelligence. Their socioeconomic status was judged to be middle or upper class. Twelve were diagnosed as having psychotic-depressive or manic-depressive reactions, and 38 as having neurotic-depressive reactions.

To establish the diagnosis of depression, the following diagnostic indicators were employed: objective signs of depression in the facies, speech, posture, and motor activity; and a major complaint of feeling depressed or sad, and at least 11 of the following 14 signs and symptoms: loss of appetite, weight loss, sleep disturbance, loss of libido, fatigability, crying, pessimism, suicidal wishes, indecisiveness, loss of sense of humor, sense of boredom or apathy, overconcern about health, excessive self-criticism, and loss of initiative.

Patients showing evidence of organic brain damage or of a schizophrenic process, and those in whom anxiety or some other psychopathological state was more prominent than depression, were excluded from this group.

In addition to the group of depressed patients, a group of 31 nondepressed patients was also seen in psychotherapy. This group was similar to the depressed group in respect to age, sex, and social position, and constituted a control group for this study.

PROCEDURE

Face-to-face interviews were conducted when the depressions were regarded as moderate to severe and I was active and supportive during these periods. Other than during periods of severe depression, formal analysis was employed for the long-term patients; I utilized the couch, encouraged free association, and followed the policy of minimal activity. The recorded data used as the basis for this study were my notes, handwritten during the psychotherapeutic interviews. These data include retrospective reports by the patients of feelings and thoughts prior to the sessions, as well as spontaneous reports of their feelings and thoughts during the sessions. In addition, several patients regularly kept notes of their feelings and thoughts between psychotherapeutic sessions and reported these.

While these data were collected, handwritten records of the verbalizations of the nondepressed patients were also collected, and these notes were compared with the notes on the depressed group.

FINDINGS

It was found that the depressed patients differed from the nondepressed group in the preponderance of certain themes which are outlined below. Moreover, each nosological group showed an idiosyncratic ideational content that distinguished it from each of the others. Depression was characterized by themes of low self-esteem, self-blame, overwhelming responsibilities, and desires to escape; anxiety state by themes of personal danger; hypomanic state by themes of self-enhancement; hostile paranoid state by themes of accusations against others.

Although each nosological group showed particular types of thought content specific for that group, the formal characteristics and processes of distortion involved in the idiosyncratic ideation were similar for each of these nosological categories. The processes of distortion and the formal characteristics will be described.

THEMATIC CONTENT OF COGNITIONS

The types of cognitions* outlined below were reported by the depressed patients to occur under two general conditions. First, the typical depressive

---

* The term cognition refers to a specific thought such as an interpretation, a self-command, or a self-criticism. The term is also applied to wishes (such as suicidal desires) that have a verbal content.

cognitions were observed in response to particular kinds of external stimulus situations. These were situations that contained an ingredient, or combination of ingredients, whose content had some relevance to the content of the idiosyncratic response. This stereotyped response was frequently irrelevant and inappropriate to the situation as a whole. For instance, any experience that touched in any way on the subject of the patient's personal attributes might immediately make him think he was inadequate.

A young man would respond with self-derogatory thoughts to any interpersonal situation in which another person seemed indifferent to him. If a passerby on the street did not smile at him, he was prone to think he was inferior. Similarly, a woman consistently had the thought she was a bad mother whenever she saw another woman with a child.

Second, the typical depressive thoughts were observed in the patients' ruminations or free associations, i.e., when they were not reacting to an immediate external stimulus and were not attempting to direct their thoughts. The severely-depressed patients often experienced long, uninterrupted sequences of depressive associations, completely independent of the external situation.

Low Self-Regard

Low self-evaluation formed a prominent part of the depressed patients' ideation. This generally consisted of an unrealistic downgrading of themselves in areas that were of particular importance to them. A brilliant academician questioned his basic intelligence, an attractive society woman insisted she had become repulsive-looking, and a successful businessman believed he had no real business acumen and was headed for bankruptcy.

The low self-appraisal was applied to personal attributes such as ability, virtue, attractiveness, and health; to acquisitions of tangibles or intangibles (such as love or friendship); or to past performance in one's career or in one's role as a spouse or parent. In making these self-appraisals, the depressed patient was prone to magnify any failure or defects and to minimize or ignore any favorable characteristics.

A common feature of many of the self-evaluations was the unfavorable comparison with other people, particularly those in his own social or occupational group. Almost uniformly, in making his comparisons, the depressed patient rated himself as inferior. He regarded himself as less intelligent, less productive, less attractive, less financially secure, or less successful as a spouse or parent than those in his comparison group. These types of self-ratings comprise the feeling of inferiority, which has been noted in the literature on depressives.

Ideas of Deprivation

Allied to the low self-appraisals are the ideas of destitution seen in certain depressed patients. These ideas were noted in the patient's verbalized thoughts that he is alone, unwanted, and unlovable, often in the face of overt demonstrations of friendship and affection. The sense of deprivation was also applied to material possessions, despite obvious contrary evidence.

Self-Criticisms and Self-Blame

Another prominent theme in the reported thoughts of the depressed patients was concerned with self-criticism and self-condemnation. These themes should be differentiated from the low self-evaluation already described. The low self-evaluation refers simply to the appraisal of themselves relative either to their comparison group or to their own standards, but the self-criticism represents the reproaches they levelled against themselves for their perceived shortcomings. It should be pointed out, however, that not all patients with low self-evaluation showed self-criticism.

The self-criticisms, just as the low self-evaluations, were usually applied to those specific attributes or behaviors most highly valued by the individual. A depressed woman, for example, condemned herself for not having breakfast ready for her husband. She reported a sexual affair with one of his colleagues, however, without any evidence of regret, self-criticism, or guilt. Competence as a housewife was one of her expectations of herself but marital fidelity was not.

The patients' tendency to blame themselves for their mistakes or shortcomings generally had no logical basis. This was demonstrated by a housewife who took her children on a picnic. When a thunderstorm suddenly appeared, she blamed herself for not having picked a better day.

Overwhelming Problems and Duties

The patients consistently magnified problems or responsibilities that they considered minor or insignificant when not depressed.

A depressed housewife, confronted with the necessity of sewing name tags on her children's clothes in preparation for camp, perceived this as a gigantic undertaking that would take weeks to complete. When she finally got to work at it she finished in less than a day.

Self-Commands and Injunctions

Self-coercive cognitions, although not prominently mentioned in the literature on depression, seemed to form a substantial proportion of the verbalized thoughts of the patients in the sample. These cognitions consisted of constant nagging or prodding to do things. The prodding would persist even when it was impractical, undesirable, or impossible for the person to implement these self-instructions.

The "shoulds" and "musts" were often applied to an enormous range of activities, many of which were mutually exclusive. A housewife reported that in a period of a few minutes, she had compelling thoughts to clean the house, to lose some weight, to visit a sick friend, to be a den mother, to get a full-time job, to plan the week's menus, to return to college for a degree, to spend more time with her children, to take a memory course, to be more active in women's organizations, and to start putting away her family's winter clothes.

Escapist and Suicidal Wishes

Thoughts about escaping from the problems of life were frequent among all the patients. Some had daydreams of being a hobo, or of going to a tropical paradise. It was unusual, however, that evading the tasks brought any relief. Even when a temporary respite was taken on the advice of the psychiatrist, the patients were prone to blame themselves for shirking responsibilities.

The desire to escape seemed to be related to the patients' viewing themselves at an impasse. They not only saw themselves as incapable, incompetent, and helpless, but they also saw their tasks as ponderous and formidable. Their response was a wish to withdraw from the "unsolvable" problems. Several patients spent considerable time in bed; some hiding under the covers.

Suicidal preoccupations seemed similarly related to the patient's conceptualization of his situation as untenable or hopeless. He believed he could not tolerate a continuation of his suffering, and he could see no solution to the problem: The psychiatrist could not help him, his symptoms could not be alleviated, and his problems could not be solved. The suicidal patients generally stated that they regarded suicide as the only possible solution for their desperate or hopeless situations.

TYPOLOGY OF COGNITIVE DISTORTIONS

The preceding section attempts to delineate the typical thematic content of the verbalizations of the depressed patients. A crucial characteristic of these cognitions is that they represent varying degrees of reality distortion. Although some degree of inaccuracy and inconsistency is expected in the cognitions of any individual, the distinguishing characteristic of the cognitions of the depressed patients is that they show a *systematic error,* viz., a bias against themselves. Systematic errors were also noted in the idiosyncratic ideation of the other nosological groups.

The typical depression cognitions can be categorized according to the ways in which they deviate from logical or realistic thinking. The processes may be classified as paralogical (arbitrary inference, selective abstraction, and overgeneralization), stylistic (exaggeration), or semantic (inexact labelling). These cognitive distortions were observed at all levels of depression, from the mild neurotic depression to the severe psychotic. Although the thinking disorder was most obvious in the psychotic depressions, it was observable in more subtle ways among all the neurotic depressed.

Arbitrary inference is defined as the process of drawing a conclusion from a situation, event, or experience, when there is no evidence to support the conclusion or when the conclusion is contrary to the evidence.

A patient riding on an elevator had the thought, "He (the elevator operator) thinks I'm a nobody." The patient then felt sad. On being questioned by the psychiatrist, he realized there was no factual basis for this thought.

Such misconstructions are particularly prone to occur when the cues are ambiguous. An intern became quite discouraged, for example, when he received an announcement that all patients worked-up by the interns should be examined subsequently by the resident physicians. His thought on reading the announcement was, "The chief doesn't have faith in my work." In this instance, he personalized the event, although there was no reason to suspect that his performance had anything to do with the policy decision.

Intrinsic to this thinking is the lack of consideration of alternative explanations that are more plausible and more probable. The intern, when questioned about other possible explanations for the policy decision, then recalled a previous statement by his chief that he wanted the residents to have more contact with the patients as part of their training. The idea that this explicitly stated objective was the basis for the new policy had not previously occurred to him.

Selective abstraction refers to the process of focusing on a detail taken out of context, ignoring other more salient features of the situation, and conceptualizing the whole experience on the basis of this element.

A patient was praised by her employer about aspects of her work. At one point, the employer asked her to discontinue making extra carbon copies of his letters, and her immediate thought was, "He is dissatisfied with my work." This idea became paramount despite all his positive statements.

Overgeneralization is the patients' pattern of drawing a general conclusion about their ability, their performance, or their worth on the basis of a single incident.

A patient reported the following sequence of events occurring within a period of half an hour: His wife was upset because the children were slow in getting dressed. He thought, "I'm a poor father because the children are not better disciplined." He then noticed a leaky faucet, and thought that this showed he was also a poor husband. While driving to work, he thought, "I must be a poor driver or other cars would not be passing me." As he arrived at work, he noticed some other personnel had already arrived. He thought, "I can't be very dedicated or I would have come earlier." When he noticed folders and papers piled up on his desk, he concluded, "I'm a poor organizer because I have so much work to do."

Magnification and minimization refer to errors in evaluation so gross as to constitute distortions. As described in the section on thematic content, these processes were manifested by underestimation of the individuals' performance, achievement, or ability, and inflation of the magnitude of his problems and tasks. Other examples were the exaggeration of the intensity or significance of a traumatic event. It was frequently observed that the patients' initial reaction to an unpleasant event was to regard it as a catastrophe. It was generally found on further inquiry that the perceived disaster was often a relatively minor problem.

A man reported that he had been upset because of damage to his house as the result of a storm. When he first discovered the damage, his thought sequence was, "The side of the house is wrecked. . . . It will cost a fortune to fix it." His immediate reaction was that his repair bill would be several thousand dollars. After the initial shock had dissipated, he realized that the damage was minor and that the repairs would cost around fifty dollars.

Inexact labelling often seems to contribute to this kind of distortion. The affective reaction is proportional to the descriptive labelling of the event, rather than to the actual intensity of a traumatic situation.

A man reported during his therapy hour that he was very upset because he had been "clobbered" by his superior. On further reflection, he realized that he had magnified the incident and that a more adequate description was that his supervisor "corrected an error" he had made. After reevaluating the event, he felt better. He also realized that whenever he was corrected or criticized by a person in authority he was prone to describe this as being "clobbered."

FORMAL CHARACTERISTICS OF DEPRESSIVE COGNITIONS

The previous sections have attempted to categorize the typical thematic contents of the verbalized thoughts of depressed patients and to present observations regarding the processes involved in the conceptual errors and distortions.

The inaccurate conceptualizations with depressive content have been labelled *depressive cognitions*. This section will present a summary of the specific formal characteristics of the depressive cognitions as reported by the patients.

One of the striking features of the typical depressive cognitions is that they were generally experienced by the patients as arising as though they were *automatic* responses, i.e., without any apparent antecedent reflection or reasoning.

A patient, for example, observed that when he was in a situation in which somebody else was receiving praise, he would automatically have the thought, "I'm nobody. . . . I'm not good enough." Later, when he reflected on his response, he would then regard it as inappropriate. Nonetheless, his immediate response to such situations continued to be a self-devaluation.

The depressive thoughts not only appeared to be automatic, in the sense just described, but they seemed, also, to have an *involuntary* quality. The patients frequently reported that these thoughts would occur even when they had resolved "not to have them" or were actively trying to avoid them. This involuntary characteristic was clearly exemplified by repetitive thoughts of suicidal content, but was found in a less dramatic way in other types of depressive cognitions. A number of patients were able to anticipate the kind of depressive thoughts that would occur in certain specific situations and would prepare themselves in advance to make a more realistic judgment of the situation. Nevertheless, despite the intention to ward off or control these thoughts, they would continue to preempt a more rational response.*

Another characteristic of the depressive thoughts is their *plausibility* to the patient. At the beginning of therapy the patients tended to accept the validity of the cognitions uncritically. It often required considerable experience in observing these thoughts and attempting to judge them rationally for the patients to recognize them as distortions. It was noted that the more plausible the cognitions seemed (or the more uncritically the patient regarded them), the stronger the affective reaction. It was also observed that when the patient was able to question the validity of the thoughts, the

---

* The foregoing features may suggest that the depressive thoughts are essentially a type of obsessional thinking. The depressive thoughts, however, differ from classical obsessional thinking in that their specific content varies according to the particular stimulus situation and also in that they are associated with an affective response. Obsessional thoughts, on the other hand, tend to retain essentially the same wording with each repetition, are generally regarded by the patient as a "strange" or "alien" idea, and are not associated with any feeling.

affective reaction was generally reduced. The converse of this also seemed to be true: When the affective reaction to a thought was particularly strong, its plausibility became enhanced, and the patient found it more difficult to appraise its validity. Furthermore, once a strong affect was aroused in response to a distorted cognition, any subsequent distortions seemed to have an increased plausibility. This characteristic appeared to be present irrespective of whether the affect was sadness, anger, anxiety, or euphoria. Once the affective response was dissipated, however, the patient could then appraise these cognitions critically and recognize the distortions.

A final characteristic of the depressive cognitions is their *perseveration*. Despite the multiplicity and complexity of life situations, the depressed patient was prone to interpret a wide range of his experiences in terms of a few stereotyped ideas. The same type of cognition would be elicited by highly heterogenous experiences. In addition, these idiosyncratic cognitions tended to occur repetitively in the patients' ruminations and stream of associations.

RELATION OF DEPRESSIVE THOUGHTS TO AFFECTS

As part of the psychotherapy, the author encouraged the patients to attempt to specify as precisely as possible their feelings and the thoughts they had in relation to these feelings.

A number of problems were presented in the attempt to obtain precise description and labelling of the feelings. The patients had no difficulty in designating their feelings as pleasant or unpleasant. Additionally, they were readily able to specify whether they felt depressed (or sad), anxious, angry, and embarrassed. When they were asked to discriminate further among the depressed feelings, there was considerable variability. Most patients were able to differentiate with a reasonable degree of certainty among the following: sad, discouraged, hurt, humiliated, guilty, empty, and lonely.

To determine the relation of specific feelings to a specific thought, the patients were advised to develop the routine of trying to focus their attention on their thoughts whenever they had an unpleasant feeling or whenever the feeling became intensified. This often meant thinking back after they were aware of the unpleasant feeling to recall the content of the preceding thought. They frequently observed that an unpleasant thought preceded the unpleasant affect.

The most noteworthy finding was that when the thoughts associated with the depressive affects were identified, they were generally found to contain the type of conceptual distortions or errors already described, as well as the typical depressive thematic content. Similarly, when the affect was anxiety, anger, or elation, the associated cognitions had a content congruent with these feelings.

An effort was made to classify the cognitions, to ascertain whether there were any specific features that could distinguish among the types of cognitions associated respectively with depression, anger, or elation. It was found, as might be expected, that the typical thoughts associated with the depressive affect centered around the idea that the individual was deficient in some way. Furthermore, the specific types of depressive affect were generally consistent with the specific thought content. Thus, thoughts of being deserted, inferior, or derelict were associated respectively with feelings of loneliness, humiliation, or guilt.

In the nondepressed group, the thoughts associated with the affect of anxiety had the theme of anticipation of some unpleasant event. Thoughts associated with anger had an element of blame directed against some other person or agency. Finally, feelings of euphoria were associated with thoughts that were self-inflating in some way.

DISCUSSION

It has been noted that "the schizophrenic excels in his tendency to misconstrue the world that is presented. . . ." (Kasanin, 1944). Although the validity of this statement has been supported by numerous clinical and experimental studies, it has not generally been acknowledged that misconstructions of reality may also be a characteristic feature of other psychiatric disorders. The present study indicates that, even in mild phases of depression, systematic deviations from realistic and logical thinking occur. A crucial feature of these cognitive distortions is that they appeared consistently only in the ideational material that had a typically depressive content, e.g., themes of being deficient in some way. The other ideational material reported by the depressed patients did not show any systematic errors.

The thinking-disorder typology outlined here is similar to that described in studies of schizophrenia. Although some of the most flagrant schizophrenic signs (such as word-salad, metaphorical speech, neologisms, and condensations) were not observed, the kinds of paralogical processes in the depressed patients resembled those described in schizophrenics (Kasanin, 1944). Moreover, the same kind of paralogical thinking was observed in the nondepressed patients in the control group.

Although each nosological category showed a distinctive thought *content,* the differences in terms of the *processes* involved in the deviant thinking appeared to be quantitative rather than qualitative. These findings suggest that a thinking disorder may be common to all types of psychopathology. By applying this concept to psychiatric classification, it would be possible to characterize the specific nosological categories in terms of the degree of cognitive impairment and the particular content of the idiosyncratic cognitions.

The failure of various psychological tests to reflect a thinking disorder in depression warrants consideration. It is suggested that the tests employed are not specifically designed for detecting the thinking deviations in depression. Since clinical observation indicates that the typical cognitive distortions in depression are limited to particular content areas (such as self-devaluations), the various object-sorting, proverb-interpreting, and projective tests may miss the essential pathology. Even in studies of schizophrenia, the demonstration of a thinking disorder is dependent on the type of test administered and the characteristics of the experimental group. Cohen and his coworkers (1956), for example, found that the only instrument eliciting abnormal responses in acute schizophrenics was the Rorschach test, whereas chronic schizophrenics showed abnormalities on a Gestalt completion test as well as on the Rorschach.

The clinical finding of a thinking disorder at all levels of depression should focus attention on the problem of defining the precise relationship of the cognitive distortions to the characteristic affective state in depression. The diagnostic manual of the American Psychiatric Association (1952) defines the psychotic affective reactions in terms of "a primary, severe disorder of mood with resultant disturbance of thought and behavior, in consonance with the affect." Although this is a widely accepted concept, the converse would appear to be at least as plausible, viz., that there is primary disorder of thought with resultant disturbance of affect and behavior in consonance with the cognitive distortions. This latter thesis is consistent with the conception that the way an individual structures an experience determines his affective response to it: If, for example, he perceives a situation as dangerous, he may be expected to respond with a consonant affect, such as anxiety.

It is proposed, therefore, that the typical depressive affects are evoked by the erroneous conceptualizations: If the patient incorrectly perceives himself as inadequate, deserted, or sinful, he will experience corresponding affects such as sadness, loneliness, or guilt. On the other hand, the possibility that the evoked affect may, in turn, influence the thinking should also be considered. It is conceivable that once a depressive affect has been aroused, it will facilitate the emergence of further depressive-type cognitions. A continuous interaction between cognition and affect may, consequently, be produced and, thus, lead to the typical downward spiral observed in depression. (The theoretical implications of this study are discussed more fully in Chapter 18.) Since it seems likely that this interaction would be highly complex, appropriately designed experiments would be warranted to clarify the relationships.

A few methodological problems should be mentioned. A question could be raised, for example, regarding the generalizing of the observations. Since the sample consisted largely of psychotherapy patients of a relatively narrow range of intelligence and social index, there may be some uncertainty as to whether the findings are applicable to the general population of depressed patients. In view of the obvious problems associated with using data from handwritten notes of psychotherapy sessions, it is apparent that the findings of the present study will have to be subjected to verification by more refined and systematic studies. One promising approach has been developed by Gottschalk, Gleser, and Springer (1963), who utilized verbatim recordings of five minute periods of free association by depressed patients, and subjected this material to blind scoring by trained judges. Such a procedure circumvents the hazards of therapist bias and suggestion associated with verbal material recorded in psychotherapy interviews.

SUMMARY AND CONCLUSIONS

A group of 50 depressed patients in psychotherapy and a control group of 31 nondepressed patients were studied to determine the prevalence and types of cognitive abnormalities. Evidence of deviation from logical and realistic thinking was found at every level of depression from mild neurotic to severe psychotic.

The ideation of the depressed patients differed from that of the nondepressed patients in the prominence of certain typical themes, viz., low self-evaluation, ideas of deprivation, exaggeration of problems and difficulties, self-criticism and self-commands, and wishes to escape or die. Similarly, each of the nondepressed nosological groups could be differentiated on the basis of their idiosyncratic thought content.

Abnormalities were detected consistently only in those verbalized thoughts that had the typical thematic content of the depressed groups. The other kinds of ideation did not show any consistent distortion. Among the deviations in thinking, the following processes were identified: arbitrary inference; selective abstraction; overgeneralization; and magnification and minimization.

Part IV.
THEORETICAL ASPECTS OF DEPRESSION

Chapter 16.
Theories of Depression

NEUROLOGICAL THEORY OF DEPRESSION

Kraines (1965) has written extensively on the possible biological explanations of depression. He bases his theory on the following assumptions. There is frequently a history of "hereditary susceptibility," especially in identical twins. He infers that the occurrence of postpartum depressions, premenstrual depressions, and the greater frequency of manic attacks in youth and depressive attacks later in life are due to hormonal changes. (For a critique of the hereditary and endocrine studies, see Chapter 9).

The course of the illness suggests a physiological basis because of its onset in personalities that are presumably well adjusted; its onset in the absence of significant precipitating stress; and the "basically identical onset, symptoms, and course in the majority of patients despite their otherwise radical differences in culture, status, etc."

The therapeutic results which suggests a physiological basis include the "spontaneous remission of the illness in the absence of any therapy; failure of psychotherapy to shorten the illness or to prevent recurrences; beneficial results of such physical therapies as drugs and electric shock."

Kraines offers as confirmatory evidence "seasonal influences with peak periods of onset in the spring or fall of the year;" and the precipitation of a depressive syndrome in vulnerable persons by the administration of large doses of phenothiazines.

Kraines presented an elaborate theory in which the hypothalamus plays a significant role. The schematic outline is as follows. A stimulus from the cerebral cortex excites the hypothalamus. This in turn produces a stimulation of the somato-visceral system. The feedback from this system stimulates the reticular system and is further integrated and elaborated in the thalamus and limbic system. The impulses finally terminate in the cerebral cortex. According to the author, the complex circuit thus traversed is an "emotional circuit." Kraines believes that the sensory experience thus derived from the emotional circuit is mood. He asserts that pathology of the hypothalamus is responsible for the manic-depressive illness. He regards psycho-pathological symptoms as secondary; they are psychodynamic defenses against the state of alarm induced by the physiopathology of the diencephalon.

The evidence upon which Kraines bases his theory is fragmentary and subject to question. As pointed out in Chapter 9, the familial and identical twin studies have not clearly established the role of hereditary transmission of depression; also no consistent hormonal abnormalities, except for a nonspecific increase in steroid excretion, have been found. Furthermore, much of the evidence he cites to support a biological etiology may be interpreted in a way as to support a psychogenic explanation of depression. Despite this objection, however, Kraines' theory should stimulate further investigations to elucidate the physiological correlates of depression.

BIOCHEMICAL THEORY OF DEPRESSION

The current belief in the effectiveness of the MAO inhibitors and the tricyclic compounds has led to research on their biochemical effects. The evidence which has been obtained is sparse, but it has resulted in an interesting supposition called "the catecholamine hypothesis of affective disorders." The strength of this hypothesis has received an excellent discussion in the review by Schildkraut (1965). His conclusion is that the hypothesis can neither be definitely accepted nor eliminated, given the currently available data, but it is useful as a guide to further experimentation.

The essential idea of the catecholamine hypothesis is that in depression the supply of active norepinephrine (at central adrenergic receptor sites) is depleted. The major evidence for this statement comes from the study of drug effects on experimental animals. In these animals, both the MAO inhibitors and imipramine may serve to increase the availability of active norepinephrine. The MAO inhibitors probably act by directly inhibiting the enzymatic oxidative deamination of norepinephrine. Imipramine, on the other hand, may act by decreasing membrane permeability that blocks the intracellular release (and hence deamination) of the storage norepinephrine; and by increasing cellular re-uptake and thus diminishing the inactivation of free extracellular norepinephrine. Furthermore, it is possible that reserpine-induced sedation in animals is associated with catecholamine depletion, though some investigators believe that other amines, most importantly serotonin, are critical here. In any case, the probable increase of active norepinephrine following antidepressant administration, and decrease of norepinephrine in reserpine sedation (both in animals) are consistent with the catecholamine hypothesis.

The hypothesis, thus, has a definite quantity of consistent evidence supporting it. However, this evidence does not, in general, come from studies of depressed patients but from other sources. The hypothesis, of course, does not contain an explanation for the large number of patients in whom the drugs do not work. As Schildkraut stated, "It must be stressed, however, that this hypothesis is undoubtedly, at best, a reductionistic over-simplification of a very complex biological state. . . ." This does not deny the usefulness of the supposition in guiding investigators in the search for a more sophisticated biochemical basis for depressive disorders.

PSYCHOANALYTIC THEORIES OF DEPRESSION

In his papers of 1911 and 1916, Abraham discusses the significance of hostility and orality in depression. Ungratified sexual aims bring about feelings of hatred and hostility which reduce the depressed patient's capacity for love. He projects this hatred externally, and the repressed hostility manifests itself in dreams and abnormal behavior, in a desire for revenge, in a tendency to annoy other people, in ideas of guilt, and in emotional impoverishment. In his later article, Abraham presented clinical evidence to support Freud's description of the stages of pregenital sexuality. He cited several cases of patients for whom sexual gratification was still associated with the nutritive act. Auto-eroticism functioned to both prevent and relieve depression. The patient may further wish to eat up or incorporate the loved object, sometimes abstaining from food as if to prevent this.

Abraham's paper of 1924 discussed the relationship between manic-depressive psychosis and obsessional neurosis. Both anal eroticism and sadistic impulses, he wrote, exhibit opposite tendencies to expel or destroy and to retain or control what is perceived as personal property—the feces or the loved object. While the obsessional tries to retain and control his object, the melancholic has regressed to the stage of anal expulsion and rejects the object which has frustrated him. He is then ambivalent in his feelings for the lost object and may try to repossess it orally. This marks a further regression beyond the anal-sadistic level. Abraham concluded that an inherited predisposition toward oral eroticism fixed the melancholic's psycho-sexual development at the oral stage. Childhood disappointments in love, especially when occurring before the Oedipal wishes have been resolved, and the repetition of these disappointments in later life, were further factors in the origins of melancholia.

In *Mourning and Melancholia* (1917), Freud compared melancholia to normal grief. While both may occur as a reaction to loss of a loved object, melancholia may occur in specially predisposed people in reaction to an imaginary or vaguely perceived loss that deprives the ego. The melancholic's self-accusations were seen as manifestations of his hostility toward the lost loved object. Freud explained this phenomenon as the narcissistic identification of the ego with the object through introjection, a regression to the oral stage of erotic development. (In his further consideration of psychic introjection, Freud referred to the "self-criticizing faculty" of the ego, the foundation for his later concept of superego. He hesitated to generalize too widely in this regard, because of his uncertainty as to the somatic aspects of melancholia.)

Rado (1928), considering predispositional factors in depression, stated that the depressive is a person with intense narcissistic needs and precarious self-esteem who, when he loses his love object, reacts first with angry rebellion and then tries to restore his self-esteem by the punishment of his ego (which includes the introjected bad part of his object) by his superego.

Rado saw the melancholic process as an attempt at reparation played out in the psychic plane rather than in relation to the object world. In this drama, self-vilification functions as an attempt at expiation undertaken in order to win back love. The obsessional character of the melancholic was considered by Rado to be a defense mechanism used to draw off the depressive's aggressive impulses into social channels. In this concept, Rado differed slightly from his predecessors.

Gero (1936) outlined in great detail his therapeutic work with two cases of neurotic depression. Gero disagreed with former writers concerning the universality of the obsessional character structure in depression; neither of his depressives used an obsessive character defense, but both demonstrated an underlying narcissistic hunger, intolerance of frustration, and the introjection of the love objects.

Gero also contributed a broadened interpretation of the concept of orality in depressives. He agreed with Abraham and Rado in saying that "oral eroticism is the favorite fixation point in the depressive." However, his detailed case studies gave no clinical confirmation of Rado's theory of intrapsychic propitiation in depression.

Melanie Klein (1934) believed that the predisposition to depression depended not on a series of traumatic incidents, but on the mother-child relation in the first year of life. Her contribution pushed psychoanalytic speculations back to the infant's first year to explain the effects of introjection and projection on his psychic development. She maintained that the infant reacts to frustration and lack of gratification with rage and sadistic fantasies corresponding to his phase of development. The infant's weakness of ego gives rise to feelings of helplessness, sadness, guilt and regret in the face of these tensions (the depressive position). The weakness of the infantile ego also stimulates the fear of being exterminated by these impulses. The external persecutor is now introjected, and the child has fears even when the external object is not present and distorts the dangers when it is present (the persecutory or paranoid position). Children experience these feelings until they become fully assured of their mother's love for them. Those children who do not meet with sufficient love, Melanie Klein presumes to be always predisposed to return to the depressive position, i.e., to feelings of loss, sorrow, guilt, and lack of self-esteem.

Melanie Klein felt that the child, as a defensive technique, denies the complexity of his love object and sees it as either all good or all bad. This tendency is a characteristic of the adult manic depressive.

Bibring (1953) departed from classical theory and allied himself with those who viewed depression as an affective state characterized by a loss of self-esteem. Like the earlier writers, he felt that a predisposition to depression stemmed from early childhood traumatic experiences. However, he added that self-esteem may be decreased, not only by frustration of need for love and affection, but also by frustration of other aspirations. He indicated that all depressive reactions have something in common although they exhibit a multiplicity of forms.

Another deviation was his concept that all depression stems from conflict or tension within the ego itself rather than from a conflict between the ego and superego. He indicated that the depression was the expression of the feeling or awareness of the ego of its helplessness and powerlessness.

As did Bibring, Jacobson (1953, 1954) proposed that the loss of self esteem is the central psychological problem in depression. She postulated the goals of the development of self-esteem, superego, and ego ideal as the firm establishment of one's own identity, the differentiation of one's self from others, the maintenance of self-esteem and the capacity to form satisfactory object-relationships. She considered that self-esteem "represents the degree of discrepancy or harmony between the self-representations and the wished-for concept of the self." She regarded all the determinants of self-esteem as having relevance for depression.

Jacobson distinguished between neurotic and psychotic depressions and attempted to clarify the nature of ego regression in psychotic depression. She proposed that the premature and excessive disappointment in the parents with the accompanying devaluation of them—and the self—occurs in the early life of depressive patients. The prepsychotic manic depressive exhibits an unusual degree of dependency and an extreme intolerance to hurt, frustration, or disappointment. The characteristic defense used by the prepsychotic manic depressive to feelings of hurt or disappointment is denial. The denial mechanism may be so augmented that the patient may lose touch with reality and go into a manic state. If this phase does not occur, the patient makes other attempts at defense and restitution. The manic depressive's last restitutive maneuver is the final withdrawal from reality. Jacobson emphasized the continuity of the restitutive process with the earlier methods used by the patient to maintain self-esteem.

Jacobson regarded the melancholic psychotic process as a process of regressive dissolution of the identifications which had been previously precariously built up. This dissolution results in the fusions "of bad or good love object images with the self image and with the superego and leads to a pathological conflict between the self and the superego."

Hammerman (1962) differentiated between depression in which the role of "sadistic superego" is prominent and self-esteem collapses due to guilt in transgressing superego standards and the depression due to defective ego organization. The sadism of the superego presupposes the existence of a comparatively well-developed ego organization and psychic structure formation; faulty ego development due to very early trauma, early loss, or defective relationship results in a distorted self-image and lack of self-esteem because of failure to measure up to a narcissistic ego ideal.

According to Zetzel (1966), psychological maturity consists in passively accepting the limitations of reality and actively working toward realistic goals. In view of the reality principle, the recognition, tolerance, and mastery of depression, like that of anxiety, must be regarded as a developmental challenge in preparation for the stress of normal adult life. Failure in this respect may lead to symptom formation, inhibition, and adaptive failures and may be caused by mechanisms such as projection and denial which prevent the subjective experience of threat, loss, and personal limitations. Such failure may also predispose an individual to chronic and psychotic depressions.

AGGRESSION IN DEPRESSION

Psychoanalysts since Abraham (1911) have ascribed a central role to aggression in the development of depression. Four writers have challenged the universality of this association. Balint (1952) considered the depressive's feelings of bitterness and resentment as reactions to, rather than essential elements of, depression. Bibring (1953) also regarded aggression as a secondary phenomenon due to the breakdown of self-esteem. Cohen and her group (1954) posited that the hostility exhibited by the patient is due to his "annoying impact upon others, rather than of primary motivation to do injury to them." Gero also challenged the view that self-devaluation can be considered self-directed aggression.

Mendelson (1960) regards these differences of opinion as due to a lack of clear definitions of depression and of aggression. He states that psychoanalysts have often constructed theoretical models based on limited definitions which have little relation to clinical reality and that later authors attempt to justify these constructions or to apply them universally and uncritically to all depressive phenomena. There is little consensus on the relation of aggression to depression or whether aggression is primary or secondary to the problem of depression. There is no agreement as to whether aggression is an innate drive or merely a reaction to frustration. Finally, the word *aggression* is used in so many different ways that it has led to semantic confusion.

ORALITY IN DEPRESSION

Since Abraham (1916) theorized that oral eroticism in neurotic depressives has the function of preventing episodes of depression, other authors have broadened the concept of orality and concluded that the depressive person, because of his excessive dependence upon external supplies of love, affection, and attention to maintain his self-esteem, is an orally dependent person who lacks these vital supplies.

Bibring (1953) first questioned the universality of oral fixation in depression. He called attention to the clinical fact that while one person may depend upon the attainment of narcissistic supplies from an outside source, another's equilibrium may depend upon supplies from an internalized source, that is, by the fulfillment of certain aspirations and ideals.

Jacobson (1953) conceived of the mechanism in depression, not as an identification achieved through oral means, but as a regressive breakdown of ego identifications in which reality testing is lost and the self images are confused with object representations. The object representations no longer adequately reflect the actual objects.

PSYCHODYNAMIC AND PSYCHOLOGICAL THEORIES

Cohen and her coworkers (1954) studied the family backgrounds of 12 manic-depressive patients. (See Chapter 10 for a review of the systematic research related to this study.) The authors described the typical family situation as one in which the mother was the stronger and more stable parent and tended to deprecate her husband. The typical parent-child relationship was one in which the parent's approval of the children was contingent on the children's accomplishments in the form of grades and other prestige symbols. The child destined to be a manic depressive was often selected as the family's standard bearer in the battle for social status.

The writers delineated a typical personality structure characterized by denying the complexity of people and seeing them as "either all white or all black." This inability to view people as complex, multi-faceted individuals was viewed as a distinguishing characteristic of the adult manic depressive's interpersonal relationships. Cohen and her group regarded this denial of the complexity of people as a defense and attributed it to the difficulty these patients had as children in integrating the different aspects of their mothers into a unified picture.

Cohen *et al.* asserted that the manic depressive's hostility has been overstressed as a dynamic factor in his illness; the patient's hostile feelings arise not primarily from the frustration of his needs, but are the result of the annoyance he arouses in others by his demanding behavior. The manic depressive does not suffer genuine guilt or feelings of regret, but expresses feelings of guilt and self-reproach as an exploitive technique "to placate authority."

According to Lichtenberg (1957), depression results when a person feels responsible for his hopelessness in regard to the attainment of goals. The author distinguishes three forms of depression, which vary with the kind of goal—a specific situation, a behavior style, or a generalized goal—to which the person directs his expectancy. Associated with each form are particular classes of events to which the feeling of hopelessness is related: distortions of time; of interpersonal relations; of valuation of personal responsibility; and of secondary gains and losses. As a person's hope in fulfilling a more differentiated goal diminishes, he directs his expectancy to a more generalized goal. The three forms of depression correspond to the neurotic, agitated, and retarded depressions. This conceptualization of depression is particularly well-suited to further clinical and experimental research.

Schwartz (1961) attempted to construct a unitary formulation of the manic-depressive reactions. He suggested that manic-depressive reactions occur when a person with excessive, unsatisfied narcissistic needs introjects the attitudes of those responsible for his "deprivation." In adult life, increased stress creates a sense of loss that is identified with the earlier deprivation. Retaliatory aggression is then directed against the introjected parental figures but the ego defends against this. In mania, ceaseless activity blocks the perception of hostility and deprivation. In depression, inhibition and immobilization are a denial of the capacity to carry out the aggressive impulses.

THE EXISTENTIAL THEORIES OF DEPRESSION

The existential theories of depression are summarized by Arieti (1959). He points out that according to the existentialists, the ambivalence of the manic-depressive patient is different from that of the schizophrenic. Whereas the schizophrenic may hate and love at the same time, the manic depressive alternates between love and hate.

According to Arieti, Henry Ey considered the depressed state to be an arrest or insufficiency of all the vital activities. Ey viewed depression as a "pathetic immobility, a suspension of existence, a syncope of time." As a result, the patient experiences a sense of incompleteness, of impotence, and of unreality.

The question of the depressed patient's attitude toward time has occupied the attention of many existential writers. They emphasized that time seems to have slowed down for the depressed patient. In his subjective experience, only the past matters. Painful memories dominate his thinking and remind him of his unworthiness and inability to accomplish.

Hubert Tellenbach in his book, *Melancholie* (1961), offered a thorough analysis of depression which in many respects is representative of existential thinking.* Tellenbach presented an analysis of the case histories of 140 melancholics. He asserted that they all have a relatively uniform premorbid personality structure. The life and work of the melancholic is dominated by a strict order: orderliness in dealing with things, conscientiousness in his work, and an overriding need to do right to those close to him. He has a great sensitivity to the dos and don'ts, the shoulds and should nots. At the same time, he has great sensitivity to guilt. The melancholic devotes his life to fulfilling his sense of order and to avoiding situations of guilt. He prefers the security of steady employment to the risk involved in free self-propelled work.

Tellenbach described a series of specific situations in which the melancholic sense of orderliness and guilt is threatened. The interplay of these situations and the melancholic's personality results in his getting increasingly tangled. The basic paradox is this: On the one hand, he is so sensitive to guilt that he will do everything to keep abreast of his obligations while on the other hand, he gives such an exacting interpretation to his obligations that he is close to the brink of getting behind in his own aspirations. In such a precariously balanced way of living, any accidental situation may throw him over the brink into being behind in his obligations or into being

---

* Dr. Egbert H. Mueller was of great help in translating this book from the German and in summarizing its contents.

behind in his sense of fulfillment. In the depressive psychosis, the distance between being and aspiration becomes an abyss.

Schulte (1961) considered the inability to be sad as the crux of the melancholic experience. According to the author, a person who can still be sad is not really melancholic, and the improvement in the state of melancholy starts when the individual can't experience sadness. Schulte stated that the melancholic has lost the ability to sympathize and to be moved. He experiences a need for an emotion which is tormenting to him. The author cautioned that the use of the word sad by the patients should be regarded as a metaphor by which they try to make some sense out of something that cannot really be expressed and explained and that is not comparable to other things.

Chapter 17.
Cognition and Psychopathology

Most contemporary writers on the psychological aspects of depression have utilized a motivational or adaptational model. Some authors view depressive symptomatology in terms of the gratification or discharge of certain needs or drives (Abraham, 1916; Rado, 1928). Others emphasize the role of the defenses against these drives (Freud, 1917). Still others emphasize the adaptive aspects of the symptomatology (Rado, 1928; Adler, 1961).

Most attempts to explain the symptoms of depression in psychological terms have introduced troublesome conceptual or empirical problems. First, many writers have a tendency to ascribe some purpose to the symptoms. Rather than looking upon the symptoms simply as a manifestation of a psychological or physiological disorder, these writers view the symptoms as serving an important intrapsychic or interpersonal function. The sadness of the depressed person, for example, has been explained by some writers (i.e., Rado and Adler) as an attempt to manipulate other people. Although such functionalist interpretations sometimes seem to fit a particular case, they have strong teleological overtones. As the history of science demonstrates, theories that ascribe some design or purpose to natural phenomena have generally been superseded as basic knowledge increased.

Second, in attempting to account for paradoxical aspects of depression, some writers have presented formulations that are so elaborate or abstract that they cannot be correlated with clinical material. Freud's conceptualization of depression in terms of the attack of the sadistic part of the ego on the incorporated loved-object within the ego is so remote from any observables in clinical data that it defies systematic validation. Similarly, Melanie Klein's (1934) formulation of adult depression as a reactivation of an early infantile depression does not provide any bridge to observable behavior.

Third, most writers have skirted the problem of the specificity of their formulations. Many of the most popular psychodynamic formulations of depression, such as the concepts of increased orality or of repressed hostility, have also been attributed to a multiplicity of other psychiatric and psychosomatic disorders. Hence, the particular formulations, if valid, might be characteristic of psychiatric disorders in general and not exclusively applicable to depression.

Finally, the various theories have offered, at best, explanations for only circumscribed aspects of the diversified clinical picture of depression. Explanations that seem to fit certain specific groups of phenomena often seem irrelevant or incongruous when applied to other phenomena.

In undertaking a conceptualization of the psychological processes in depression, writers must account for a wide variety of psychopathological phenomena (Grinker *et al.* 1961). As described in Chapter 2, we found 21 different symptom-categories that occurred significantly more frequently in depressed than in nondepressed patients. The various symptoms of depression fell into certain clusters and were grouped under the following headings. The *affective* group includes the various adjectives and phrases employed by patients to describe their feelings: sad, lonely, empty, bored, and hopeless. The *motivational* group includes intensified wishes for help, yearning to escape, desire to commit suicide, and the phenomenon of loss of spontaneous motivation (paralysis of the will). The *cognitive* group includes negative self-concept, pessimism, and negative interpretations of experience. The *physical and vegetative* symptoms include retardation, fatigability, loss of appetite, loss of libido, and sleep disturbance.

These groupings of symptoms may not seem to bear much relationship to each other. Many previous writers have attempted to present a unifying theory that would establish understandable connections among these groupings. Freud's theory of retroflected hostility, for instance, may be used to interrelate negative self-concept, self-criticism, and suicidal wishes, but falls short in providing plausible connections with the other symptoms. His complementary concept of depression as a grief reaction provides a thread between affects (especially sadness and loneliness), loss of outside interests, and loss of appetite but does not offer a rational explanation for other major symptoms such as loss of self-esteem and suicidal wishes. The concept of depression as an attempt to gain love (Rado) does not explain such behaviors as seclusiveness, or the physical and vegetative symptoms. The theories of autonomic or hypothalamic dysfunction (Campbell, 1953; Kraines, 1965) may provide a possible explanation of the physical and vegetative phenomena but offer no plausible explanations of the other symptoms.

In an attempt to find some alternative explanations for the behavioral characteristics of depression, I reviewed the clinical material of 50 depressed patients in psychotherapy and selected those themes which differentiated these patients from a control psychotherapy group (Chapter 15). These themes were regarded as derivatives of certain basic cognitive patterns which are activated in depression. Similar thematic contents were observed in the dreams, early memories, and responses to projective tests in several systematic studies of depression (Chapter 11).

In this chapter I will present a paradigm which is intended to show the connections between the cognitive aspects described previously and the affective, motivational, and physical phenomena of depression. The formulations to be presented are applicable to the various types of depression, including those that might be classified as neurotic or psychotic, endogenous or reactive, involutional or manic depressive. Finally, I will present a system of classification to demonstrate how the various psychiatric disorders may be differentiated on the basis of cognitive content.

THE PRIMARY TRIAD IN DEPRESSION

The disturbances in depression may be viewed in terms of the activation of a set of three major cognitive patterns that force the individual to view himself, his world, and his future in an idiosyncratic way. The progressive dominance of these cognitive patterns leads to the other phenomena that are associated with the depressive state.

The first component of the triad is the pattern of construing experiences in a negative way. The patient consistently interprets his interactions with his environment as representing defeat, deprivation, or disparagement. He sees his life as filled with a succession of burdens, obstacles, or traumatic situations, all of which detract from him in a significant way.

The second component is the pattern of viewing himself in a negative way. He regards himself as deficient, inadequate, or unworthy, and tends to attribute his unpleasant experiences to a physical, mental, or moral defect in himself. Furthermore, he regards himself as undesirable and worthless because of his presumed defect, and tends to reject himself because of it.

The third component consists of viewing the future in a negative way. He anticipates that his current difficulties or suffering will continue indefinitely. As he looks ahead, he sees a life of unremitting hardship, frustration, and deprivation.

The relationship between the cognitive patterns and the affective and motivational symptoms is illustrated in Figure 17–1. This relationship will be described in detail in later sections.

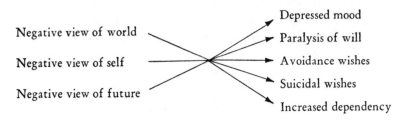

Figure 17–1.

THE EFFECT OF COGNITIVE PATTERNS ON AFFECTS AND
MOTIVATIONS IN DEPRESSION

NEGATIVE INTERPRETATION OF EXPERIENCE

The depressed patient selectively or inappropriately interprets his experiences as detracting from him in some substantive way. Whereas the manic sees neutral or ambiguous life situations as self-enhancing, the depressive regards them as self-deflating. The manic, for instance, may interpret a neutral attitude on the part of a friend as indicating overwhelming approval; the depressive may regard the same attitude as a rejection. This is particularly evident in patients with manic-depressive cycles who show completely opposite reactions to the same set of external conditions when they are in different phases of the cycle.

As was pointed out in Chapter 15 the distorted conceptualizations may range from mild inaccuracies to total misinterpretations. The typical cognitions show a variety of deviations from logical thinking, including arbitrary inferences, selective abstractions, overgeneralizations, and magnifications. The patient automatically makes a negative interpretation of a situation even though more obvious and more plausible explanations exist. He tailors the facts to fit his preformed negative conclusions. He may, furthermore, exaggerate the significance of any actual loss, thwarting, or depreciation he encounters.

Thwarting or Defeat

The depressed patient is peculiarly sensitive to any impediments to his goal-directed activity. An obstacle is regarded as an impossible barrier; difficulty in dealing with a problem is interpreted as a total failure. His cognitive response to a problem or difficulty is likely to be an idea such as "I'm licked," "I'll never be able to do this," or "I'm blocked no matter what I do."

A depressed woman, for example, having some difficulty finding a pencil she knew she had placed in her purse, had the thought, "I'll never be able to find it." She experienced a strong sense of frustration even though she was able to find it in a few seconds. Any problem seemed insoluble, and any delay in reaching a goal seemed interminable. Similarly, a depressed man discovered his car had a flat tire. Although he was a good mechanic he was overwhelmed by the idea that there was nothing he could do about the tire. In consonance with his sense of defeat, he abandoned the car.

In achievement-oriented situations the depressed patients are particularly prone to react with a sense of failure. As shown in certain controlled experiments (Chapter 10) they tend to underestimate their actual performances. Furthermore, if their actual performance falls short of the high standards they set for themselves, they are likely to regard their work as a total failure. A mildly depressed student, for example, barely missed making the honor roll at school. He looked upon this as a complete defeat and considered dropping out of school.

Deprivation

The depressed patient is apt to interpret relatively trivial events as constituting a substantial loss. A patient on the way to see his psychiatrist reacted to a large number of incidents as though he had lost something of value. First, he had to wait about 30 seconds for the elevator and thought, "I'm losing valuable time." As he rode up alone on the elevator, he regretted having no one to ride with and thought, "I'm missing out on the companionship of other people." When he discovered that another patient had an earlier appointment, he regretted that he was not the first patient the psychiatrist would see that day. When he had to wait a few minutes in the waiting room, he had the thought that the psychiatrist did not care for him. He started to read a magazine and when he had to put it down to start his appointment he felt deprived of the opportunity of finishing the magazine.

The sense of loss often centers around money. Many depressed patients regard any expenditure of money as a loss; e.g., a very wealthy man felt deprived when he had to pay fifteen cents to ride on the subway. The opposite reaction is sometimes observed. One man felt deprived whenever he was prevented from spending money. This occurred when the stores were closed or when a store did not have a particular item he wanted to buy. The act of buying tended to ward off the sense of deprivation. When he wasn't able to make purchases, he felt sad and empty.

Making comparisons with other people is especially likely to activate feelings of deprivation. Many depressed patients reported having thoughts such as "I don't have anything" when one of their friends acquired something new. A well-to-do businessman was prone to regard himself as poor whenever he heard that someone made more money than he. A wealthy woman regarded herself as deprived whenever one of her friends made a new acquisition, whether it was a hat, a dress, or a house.

Depreciation

The depressed patient is prone to read insults, ridicule, or disparagement into what other people say to him. He often interprets neutral remarks as directed against him in some way. He may even twist a favorable comment so that it seems unfavorable. An employer, for instance, praised an employee for her work. The entire time he was talking, she had the repetitive thought, "He's criticizing me."

Often the patient believes that other people have derogatory ideas about him (negative attributions). He may attribute such negative judgments to others only in certain limited situations, or in severe cases he may succumb to them in every personal contact. One woman, for example, regarded practically every statement, change of facial expression, or movement by the psychiatrist as indicative of a criticism of her. Even when he asked her questions, she thought he was criticizing her. While she was talking and he was listening, she also attributed negative judgments to him, such as "He thinks I'm a bore," or "He must think I'm awfully childish."

Some patients tend to make negative attributions whenever they are in a competitive situation. One patient had the highest standing in class, but whenever the teacher called on another student to answer a question, the patient thought, "He doesn't really think I'm smart or he would have called on me." If the professor complimented other students, he would have the thought that the professor had a low opinion of him. Another patient would make a characteristic negative attribution while driving. If another driver passed him, he would think, "He thinks I'm the kind of person who can be pushed around." He would have the same thought if he was kept waiting by a salesman or by a waitress.

Similar negative attributions are often aroused in group situations. One patient participating in group therapy thought, "They must think I'm an awful dunce because I don't talk more." When somebody told a joke, he thought, "They must think I am not amusing because I didn't tell a joke." When he did speak, he had the thought, "They think I talk too much." When a group member agreed with another patient's opinion, he thought, "They think I'm not worth listening to because nobody agrees with me."

NEGATIVE VIEW OF SELF

The depressed patient not only interprets his experiences as detracting from himself in some way, but he concurrently devalues himself. If he does not do as well as he expected on a test or a business venture, he regards himself as socially undesirable. If his children seem boisterous, he views himself as a poor parent.

To sharpen the distinction between negative interpretation of experience and the negative view of the self, we can compare the paranoid with the depressed patient. Like the depressed patient, the paranoid patient may see others as thwarting or rejecting him, but unlike the depressed patient, the paranoid maintains a positive concept of himself. He tends to blame others for his fantasied thwarting, depreciation, or deprivation; the depressed patient tends to blame himself.

A striking feature of the depressed patient is his tendency to generalize from a particular behavior to a character trait. Any single deviation from a high level of performance is assumed to represent a major shortcoming. If he does not do as well as somebody else financially, socially, or academically, he tends to regard himself as a generally inferior person. A student, for example, who had difficulty getting a date on a single occasion thought, "I must be repulsive to girls." A highly successful businessman who made one transaction that lost money became obsessed by the idea that he was stupid. A mother whose child was untidy on one occasion thought, "I'm a terrible parent."

The supposed deficiency becomes so magnified that it occupies the individual's total self-concept. The patient seems incapable of viewing himself in any way other than in terms of this deficiency. A woman who thought she was losing her beauty could describe herself only as unattractive and automatically excluded any other traits or characteristics. She tended to equate herself with her superficial physical characteristics.

The negative self-concept is associated with self-rejection. The patient not only sees himself as inferior, but he dislikes himself for it. He criticizes, reproaches, and castigates himself for being so inferior. If he recognizes that he is depressed, he criticizes himself for being ill. He regards it as an inexcusable weakness to "let himself" become ill.

NEGATIVE EXPECTATIONS

The depressed patient generally shows considerable preoccupation with ideas of the future. His expectations usually have a negative cast and may occur in the form of pictorial fantasies or as obsessive ruminations. His anticipations of the future are generally an extension of what he views as his present state. If he regards himself as currently deprived, immobilized, or rejected, he visualizes a future in which he is continually deprived, immobilized, or rejected. He seems to be unable to view his current state as having any time limits or to consider the possibility of any improvement.

Not only are the patient's long range forecasts of a negative nature, but his short term predictions are similarly negative. When he awakens in the morning, he anticipates that every experience during the day will pose great difficulties. When he contemplates undertaking a task, he predicts that he will make a mess of it. When a suggestion is made to engage in an activity that he ordinarily enjoys when not depressed, he automatically assumes he will not have a good time. One patient frequently would have an elaborate fantasy before engaging in any activity. When she thought of driving to the psychiatrist's office for an appointment, she pictured herself making a wrong turn and getting lost. When she considered calling a friend on the phone, she had a daydream of getting no answer or a busy signal. If she decided to go marketing, she imagined herself losing her purse or making the wrong purchases. When the doorbell rang, she would have a fantasy of receiving a telegram or special delivery letter with bad news.

It is useful to make a distinction between the negative predictions of the depressed patient and the fears of the anxious patient. This may be illustrated by the following example. A student preparing for an examination experienced continual thoughts that he might fail. Each time he thought of failing, he experienced anxiety. Questioned as to what he thought would happen if he failed, he responded that everybody would think he was stupid. His apprehension continued until he completed the examination. Up to this point, his thinking was similar to that observed in an anxiety neurotic. He was reacting to a situation which he perceived as a source of harm. The threatening situation was distinct from him—it had not yet inflicted its damage and his concept of himself was still intact.

After taking the examination, the student thought he had performed poorly and reached the conclusion that he had failed. He no longer felt anxious—he felt depressed. The change in his feeling may be explained as being consonant with a change in his conceptualizations. Before he took the examination the harm to his self-esteem was only potential; now it was actual. Once the injury had been inflicted, he suffered from the psychic pain it had produced. Before the examination, he could see himself as a person with many attributes, some positive and some negative. Now he could see himself in only one way: as a failure. When he looked ahead to the future, he could foresee a procession of future failures; this prospect did not produce any apprehension because he did not expect them to make him feel any worse than he now felt. The anticipated failures merely represented to him the impossibility of ever feeling better and the futility of trying.

The difference between the fears of the anxious patient and the gloomy outlook of the depressed patient may be summarized as follows: The anxious patient is concerned with the possibility of being hurt (either physically or emotionally) but sees the trauma as something in the future. The depressed patient perceives himself as already damaged (defeated, deprived, or depreciated). When he thinks of the future, it is in terms of a continuation of his present pain. There is no stimulus to alarm him because the dreaded event has already occurred. He anticipates future failures in terms of a replication of the failure that he has already experienced.

THE AFFECTIVE RESPONSE

The affective state can be regarded as the consequence of the way the individual views himself or his environment. I have noted that there is a predictable relationship between an antecedent event and the affective response (Chapter 15). If the patient was rejected, he would experience a negative affect. Similarly, if he simply *thought* he was rejected, he would experience the same negative affect. I concluded that the way an individual structures his experiences determines his mood. Since the depressed person consistently makes negative conceptualizations, he is prone to have a consistently negative mood.

I also noted that there was a similar consistency between the ideation and the affect in the patients' free associations. If a patient had the thought that he was a social outcast, he would feel lonely. If he had the thought that he would never get well, he would feel sad and hopeless.

The conception that the mood disorder in depression is secondary to the cognitive disorder is not new. Robert Burton, writing in the seventeenth century, quoted a number of writers from antiquity to the seventeenth century who held that the "afflictions of the mind" produced the affective disturbance. In 1602, Felix Platter described melancholia as "a kind of mental alienation, in which imagination and judgment are so perverted that without any cause the victims become very sad and fearful." (Diethelm and Hefferman, 1965). He emphasized that the whole illness "rests upon a foundation of false conceptions." (Jelliffe, 1931).

Among contemporary writers there has been an increasing emphasis on the role of cognitive processes in psychiatric disorders (Kelly, 1955; Harvey, Hunt, and Schroder, 1961; Ellis, 1962; Arieti, 1963). Ellis, within the framework of his concept of psychotherapy, stresses the primacy of irrational thinking in depression, anxiety reactions, and other neuroses.

In the moderate and severe depressions, in which the depressive feeling is constantly present, there may be some argument as to which comes first: the cognition or the affect. In my clinical studies I noted that changes in the intensity of the depressed feeling followed changes in the patient's cognition. This principle was borne out in a controlled experimental manipulation. We found that we were able to reduce or accentuate patients' negative affect by exposing them to situations in which they were induced to regard themselves as having succeeded or failed, respectively, in a task (Loeb *et al.*, 1964).

The following example is presented to illustrate the interplay of cognition and affect. A student was informed by a classmate that he had failed the final examination in one of his courses. He realized that he would fail the course as a consequence, and he felt discouraged and hopeless. Later, he checked his grade on the bulletin board and discovered that he had actually passed the examination. He verified that the initial information was incorrect, and his mood changed from sadness to jubilation. In this example, the relationship between the conceptualization of the experience and the consequent affect is clear-cut.

In the case of the depressed patient a similar consistency is found between the conceptualization and the affect. He perceives that he has failed or lost something of value, and he consequently feels sad or apathetic. The clinically-depressed patient differs from the example of the student who received false information about his grade—and this difference is crucial in distinguishing between normal and abnormal reactions—in that the source of his error is internal rather than external. The depressive's reaction is based on a faulty interpretation of the available data rather than on incorrect data. Sometimes, an event that precipitates a depression may indeed be noxious, but once the depressive machinery is in operation, neutral or even favorable events are processed in such a way as to produce a negative conclusion. The presentation of new information to correct this erroneous conclusion is subjected to the same distorting procedure, and consequently it frequently fails to change the patient's conceptualization. As the erroneous conceptualizations become more refractory to modification by external information, the negative mood becomes more intractable.

A wide range of unpleasant feelings has been reported by patients diagnosed as depressed. A careful scrutiny of the detailed descriptions of the feeling states indicate that these are not the same for all patients. Some complain of a sad feeling, which they liken to grief; some describe feelings of shame or humiliation; some emphasize a feeling of being bored. It is possible to establish a plausible connection between the experienced affect and the predominant cognitive pattern. A patient, for example, who believes he has lost his friends complains of feeling lonely. The patient who sees the future as bleak and hopeless emphasizes feelings of discouragement. The patient who perceives himself as constantly thwarted complains of feeling frustrated. The patient who believes he appears stupid or inept feels humiliated. The patient who regards his life as devoid of any possibility of gratification complains of feeling apathetic or bored.

CHANGES IN MOTIVATION

The motivational changes in depressed patients may be considered under four groupings: paralysis of the will, escapist and avoidance wishes, suicidal wishes, and intensified dependency wishes. The sequential relationship between cognition and motivation may be observed under two conditions. First, by knowing an individual's cognitions one can predict his motivation or lack of motivation. Second, by changing the cognition one can change the motivation.

The loss of spontaneous motivation, or paralysis of the will, has been considered a symptom *par excellence* of depression in the classical literature. The loss of motivation may be viewed as the result of the patient's hopelessness and pessimism: as long as he expects a negative outcome from any course of action, he is stripped of any internal stimulation to do anything. Conversely, when he is persuaded that a positive outcome may result from a particular endeavor, he may then experience an internal stimulus to pursue it.

An example may illustrate this point. I was searching for some way to induce a retarded, depressed woman to go to occupational therapy. When I first recommended this activity, she remained immobile. Then I suggested that she could make something pretty for her granddaughter, and that this would please her granddaughter. At this point, she became more animated and expressed a desire to start the project. She got up from her chair with some vigor. All at once, she slumped back, an expression of despair on her face. Questioned about her reaction, she told me that the following sequence had occurred: At first when she thought of pleasing her grandchild, she experienced a desire to work on the project. Then, she pictured herself making a mess of it. She then had an image of herself feeling humiliated and disappointed at the failure. Interestingly, she actually experienced the humiliated feeling while she was having the fantasy. Once she had fantasied this unfavorable outcome, she lost all desire to start the project and returned to her immobile position in the chair. Further questioning brought out her deep sense of futility: She felt that nothing she did could turn out right or could give her any satisfaction.

Avoidance and escapist wishes are similarly related to expectations of a negative outcome. A moderately depressed student had a strong desire to avoid studying. He felt that he would find the material dull and boring. I pointed out to him that he had always enjoyed studying this particular material once he became absorbed in it. When he could see the possibility of some gratification, he experienced a desire to study. With the change in his expectancy came a consequent change in his motivation.

Another patient wanted to stay home from work. He gave as his reason that the responsibilities at work were too great and that he would not be able to cope with them. As he thought of the things he had to do, he envisioned himself failing at each task. I suggested that we examine the specific responsibilities that he had to encounter that day and some of the problems that might arise. As the responsibilities were reviewed, the patient acknowledged that he had taken care of these many times in the past. We then discussed the difficult problems that might arise and I induced the patient to verbalize the steps he would take to solve them. Following this discussion, the patient changed from an expectation of being overwhelmed to an expectation that he would probably be able to handle things adequately. At this point his desire to escape from work was superseded by a desire to go to work.

The suicidal wishes may be regarded as an extreme expression of the desire to escape. The suicidal patient sees his future as filled with suffering. He cannot visualize any way of improving things. He does not believe it is possible to get better. Suicide under these conditions seems to the patient to be a rational solution. It promises an end to his own suffering and a relief of the supposed burden on his family. Once suicide appears as a reasonable alternative to living, the patient feels attracted to it. The more hopeless and painful his life seems, the stronger his desire to escape from that life.

The wish to escape from life via suicide because of suffering and hopelessness is illustrated in the following quotation from a patient who had been rejected by her boy friend. "There's no sense in living. There's nothing here for me. I need love and I don't have it any more. I can't be happy without love—only miserable. It will just be the same misery, day in and day out. It's senseless to go on."

The desire to escape from the apparent futility of his existence was expressed by another patient. "Life is just to go through another day. It doesn't make any sense. There's nothing here that can give me any satisfaction. The future isn't there. I just don't want life any more. I want to get out of here. It's stupid just to go on living."

Another false premise that underlies the suicidal wishes is the patient's belief that everybody would be better off if he were dead. Since he sees himself as worthless and as a burden, arguments that his family would be hurt if he died seem hollow. How can they suffer from losing a burden? One patient envisioned killing herself as doing her parents a favor. She would not only end her own suffering but would relieve them of psychological and financial responsibilities. "I'm just taking money from my parents. They could use it to better advantage. They wouldn't have to support me. My father wouldn't have to work so hard and they could travel. I'm unhappy taking their money and they could be happy with it."

In a number of cases, the suicidal wishes were ameliorated by examining the underlying premises and considering alternative solutions. A patient became depressed because he had lost his job. He said, "I want to shoot myself. Nobody thinks I'm capable of doing anything. I don't think so either. I'll never get another job. I don't have any friends or dates. I'm isolated. I'm just completely stuck for all time. If I shot myself, it could solve all my problems."

In this case, I had a detailed discussion with the patient of all the job opportunities which were available to him. His professional training was in high demand, and in the course of the discussions he was able to see many means of getting another position, e.g., through a placement bureau or an employment agency. His attitude that it would be impossible to get further employment changed to an expectation that he probably would get a job. Concurrently, his suicidal wishes disappeared.

The increased dependency that is so characteristic of many depressions may be attributed to a number of factors. The patient sees himself in negative terms—as being inept, inadequate, and undesirable. Furthermore, he tends to overestimate the complexity and difficulty of the normal details of living. In addition, he expects everything to turn out badly. Under these conditions, many depressed patients yearn for somebody strong to take care of them and to help them with their problems. They often tend to magnify the strength of the person on whom they are dependent. One woman who generally disparaged her husband when she was not depressed regarded him as a kind of superman when she was depressed.

As with the other motivations, I have found that the dependency wishes may be attenuated if the patient can view himself and his problems more objectively. As his self-esteem improves and he sees ways of coping with his problems, he feels less driven to seek help from others.

The relation between cognition and motivation has also been demonstrated in a controlled experimental situation. We found that patients who (as the result of the experimenter's manipulation of the degree of difficulty of an assigned task) viewed their performance on a task as inferior were less motivated to volunteer for a new experiment than those who believed their performance was superior.

PHYSICAL SYMPTOMS

The explanation of the physical and vegetative symptoms of depression in the framework of a psychological model presents certain difficulties. The introduction of physiological variables requires the mixing of different conceptual levels and entails the risk of confounding rather than clarifying the problem. Furthermore, whereas the patients' verbal material has been a rich source of information for establishing meaningful connections among the psychological variables, it has provided scanty data for determining psychophysiological relationships.

With these reservations in mind, I have attempted to relate the cognitive patterns to some of the physical correlates of depression, viz., retardation, fatigability, and agitation. The retarded patients that I have observed have generally expressed attitudes of passive resignation to their supposedly terrible fate. The attitude is expressed in such statements as "There's nothing I can do to save myself." In the most severe cases, such as the benign stupors, the patient may believe that he is already dead. In any event, the profound motor inhibition appears to be congruent with the patient's negative view of himself, his sense of futility, and his loss of spontaneous motivation. When I have been able to stimulate the patient's desire to do something (as described in the section on motivation), I found that the retardation became reduced or temporarily disappeared. Moreover, when the patient could entertain the idea of gaining some gratification from what he was doing, there was a reduction in the subjective sense of fatigue.

The influence of psychological factors on inertia, retardation, and fatigability in depression has been confirmed by several systematic studies. We found that when depressed patients are given a concrete task, such as the Digit-Symbol Substitution test, they mobilize sufficient motivation to perform as well as nondepressed patients of similar severity of illness (Chapter 10). Since this test is essentially a speed test, it should be particularly sensitive to psychomotor retardation. Similarly, Friedman (1964) found that depressed patients showed either no impairment or only minimal impairment when engaged in a variety of psychological tests.

The thought content of the agitated depression is congruent with the overt behavior. Unlike the retarded patient, the agitated patient does not accept his fate passively and does not believe that it is futile to try to save himself. He desperately seeks some way to ease his distress or escape from his problems. Since there is no apparent method for achieving this, his frantic search drives him into aimless motor activity such as pacing the floor, scratching his skin, or tearing his clothes. These behaviors reflect ideas such as "I can't stand this;" "I've got to do something;" or "I can't go on any longer this way." He also manifests these attitudes in his frenzied entreaties for help.

RELATIONSHIP TO OTHER DISORDERS

Psychiatric disorders other than depression also show an idiosyncratic thought content that is specific for the particular disorder. This holds true for the neuroses as well as the psychoses (Editorial, 1963). The cognitive patterns peculiar to the manic phase of the manic-depressive reaction have a content that is directly opposite to that observed in depression. It is possible, in fact, to delineate a *manic triad* that corresponds to the depressive triad. The manic triad consists of an unrealistically *positive* view of the world, of the self, and of the future. The affective and motivational characteristics of the manic phase may be viewed as a consequence of the operation of these cognitive patterns.

The relationship between the depressive and manic phases may be illustrated by the following case history. A 40-year-old man was admitted to the hospital following a serious suicidal attempt. At the time of admission to the hospital, he believed the following: He thought that his friends and relatives had contempt for him, and that everybody in the hospital disliked him. He attributed their low opinion of him to his personal deficiencies and worthlessness. He considered himself lacking in character and ability. He anticipated that nothing would ever improve for him and that he would fail miserably in anything he undertook. He felt sad, discouraged, and fatigued, and had no spontaneous desire to do anything. Continuous observation indicated that he appeared generally retarded in his speech and movements.

On the tenth day of hospitalization, there was a dramatic change in his behavior. He began to show typical manic symptoms—excessive volubility, overactivity, and excessive cheerfulness. His thought content showed the following themes: He believed that he was popular among the patients and that the ward personnel admired him for his helpfulness, ability, and wit. He believed that he had an unusual insight into other patients' problems which enabled him to cure them. He expressed the opinion that he was a deeply religious man who could inspire others by his example. He planned to devote his life to helping psychiatric patients and foresaw a future of happiness from being of service to others.

The various affective and motivational reactions of this patient may be attributed to the change in his cognitive patterning. His euphoria stemmed from his positive evaluations of himself and his expectations of future achievement and happiness. His greatly increased drive, energy, and activity may similarly be attributed to his positive view of himself and his expectations of success.

When the specific cognitive content of depression is compared with that of other disorders, it is found that although there are some similarities, there are important differences. For instance, the typical paranoid patient may believe that other people dislike him (negative view of the world). He tends, however, to blame others for those negative reactions and maintains a favorable view of himself. He regards the others as unfair and unjustified in their supposed mistreatment of him. His affect is in accord with this conceptualization—viz., anger.

In anxiety reactions, there is an anticipation of future unpleasantness that is similar to that seen in depressions (negative expectations of the future). As was pointed out previously, however, the depressed patient sees himself as already damaged, and his view of the future is essentially a reproduction of his image of the present. The anxious patient, on the other hand, anticipates certain potentially harmful experiences but is able to maintain a positive self-regard. Also, unlike the depressed patients, he is capable of anticipating that certain experiences in the future might be pleasant, and that at least some of his endeavors would have a favorable outcome.

Some patients may show two components of the depressive triad but not the third. They consequently may experience a few of the typical symptoms of depression but not enough to warrant the diagnosis of clinical depression. One woman, ordinarily energetic and optimistic, complained of an overwhelming feeling of lassitude and fatigability of many months' duration. She felt so exhausted that she spent most of the day in bed and engaged in minimal physical activity. On interview, the following data were elicited. She saw herself as burdened with insoluble problems: an egocentric husband, who made great demands on her but was insensitive to her needs, and a variety of household difficulties (negative view of the world). She could not see any way out of this difficult situation (negative view of the future). She was able, however, to maintain a positive view of herself, and in fact, attributed her difficulties to shortcomings in her husband. In the course of her brief psychotherapy some of the household problems were solved, and she was able to establish a more effective working relationship with her husband. At this point, her negative view of her home and of her marriage dissolved, and with it went her extreme feelings of fatigue. She once again was outgoing, cheerful, and energetic.

Other patients may manifest a negative self-concept and may tend to interpret their current experiences negatively but still maintain a positive view of the future. These patients feel sad but at the same time look forward to an improvement in their lot, and consequently are motivated to keep trying. In other words, they show some of the affective symptoms, but do not experience the motivational or physical symptoms associated with depression. Hence, they would not be diagnosed as depressed.

The psychiatric conditions described above show distorted conceptualizations. These distortions constitute one aspect of a thinking disorder. The term "thinking disorder," as commonly used, generally encompasses, in addition to cognitive distortions, broad areas of impairment that Bleuler described under the term "loosening of associations." Factor analytic studies of the verbal behavior of patients have indicated the presence of two independent factors (Overall and Gorham, 1961). One factor, related to disruption of the formal thought processes, includes such characteristics as irrelevant responses, disconnected ideas, vagueness, and peculiar word usage or syntax. This factor, which could be labelled "conceptual disorganization," is characteristic of schizophrenia. The second factor appears to be related to a distortion of thought content rather than to the disorganization of thought. This second factor appears to be characteristic of neuroses as well as psychoses and is related to the cognitive triad described in this chapter.

A COGNITIVE CLASSIFICATION OF PSYCHIATRIC DISORDERS

A thinking disorder is by no means limited to depression, but is a general characteristic of psychopathology. A sharp delineation of the specific content of the thinking disorder can help in making a differential diagnosis among the various psychiatric disorders. In addition, a careful assessment of the degree of cognitive impairment can help distinguish neurosis from psychosis.

NEUROSES

For the most part, the neuroses may be differentiated on the basis of the thought content. In some cases, additional characteristics are important; for example, whether a specific situation is necessary to produce a symptom, as in the case of phobic reaction, or whether abnormal behavior is a basic criterion, as in the compulsions (See Table 17–1).

Table 17–1.

NEUROTIC AND ALLIED DISORDERS DIFFERENTIATED ACCORDING TO COGNITIVE CONTENT

Reaction	*Idiosyncratic ideational content*
Depressive	Negative concept of self, world, and future
Hypomanic	Exaggerated positive concept of self, world, and future
Anxiety	Concept of personal danger
Phobic	Danger connected with specific, avoidable situations
Conversion (hysterical)	Concept of motor or sensory abnormality
Paranoid	Concept of abuse, persecution, injustice
Obsessive	Repetitive thought, usually a warning or doubting
Compulsive	Self-command to perform a specific act to allay obsessive doubting

Depressive Reaction

The thought content is concerned with ideas of personal deficiency, impossible environmental demands and obstacles, and nihilistic expectations. As a result, the patient experiences sadness, loss of motivation, suicidal wishes, and agitation or retardation.

Hypomanic Reaction

The thought content is opposite that of depression. The dominant cognitive patterns are exaggerated ideas of personal abilities, minimization of external obstacles, and overly optimistic expectations. These patterns lead to euphoria, to increased drive, and to overactivity.

Anxiety Reaction

The ideational content is dominated by themes of personal danger. In contrast to the phobic, who experiences a sense of danger only in specific, avoidable situations, the anxiety neurotic perceives danger continuously and, consequently, is continuously anxious.

The danger may be perceived as internal: A patient with an irritable colon had unremitting anxiety because of his idea that he might have cancer. The stimuli may be external: A patient interpreted every loud sound as a signal of catastrophe. A siren meant her house was on fire, an automobile backfiring indicated somebody shooting at her, and the noise of an airplane suggested an atomic attack. Another patient was constantly in dread of being rejected by members of her family, friends, and even strangers; she consequently had continuous anxiety.

Phobic Reaction

The phobic patient expects some physical or psychological injury in certain defined situations. If he avoids these situations, the danger is averted and he is tranquil. When exposed to the stimulus situation, he reacts with all the typical signs and symptoms of the anxiety neurotic.

The cognitive reaction to the phobic situation may be expressed in purely verbal form on in the form of imagery. A patient with a bridge phobia would have the thought, "The bridge is going to collapse." Another patient would get a visual image of the bridge collapsing and of himself drowning.

Some of the typical cognitions in the common phobic situations are: elevators—"I am starting to suffocate;" high places—"I might jump off," "I may fall off," or "It may collapse;" tunnels—"The walls may cave in," or "I don't have enough air;" boats—"It is starting to sink and I'll drown."

Conversion Reaction

In conversion (hysterical) reactions, the patient erroneously believes that he has a particular physical disorder. As a result of this belief, he experiences sensory and/or motor abnormalities that are consistent with his faulty conception of organic pathology. His symptoms are manifestations of the particular idea and are often at variance with those produced by an actual lesion.

Charcot (1890) cited the case of a patient involved in a street accident who believed (erroneously) that a carriage had run over both legs. He subsequently developed hysterical paralysis of both legs. Sometimes, the symptom is based on an incorrect diagnosis by the patient of an actual lesion. A soldier sustained a bullet wound in his leg and subsequently developed a "stocking" anesthesia: He believed the bullet had severed a nerve in his leg. When it was demonstrated to him that the nerve was intact, his anesthesia began to disappear. Patients with hysterical motor paralyses believe that a part of the body is paralyzed and therefore do not try to move it: The patient, in fact, often resists attempts by the examiner to move the "paralyzed" part.

It is possible to demonstrate that not only the hysterical sensory and motor paralyses but also the hyperalgesias and hyperkinetic reactions are based on an erroneous idea of physical pathology. When the erroneous idea is undermined through suggestion, hypnosis, or re-education, the symptom disappears.

Paranoid Reaction

The cardinal feature of the paranoid reaction is the misinterpretation of experience in terms of mistreatment, abuse, or persecution: A patient hears people whispering and he has the thought that they are jealous of him and are saying degrading things about him. A student gets a low grade on an exam and he immediately thinks the teacher was biased.

The anxious paranoid does not feel capable of coping with the sinister behavior of others. He feels the threat is too overwhelming and he wants to flee. The hostile paranoid, on the other hand, experiences anger rather than anxiety because he does not feel helpless in the face of the apparent discrimination or injustice. He wants to fight back against the persecutors and protect his rights.

Obsessions and Compulsions

The obsessions may be defined as recurrent thoughts having the same or similar content. The content is usually concerned with some risk or danger expressed in the form of a doubt or a warning: "Did I turn off the gas in the oven?" "Will I be able to speak?" "Perhaps I got some disease from the dirt," "My eyeglasses are on crooked," "I may get a speck in my eye."

Compulsions are based on obsessions, and represent attempts to allay the obsessive doubts or worries through action. A patient with a hand-washing compulsion would get the thought after each handwashing ritual, "I didn't get all the dirt off." Another patient with the obsession that he looked odd to other people would compulsively turn his head away when anybody approached. Another patient would count to nine each time he had a thought that something terrible would happen to his family; the number represented a magical device for averting disaster.

PSYCHOSES

The thought content of the psychoses is similar to that of the neuroses. The themes in the cognitive distortions of psychotic depressive reaction parallel those of neurotic depressive reaction; manic reaction parallels hypomanic; paranoia or paranoid schizophrenic reaction parallels the paranoid state. Although the general themes in neuroses and psychoses may be similar, the specific content is often more extreme or more improbable in the psychoses. A neurotic depressive may view himself as a sinner or as socially undesirable; the psychotic depressive believes he is the devil or that he emanates disgusting odors.

The major difference between neurosis as a class and psychosis as a class is the presence of more pronounced cognitive impairment in the latter. The erroneous ideas are more intense, more compelling, and more impermeable. The conceptual errors (arbitrary inference, selective abstraction, and overgeneralization) are more frequent and more extreme. On the one hand, the distortions are more fixed while on the other, the patient's ability to view them objectively is impaired. In short, the patient has a delusion.

Schizophrenic reaction may be distinguished from the other psychoses by the disruption of formal thought processes. As mentioned previously, Overall and Gorham (1961) attached the label "conceptual disorganization" to the factor characterized by irrelevant, vague, disconnected, or peculiarly formed verbal responses. On the basis of the content of his cognitive distortions, a patient is diagnosed as having psychotic depressive reaction, manic reaction, or paranoia; if conceptual disorganization is present, then the diagnosis is schizo-affective reaction or paranoid schizophrenic reaction. If there is conceptual disorganization without any consistent distortion, then the diagnosis is schizophrenic reaction, simple type.

SUMMARY

I have attempted to clarify the relationships among the variegated phenomena of depression: cognitive, affective, motivational, and physical. A primary factor appears to be the activation of idiosyncratic cognitive patterns which divert the thinking into specific channels that deviate from reality. As a result, the patient perseverates in making negative judgments and misinterpretations. These distortions may be categorized within the triad of negative interpretations of experience; negative evaluations of the self; and negative expectations of the future.

The cognitive distortions lead to the affective and motivational symptoms that are characteristic of depression. The misinterpretation of experience in terms of deprivation leads to sadness, just as in the case of an actual deprivation. Unrealistic negative expectations lead to hopelessness, just as do reality-based expectations. Similarly, the negative view of the world, of the self, and of the future strip the patient of any positive desires and stimulate desires to avoid the apparent unpleasantness, intensify dependency wishes, and evoke wishes to find an escape route via suicide.

Some of the physical symptoms of the depressed patient may be ascribed to the way he structures his experiences. Retardation may be regarded as the outcome of his passive resignation, his sense of futility, and his loss of spontaneous motivation. Agitation, on the other hand, appears to be related to the patient's frantic desire to fight his way out of a situation he regards as desperate.

The differential diagnosis of the psychiatric disorders may be sharpened by using the cognitive content and the degree of impairment as diagnostic criteria. Depression, mania, anxiety reaction, conversion reaction, and paranoid reaction may be diagnosed, respectively, according to themes of self-deflation, self-enhancement, danger, motor or sensory abnormality, and persecution. Psychosis is distinguished from neurosis on the basis of more severe cognitive impairment. Schizophrenic reaction is distinguished from other psychotic reactions on the basis of conceptual disorganization.

Chapter 18.
Development of Depression

PREDISPOSITION TO DEPRESSION

Formation of Permanent Concepts

Early in his life, an individual develops a wide variety of concepts and attitudes about himself and his world. Some of these concepts are anchored to reality and form the basis for a healthy personal adjustment. Others deviate from reality and produce vulnerability to possible psychological disorders.

An individual's concepts—realistic as well as unrealistic—are drawn from his experiences, from the attitudes and opinions communicated to him by others, and from his identifications. Among the concepts that are central in the pathogenesis of depression are the individual's attitudes towards himself, his environment, and his future. Since the formulation of all three types of concept is similar, that of the self-concepts can serve as a pattern for the other two.

The individual's self-concepts are clusters of attitudes about himself, some are favorable and others are unfavorable. These clusters consist of generalizations he has made on the basis of his interactions with his environment. He derives his self-concepts from his personal experiences, from others' judgments of him, and from his identifications with key figures such as parents, siblings, and friends.

Once a particular attitude or concept has been formed, it can influence subsequent judgments and become more firmly set. For instance, a child who gets the notion that he is inept, as a result of either a failure or of being called inept by somebody else, may interpret subsequent experiences according to this notion. Each time thereafter that he encounters difficulties in manual tasks he may have a tendency to judge himself as inept. Each negative judgment tends to reinforce the negative concept or self-image. Thus, a cycle is set up: Each negative judgment fortifies the negative self-image which in turn facilitates a negative interpretation of subsequent experiences which further consolidates the negative self-concept.

Unless this negative image is extinguished, it becomes structuralized, i.e., it becomes a permanent formation in the cognitive organization. Once a concept is structuralized, it remains permanently with the individual even though it may be dormant; it becomes a cognitive structure, or *schema*.

Among the positive (or self-enhancing) self-concepts are such attitudes as "I am capable," "I am attractive," "I can get what I want," "I can understand problems and solve them." Examples of negative (or self-diminishing) self-concepts are "I am weak," "I am inferior," "I am unlovable," and "I can't do anything right." These negative self-concepts emerge with great force in depression.

The nuclei of positive and negative self-concepts determine the direction of an individual's self-esteem. When the positive self-concepts are activated, the individual regards himself more favorably; i.e., he experiences an increase in the self-esteem. Activation of the negative self-concepts lowers the self-esteem. The role of an individual's self-esteem is regarded by Jacobson (1953) and Bibring (1953) as being of central importance in depression.

VALUE JUDGMENTS AND AFFECT

Of pertinence in the predisposition to depression are the value judgments or connotations attached to the self-concepts. When an individual makes negative generalizations about himself, such as he is inept, unpopular, or dull, he is prone to regard these attributes as bad, unworthy, or undesirable. He may extend his dislike for the particular trait to a dislike of himself; he moves from a specific rejection of the trait to a global rejection of himself.

Concepts such as good and bad are "superordinate constructs" (Kelly, 1955). A specific attribute may not be regarded initially as either good or bad but may, as the result of social learning, be organized under such a superordinate construct. Subsequently, when the person judges himself as "inept," the connotation of "bad" automatically accompanies the judgment.

Constructs such as "bad" or "undesirable" seem to be closely linked to affective responses. When an individual perceives himself as bad or undesirable he is likely to experience an unpleasant feeling such as sadness. On the other hand, when he views himself positively as admirable or desirable, he experiences a pleasant affect. Once the pathways between a certain concept such as "I am inept" and the negative affect have been established, the patient experiences the unpleasant affect each time he makes the negative judgment of himself. Similar interconnections are established between cognitions such as "Things never work out for me" or "I will never get what I want" and affects such as discouragement and hopelessness.

Specific Vulnerability

The vulnerability of the depression-prone person is attributable to the constellation of enduring negative attitudes about himself, about the world, and about his future. Even though these attitudes (or concepts) may not be prominent or even discernible at a given time, they persist in a latent state like an explosive charge ready to be detonated by an appropriate set of conditions. Once activated, these concepts dominate the person's thinking and lead to the typical depressive symptomatology.

The specific depressive constellation is composed of a network of interrelated negative attitudes. One group of attitudes consists of negative generalizations about the self such as "I am dumb," "People don't like me," "I'm a weakling," and "I don't have any personality." These generalizations are connected to negative attitudes about the attributes, such as "It's terrible to be stupid" or "It's disgusting to be weak." Hence, the linkage of the self-concept to the negative value judgment produces attitudes such as "I'm no good because I'm weak," or "I'm nothing because I'm unattractive."

In order for a negative self-concept to be pathogenic it must be associated with a negative value judgment. Not all people who regard themselves as physically, mentally, or socially deficient consider these traits bad nor are repelled by them. I have interviewed several intellectually and physically handicapped people who do not attach a negative value to their disabilities and who have never shown any depressive tendencies. Furthermore, some individuals with traits that are distasteful to most people may admire themselves for that trait, e.g., the juvenile delinquent who takes pride in being bad.

The concept of self-blame is another component of the predepressive constellation. According to his primitive notion of causality, the individual holds himself responsible for his defects and presumed deficiencies. This attitude is expressed as follows: "It's my own fault I always make mistakes. I'm to blame for being so weak."

Another group of attitudes in the predepressive constellation revolves around the theme of negative expectations. The pessimistic view of the future is expressed in attitudes such as "Things will never get any better for me." "I will always be weak and get pushed around." "I'm basically unlucky and always will be." When these attitudes are mobilized, they produce the feeling of hopelessness characteristic of depression. Many individuals confronted with adversity face the future with equanimity and are not gripped by negative attitudes about the future. Many patients with chronic or fatal medical illnesses are optimistic about the future, in contrast to manic-depressive patients, who have a good prognosis for recovery, but who uniformly expect to remain ill (Cassidy, Flanagan, and Spellman, 1957).

When all the components of the depressive constellation are activated, a sequence such as the following occurs: The individual interprets an experience as representing a personal defeat or thwarting; he attributes this defeat to some defect in himself; he regards himself as worthless for having this trait; he blames himself for having acquired the trait and dislikes himself for it; and since he regards the trait as an intrinsic part of him, he sees no hope of changing and views the future as devoid of any satisfaction or filled with pain.

PRECIPITATION OF DEPRESSION

An individual who has incorporated the constellation of attitudes just described has the necessary predisposition for the development of clinical depression in adolescence or adulthood. Whether he will ever become depressed depends on whether the necessary conditions are present at a given time to activate the depressive constellation.

SPECIFIC STRESS

In childhood and adolescence, the depression-prone individual becomes sensitized to certain types of life situations. The traumatic situations initially responsible for embedding or reinforcing the negative attitudes that comprise the depressive constellation are the prototypes of the specific stresses that may later activate these constellations. When a person is subjected to situations reminiscent of the original traumatic experiences, he may then become depressed. The process may be likened to conditioning in which a particular response is linked to a specific stimulus; once the chain has been formed, stimuli similar to the original stimulus may evoke the conditioned response.

The association of stimulus situation and response may be illustrated by the following: A successful businessman stated that he had always felt inferior to his classmates who came from prosperous families because he was from a poor family. He always felt distinctly different and unacceptable. When, as an adult, he was with people wealthier than he, this caused him to have thoughts that he did not belong, that he wasn't as good as the others, and that he was a social outcast. These ideas were associated with transient feelings of sadness. At one point in his career, he was elected to the board of directors of a corporation. He viewed the other directors as coming from the "right side of the tracks" and himself as from "the wrong side." He felt he could not measure up to the other directors and slipped into a depression lasting several days.

Situations that might be expected to lower an individual's self-esteem are frequent precipitators of depression. Some that I have observed in clinical practice include failing an examination, being jilted by a lover, being rejected by a fraternity, and being fired from a job.

Another type of situation that may precipitate a depression is one involving a thwarting of important goals or posing an insoluble dilemma. A man became depressed when his summons to military service forced him to relinquish his plans to enter medical school. A soldier assigned to duty in a remote portion of Canada, confronted with the prospect of an unlimited period of time devoid of any satisfactions, slipped into a depression. A girl was trapped between her fiancé, who insisted that they get married or break the engagement, and her parents, who adamantly refused to give their permission for the marriage; she reacted by feeling hopeless and suicidal.

Sometimes the precipitating event is a physical disease or an abnormality that activates ideas of physical deterioration and death. A woman observed a red coloration in her urine and developed the idea that she had cancer. Despite reassurances by her physicians after an exhaustive series of tests, she became more convinced that she had cancer and became increasingly depressed. She anticipated steady deterioration and felt she was worthless and a burden to everyone.

Another woman developed mild arthritis. She saw it as a disabling illness and visualized herself as completely bedridden. She predicted a hemmed-in, pleasureless existence for herself and she became increasingly hopeless and agitated.

These circumstances might produce feelings of pain or frustration in most people but they would not cause a depression. A person must be peculiarly sensitive to the situation and must have a predepressive constellation to react with a clinical depression. A nondepressive person who has experienced a trauma such as a financial reversal or the news that he has a chronic illness may still be able to maintain his interest in all aspects of life. The depression-prone person, on the other hand, experiences a *constriction of his cognitive field* and he is bombarded by negative self-judgments and negative ideas about the future.

I have noticed that the depression often seems to arise from a *series* of stressful situations that impinge on the specific vulnerability rather than from a single situation. A number of blows in rapid succession to the sensitive areas may be sufficient to exceed the patient's tolerance, although he might be able to absorb a single trauma.

One of the problems in assessing the contribution of external factors to the precipitation of depression is that these factors are often insidious. The patient may not be aware of their operation, and may pass through several depressive episodes without identifying the pairing of the depression with a recurrent set of traumatic conditions. One woman experienced depressions on three consecutive summers. These started in July and August and did not begin to subside until the end of September. It was not until the third episode that I ascertained that each depression began about five weeks after her son came home from college for a summer vacation. It was then established that her son had a contemptuous attitude towards her and that, without her realization, constantly undermined her self-esteem. His incessant but subtle grinding away at her slid her into a depression which persisted until he returned to school.

NONSPECIFIC STRESS

An individual may develop some form of psychological disturbance when exposed to any overwhelming stress, even if it does not strike at the specific sensitivity. A woman became depressed when her husband and all her children were killed in an automobile accident. A man was precipitated into a depression when he was wrongfully accused of a crime and discharged from his job as a result of the notoriety.

Sometimes a depression is precipitated, not by a single overwhelming incident, but by a series of traumatic events. A law professor was able to maintain his equilibrium even after being passed over for a promotion he felt he deserved and after losing his most important court case but when he discovered that his wife was having an affair, however, he was unable to ward off his feelings of despair and slipped into a depression.

These nonspecific stress situations do not necessarily produce depression. Other types of pathological reaction may be produced, depending on the specific predispositions of a particular person. Other individuals subjected to the same traumatic situations might have totally different disturbances such as paranoid reactions, anxiety reactions, or psychosomatic disorders—or no psychiatric disorder at all.

OTHER CONTRIBUTING FACTORS

The predispositional and precipitating factors probably do not include all the conditions necessary for the development of depression. It is likely that there are other, not readily identifiable, contributing factors.

One such factor I call *psychological strain.* I have observed that a number of patients who have been overtaxed or overstimulated for long periods are especially susceptible to specific stress. The same patients, on the other hand, can sustain the same stress if it comes at a time when they have not been strained.

PERSONALITY ORGANIZATION IN DEPRESSION

In the preceding discussion, the characteristics of depression have been described primarily in terms of phenomena introspectively identified by the patient and reported to the investigator. Constructs such as self-concept and specific sensitivities are *close to the data,* i.e., they are easily inferred from the clinical material and do not represent a high level of abstraction.

There are a number of questions still unanswered. How does the peculiar depressive thinking become dominant? Why does the depressed patient cling so tenaciously to his painful ideas, even when he is confronted with contradictory evidence? What is the relationship between thinking and affect?

To answer these questions, it is necessary to provide more abstract and more speculative formulations. The theory I will present in this section deals with entities (hypothetical constructs) not experienced by the patient as such, but whose existence is postulated to account for the regularities and predictabilities in his behavior. These hypothetical constructs include cognitive structures and energy. The formulations are not intended to present a comprehensive explanation of depression, but will be limited to a few broad areas in which the relevant clinical material was adequate to warrant a formal theoretical exposition.

LITERATURE ON COGNITIVE ORGANIZATIONS

The study of cognitive systems has received increasing attention during the past 15 years. The relevant psychoanalytic literature, particularly in the area of ego psychology, has been systematically reviewed and integrated by Rapaport (1951). The contemporary psychological literature on cognition has been more diverse, as indicated by the disparate approaches of writers such as Allport (1955), Bruner, Goodnow, and Austin (1956), Festinger (1957), Osgood (1957), Sarbin, Taft, and Bailey (1960), Harvey, Hunt, and Schroder (1961), and Ellis (1962).

There has been a notable lag in applying the structural concepts generated by studies of normal thinking to the thinking disorder associated with various psychiatric syndromes. There have been few attempts to formulate the particular cognitive organizations in these syndromes. A number of clinicians, however, have provided constructs that, although not explicitly defined as such, have the earmarks of cognitive structures. Among these are Freud's conceptualizations of the primary and secondary processes (1938), Horney's concept of the self image (1945), Rogers' formulation of the self concept (1951), Kelly's theory of personal constructs (1955), and Ellis's concept of self-verbalizations. Harvey, Hunt, and Schroder have presented the most complete model of the conceptual systems in specific forms of psychopathology, including depression.

DEFINITION OF SCHEMAS

In conceptualizing any life situation composed of a kaleidoscopic array of stimuli, an individual has a number of alternatives as to which aspects of the situation he extracts and how he combines them into a coherent pattern. Different people react differently to specific complex situations and may reach quite dissimilar conclusions.

A particular individual, moreover, tends to show consistencies in the way he responds to similar types of events. In many instances these habitual responses may be a general characteristic of individuals in his culture; in other instances they may represent a relatively idiosyncratic type of response derived from experiences peculiar to him. In any event, stereotyped or repetitive patterns of conceptualizing may be regarded as manifestations of cognitive organizations or structures.

A cognitive *structure* is a relatively enduring component of the cognitive organization, in contrast to a cognitive *process*, which is transient. Cognitive structures have been postulated by a number of writers to account for the observed regularities in cognitive behavior. Piaget's "schemas" (1948), Rapaport's "conceptual tools" (1951), Postman's "categories" (1951), Kelly's "personal constructs" (1955), Bruner's "coding systems" (Bruner, Goodnow, and Austin, 1956), Sarbin's "modules," (Sarbin, Taft, and Bailey, 1960) and Harvey's "concepts" (Harvey, Hunt and Schroder, 1961) are examples of such postulated structures.

In the present formulation I employ the term *schema* to designate a cognitive structure because of its relatively greater usage and familiarity than other terms. A cognitive schema has been defined by English and English (1958) as "the complex pattern, inferred as having been imprinted in the organismic structure by experience, that combines with the properties of the presented stimulus object or of the presented idea to determine how the object or idea is to be perceived and conceptualized." The term is broad and has been applied both to small patterns involved in relatively discrete and concrete conceptualizations such as identifying a shoe, and to large, global patterns such as ethnocentric prejudice (which causes one to regard the behavior of persons from another social group in an unfavorable way.) In this discussion, the focus is on the broader, more complex schemas such as the self-concepts and constellations described earlier in this chapter.

A schema is a structure for screening, coding, and evaluating the stimuli that impinge on the organism. It is the mode by which the environment is broken down and organized into its many psychologically relevant facets. On the basis of the matrix of schemas, the individual is able to orient himself in relation to time and space and to categorize and interpret his experiences in a meaningful way. (Harvey, Hunt, and Schroder, 1961). The schemas channel thought processes irrespective of whether they are stimulated by the immediate environmental situation. When a particular set of stimuli impinge on the individual a schema relevant to these stimuli is activated. The schema condenses and molds the raw data into cognitions. A cognition, in the present usage, refers to any mental activity which has a verbal content; hence, it includes not only ideas and judgments but also self-instructions, self-criticisms, and verbally-articulated wishes. In the formation of a cognition, the schema provides the conceptual framework and the particular details are filled in by the external stimuli.

Cognitive activity may proceed independently of immediate external events. The schemas pattern the stream of associations and ruminations as well as the cognitive responses to external stimuli. Hence, the notion of schemas is utilized to account for the repetitive themes in free associations, daydreams, ruminations, and dreams, as well as in the immediate reactions to environmental events.

When a verbal response consists of labelling a discrete configuration such as a shoe, the particular schema utilized may be a simple linguistic category. A more abstract conceptualization, as an individual's judgment of other people's attitudes towards him, involves a more complicated schema. Schemas include not only complex taxonomic systems for classifying stimuli, but also structuralized logical elements, consisting of premises, assumptions, and even fully developed syllogisms. An individual who, for example, has the notion that everybody hates him will tend to interpret other people's reactions on the basis of this premise. Schemas such as these are involved in the inaccuracies, misinterpretations, and distortions associated with all kinds of psychopathology.

The schemas have a content that corresponds to the constellations previously described. But since schemas are structures, they are also characterized by other qualities, such as flexibility-inflexibility, openness-closedness, permeability-impermeability, and concreteness-abstractness. They may be inactive at a given time and have no effect on the thought process, but they become active when energized and they remain active as long as they carry a specific quantity of energy. A specific schema can be energized or de-energized rapidly as a result of changes in the type of input from the environment.

Identification of Schemas

The most striking characteristic of the schemas is their content. The content is usually in the form of a generalization corresponding to the individual's attitudes, goals, values, and conceptions. The content of the idiosyncratic schemas found in psychopathology is reflected in the typical chronic misconceptions, distorted attitudes, invalid premises, and unrealistic goals and expectations.

Their content may be inferred: from an analysis of the individual's characteristic ways of structuring specific kinds of experiences; from the recurrent themes in his free associations, his ruminations, and his reveries; from the characteristic thematic content of his dreams; from direct questioning about his attitudes, prejudices, superstitions, and expectations; and from his responses to psychological tests designed to pinpoint his stereotyped conceptions of himself and his world.

How the clinician may obtain an idea of the content of a schema is illustrated in the following example. A highly intelligent patient reported that whenever she was given a problem to solve her immediate thought was, "I'm not smart enough to do it." During psychotherapy interviews, she frequently experienced the same type of reaction, as, for example, when she was asked for associations to a dream. Her free-associations showed the same theme, i.e., of not being smart. A scrutiny of her history revealed that her self-devaluation was a pattern occurring repeatedly throughout her life. Its incongruity was borne out by the fact that she was unusually successful in solving problems. When asked directly about her concept of her own intelligence, she replied that, although all the evidence indicated she was very bright, she "really believed" she was stupid. In the manifest content of her dreams she frequently appeared as stupid, inept, and unsuccessful.

In analyzing this clinical material, it may be concluded that one of the patient's characteristic modes of organizing her experiences was in terms of the notion, "I am stupid." This idea corresponds to a specific schema, which was evoked repetitively and inappropriately in response to situations relevant to her intellectual ability.

SCHEMAS IN DEPRESSION

A depressed person's ideation is tinged with certain typically depressive themes. His interpretation of his experiences, his explanation for their occurrence, and his outlook for the future, show respectively, themes of personal deficiency, of self-blame, and of negative expectations. These idiosyncratic themes pervade not only his interpretations of immediate environmental situations but also his free associations, his ruminations, and his reflections.

As the depression deepens, his thought content becomes increasingly saturated with depressive ideas. Almost any external stimulus is capable of evoking a depressive thought. There may be no logical connection between the interpretation and the actual situation. The patient reaches negative conclusions about himself based on the most scanty data, and shapes his judgments and interpretations according to his idiosyncratic preconceptions. As his distortion and misinterpretation of reality increases, his self-objectivity decreases.

This cognitive impairment may be analyzed in terms of the proposition that in depression specific idiosyncratic schemas assume a dominant role in shaping the thought processes. These schemas, relatively inactive during the nondepressed period, become progressively more potent as the depression develops. Their influence is reflected in characteristic disturbances in the patient's thinking.

Distortion and Misinterpretation

The depressed patient shows certain patterns of illogical thought. The systematic errors, leading to distortions of reality, include arbitrary interpretation, selective abstraction, overgeneralization, exaggeration, and incorrect labelling (Chapter 15). The deviant thinking may be understood in terms of the hyperactivity of the idiosyncratic schemas.

When one attempts to predict the response to a stimulus situation, it is apparent that there are a variety of ways in which the situation may be construed. Which construction is made depends on which schema is selected to provide the framework for the conceptualization. The specific steps of abstraction, synthesis, and interpretation of the stimuli depend on the specific schemas activated. Normally, a matching process occurs, so that a schema evoked by a particular external configuration is congruent with it. In such a case, although a certain amount of variation may occur from one individual to another, the cognition resulting from the interaction of the schema with the stimuli may be expected to be a reasonably accurate (veridical) representation of reality. In depression and in other types of psychopathology, however, the orderly matching of stimulus and schema is upset by the intrusion of the hyperactive idiosyncratic schemas. Because of their greater strength these schemas displace the more appropriate schemas and the resulting interpretations deviate from reality to a degree corresponding with the incongruity of the schema to the stimulus situation.

As these schemas become more active they are capable of being evoked by stimuli less congruent with them ("stimulus generalization"). Only those details of the stimulus situation compatible with the schema are abstracted, and these are reorganized in such a way as to make them congruent with the schema. In other words, instead of a schema being selected to fit the external details, the details are selectively extracted and molded to fit the schema.

Perseveration

The moderately or severely depressed patient has a tendency to brood or ruminate over a few characteristic ideas such as "I'm a failure," or "my bowels are blocked up." These repetitive ideas are generally the same as those cognitive responses to external situations described in the previous section. The idiosyncratic schemas continually grind out the depressive cognitions that crowd out the nondepressive cognitions.

As the depression progresses, the patient loses control over his thinking processes, i.e., even when he tries to focus on other subjects, the depressive cognitions continue to intrude and to occupy a central position. Furthermore, he is unable to suppress these thoughts or to be more than momentarily distracted from them. The depressive schema is so potent that the patient is unable to energize other schemas sufficiently to offset its dominance.

Loss of Objectivity

In the milder stages of depression, the patient is able to regard his negative thoughts with objectivity and, if not able to reject them completely, he is able to modify them. He can, for instance, change the idea, "I'm a complete failure" to "I may have failed at a lot of things but I also succeeded at a lot of things."

In the more severe stages, the patient has difficulty in even considering the possibility that his ideas or interpretations might be erroneous. He finds it difficult or impossible to consider contradictory evidence or alternative explanations. The idiosyncratic schema may be so strong as to interfere with recalling any events that might be inconsistent with it.

A highly successful research scientist had a chronic attitude, "I am a complete failure." His free associations were largely concerned with thoughts of how inferior, inadequate, and unsuccessful he was. When questioned regarding past performance, he was unable to recall a *single experience* that did not constitute a failure to him.

In this case, a schema with a content such as "I am a failure" worked over the raw material of his experiences and distorted the data to make it compatible with this content. Whether the particular cognitive process was recollection, or evaluation of his current status, or prediction of the future, his thoughts bore the imprint of this schema.

The loss of objectivity and reality-testing perhaps may be understood in terms of the hyperactivity of the depressive schemas. The energy attached to those schemas is substantially greater than that possessed by other structures in the cognitive organization. Hence, the idiosyncratic schemas tend to interfere with the operation of the cognitive structures involved in reasoning and reality-testing.

The cognitions produced by the hyperactive idiosyncratic schema are exceptionally compelling, vivid, and plausible. The nondepressive cognitions tend to be relatively faint in comparison with the depressive cognitions. In scanning the various possible interpretations of a situation, the individual is affected by the idea with greatest intensity rather than by that which is most realistic.

In severe cases, the cognitive processes may be likened to the situation during dreaming. When an individual is dreaming, the imagery of the dream totally occupies the phenomenal field and is accepted by the individual as reality. If he attempts to assess the reality of the dream while asleep, he is generally forced to accept that it is real.

AFFECTS AND COGNITION

In Chapters 15 and 17, I presented a summary of the characteristic thoughts and affects of depressed patients, and indicated that there is a definite temporal contiguity of thought and affect. I noted, furthermore, that there is a logical consistency between them, i.e., the specific affect is congruent with the specific thought content.

The thesis derived from these clinical observations is: *The affective response is determined by the way an individual structures his experience.* Thus, if an individual's conceptualization of a situation has an unpleasant content he will experience a corresponding unpleasant affective response.

The cognitive structuring or conceptualization of a situation is dependent on the schema elicited. The specific schema, consequently, has a direct bearing on the affective response to a situation. It is postulated, there-fore, that the schema determines the specific type of affective response. If the schema is concerned with self-depreciation, a feeling of sadness will be associated with it; if the schema is concerned with the anticipation of harm to the individual, anxiety will be produced. An analogous relationship between the content of the schema and the corresponding feeling holds for the other affects, such as anger and elation.

In clinical syndromes such as depression this relationship between cog-nitive process and affective response is easily identified. When the affective response seems inappropriate to a particular stimulus situation, the incon-gruity may be attributed to the particular schema evoked. Thus, the para-doxical gloom in depression results from the idiosyncratic schemas that are operative. This may be illustrated by the example of a depressed patient who wept bitterly whenever he was praised. His predominant attitude (schema) was that he was a fraud. Any praise or other favorable comment activated this idea about himself. Receiving praise was interpreted by him as confirmatory evidence of how he consistently deceived people.

The specific types of depressive affects are related to the specific types of thought patterns. Thus, schemas which have a content relevant to being deserted, thwarted, undesirable, or derelict in one's duties will produce, respectively, feelings of loneliness, frustration, humiliation, or guilt. The relative absence of anger among the more severely depressed patient, par-ticularly in situations that uniformly arouse anger in other people, may be attributed to their tendency to conceptualize situations in terms of their own supposed inadequacies. One currently popular explanation for the relative absence of overt anger in depression is that this affect is present and, in fact, intensified in depression but is repressed or inverted. The pres-ent explanation seems to be closer to the data. The theme of the dominant schemas is that the depressed patient is deficient or blameworthy. Proceed-ing from this assumption the patient is forced to the conclusion that in-sults, abuse, and deprivation are justifiable because of his own supposed shortcomings or mistakes. Remorse rather than anger stems from these conceptualizations.

In other clinical syndromes characterized by an abnormal intensity of a particular affect, there is a dominance of the cognitive patterns corre-sponding to that affect. The anxiety neurotic demonstrates the dominance and inappropriate use of schemas relevant to personal danger. The hostile paranoid is dominated by schemas concerned with blaming or accusing other individuals (or external agencies) for their perceived abuse of him. The manic patient is influenced by schemas of positive self-evaluation.

It could be speculated that once these idiosyncratic schemas have been mobilized and have produced an affective reaction, the schemas are in turn affected by the affects. It is possible that a circular mechanism is set up, with the schemas stimulating the affects and the affects reinforcing the activity of the schemas.

A CIRCULAR FEEDBACK MODEL

The discussion so far has viewed the connection between cognitive structure and affect as a kind of one-way street, i.e., the direction has been from cognition to emotion. But it is conceivable that there is an interaction between these, and that feelings may also influence thought content. The lack of concrete clinical data to support the concept of a reverse flow makes such theorizing highly speculative. Nevertheless, the formulation of a mutually reinforcing system (Feshbach, 1965) can provide a more complete explanation for the phenomena observed in depression. The operation of this system can be presented as follows: Let us assume that an unpleasant life situation triggers schemas relevant to loss, self-blame, and negative expectancies. As they become activated, these schemas produce a stimulation of the affective structures connected to them. The activation of the affective structures is responsible for the subjective feeling of depression. These affective structures in turn, further innervate the schemas to which they are connected and consequently reinforce the activity of these schemas. The interaction, thus, consists of schemas $\longleftrightarrow$ affective structures. This model could explain the downward spiral in depression: The more negatively the patient thinks, the worse he feels; the worse he feels, the more negatively he thinks.

It is possible to travel into still more speculative areas by incorporating the concept of energy* into this formation. Let us assume that initially the schema is energized as the result of some psychological trauma. The activation of this cognitive structure leads to the stimulation of the affective structure. The activation of the affective structure produces a burst of energy, which is experienced subjectively as a painful emotion. The energy then flows back to the cognitive structure and increases the quantity of energy attached to it. This then produces further innervation of the affective structure.

---

* In discussing structure and process it is difficult to avoid the introduction of energy concepts. Such concepts are often vague and elusive and their utility and validity in personality theory have been strongly challenged. At a 1962 symposium sponsored by the American Psychoanalytic Association there was sharp disagreement regarding the advisability of retaining energy concepts in psychoanalytic theory. On the other hand, the concept of energy is employed by many disparate schools of psychological theory. Floyd Allport (1955), for example, utilizes energy concepts extensively in his formulation of the processes of perception and cognition.

Further data are certainly required to remove this discussion from the realm of speculation and to determine whether there is any utility in the formulation.

SUMMARY

During the developmental period the depression-prone individual acquires certain negative attitudes regarding himself, the outside world, and his future. As a result of these attitudes, he becomes especially sensitive to certain specific stresses such as being deprived, thwarted, or rejected. When exposed to such stresses he responds disproportionately with ideas of personal deficiency, with self-blame, and with pessimism.

The idiosyncratic attitudes represent persistent cognitive patterns, designated as schemas. The schemas influence the way an individual orients himself to a situation, recognizes and labels the salient features, and conceptualizes the experience.

The idiosyncratic schemas in depression consist of negative conceptions of the individual's worth, personal characteristics, performance or health, and of nihilistic expectations. When these schemas are evoked, they mold the thought content and lead to the typical depressive feelings of sadness, guilt, loneliness, and pessimism. The schemas may be largely inactive during the asymptomatic periods but become activated with the onset of depression. As the depression deepens, these schemas increasingly dominate the cognitive processes and not only displace the more appropriate schemas but also disrupt the cognitive processes involved in attaining self-objectivity and reality testing.

It is suggested that the affective reactions may facilitate the activity of these idiosyncratic schemas and, consequently, enhance the downward spiral in depression. The relative absence of anger in depression is attributed to the displacement of schemas relevant to blaming others by schemas of self-blame.

Part V.

TREATMENT OF DEPRESSION

Chapter 19.
Pharmacotherapy

Pharmacotherapy for depression is at least as old as Homer, being mentioned in *The Odyssey* when Penelope takes a drug to dull her grief for her long-absent husband. The two main classes of drugs in use for the treatment of depression today were originally tested in schizophrenic patients but, as in the case of electroconvulsive therapy, were found to be more effective in treating apathy and depression than other clinical symptoms (Kline, 1964; Hordern, 1965). Iproniazid, in the first major class, was shown to prevent sedation in mice given reserpine; this drug had also been used in the treatment of tuberculosis in 1955, and it was observed to produce a euphoric effect. Interest in imipramine and certain of its derivatives was stimulated because of their structural resemblance to the phenothiazines which had been used successfully in schizophrenia. Iproniazid seemed to be effective in its first tests as an antidepressant and imipramine given to a large group of patients seemed, to the surprise of investigators, to work far better with predominantly depressive patients than with predominantly schizophrenic patients.

The two new classes of drugs were simultaneously introduced in 1957 and they have stimulated a considerable amount of research since then. They are the tricyclic imipramine and closely related compounds and the monoamine oxidase inhibitors (MAO inhibitors), which include iproniazid and several others. These drugs are listed in Table 19–1 along with a number of other compounds whose effectiveness in treating depression has been studied. Dosage data (Cole, 1964; Goodman and Gilman, 1965) are listed for the more extensively studied and more widely used compounds.

The controlled studies of the antidepressant agents have been the subject of a number of review articles. Since there is substantial disagreement among the reviewers, it is necessary to compare their evaluations of the drug studies. This review of the literature is designed to highlight the points of consensus and disagreement among the specialists regarding the current status of the antidepressants. It is also intended to map out the areas that require clarification by further research.

Table 19–1.
DRUGS USED IN TREATMENT OF DEPRESSION

Generic name	Trade name	Strength	Daily total*
TRICYCLIC COMPOUNDS			
imipramine	Tofranil	10 mg., 25 mg.	75–300 mg.
desipramine	Norpramin	25 mg.	75–200 mg.
	Pertofrane		
amitriptyline	Elavil	25 mg.	75–300 mg.
nortriptyline	Aventyl	10 mg., 25 mg.	20–100 mg.
MONOAMINE OXIDASE (MAO) INHIBITORS			
phenelzine	Nardil	15 mg.	45–75 mg.
isocarboxazid	Marplan	10 mg.	30–50 mg.
nialamide	Niamid	25 mg., 100 mg.	75–200 mg.
tranylcypromine	Parnate	10 mg.	10–60 mg.
iproniazid	Marsilid	(Withdrawn from use)	
PSYCHOMOTOR STIMULANTS			
Amphetamines			
amphetamine	Benzedrine	5 mg., 10 mg.	5–30 mg.
dextroamphetamine	Dexedrine	5 mg.	5–15 mg.
methamphetamine	Methedrine, etc.	2.5 mg., 5 mg.	7.5–15 mg.
Other			
methylphenidate	Ritalin	5 mg., 10 mg.	20–60 mg.

* Maximum dose used only in refractory cases. Minimum dose used as a starter or for slight or elderly patients. Usually dose is cut back after therapeutic change has occurred.

THE TRICYCLIC DRUGS

Imipramine is the most thoroughly studied antidepressant drug. Its effectiveness in comparison with placebo in double-blind studies has been reviewed by Brady (1963), Cole (1964), Klerman and Cole (1965), and Friedman, *et al.* (1966). The results of their review of the literature is presented in Table 19–2. It is notable that Brady's review of inpatient and outpatient studies and the review by Friedman, *et al.* of inpatient studies show an essentially even distribution of positive and negative results. The reviews by Cole (1964) and Klerman and Cole (1965), on the other hand, show a definite weighting in favor of positive results.

The differences in the findings reported by Klerman and Cole as compared with Brady may be explained partly on the basis of two factors. First, Klerman and Cole missed three negative studies included by Brady; also, Klerman and Cole included seven studies published in 1964 after Brady completed his review. Second, Klerman and Cole counted as positive re-

Table 19–2.
SURVEYS OF STUDIES COMPARING EFFICACY OF IMIPRAMINE
(TOFRANIL) WITH PLACEBO

	Outpatients		*Inpatients*		*Total*	
	Imipramine superior		*Imipramine superior*		*Imipramine superior*	
Study	*Yes*	*No*	*Yes*	*No*	*Yes*	*No*
Brady (through 1963)	4	1	8	12	12	13
Cole (through 1964)			9	6	9	6
Klerman & Cole (through 1964)*	5	0	7	6	17*	8*
Friedman, *et al.*† (through 1964)			11	11	11	11

* Total includes seven studies not classified as inpatient or outpatient.
† Includes literature review plus results of imipramine trial by authors.

sults many studies in which the superiority of imipramine was slight and fell short of statistical significance, but Brady used the 5 per cent level of significance to designate a study as positive.

Cole, reviewing the literature through 1964, found 15 studies on hospitalized inpatients. Friedman *et al.* (1966), also reviewing the literature through 1964, found 21 studies on hospitalized psychotic depressives. This is an important difference, for Friedman *et al.* found four more negative studies. This was in addition to their own study, which indicated that imipramine was no more effective than placebo in hospitalized psychotic depressives.

All the reviewers attempt to evaluate the methodological adequacy of the studies they reviewed. Cole and Brady criticize the negative studies and Friedman *et al.* and Wechsler *et al.* (1965), whose conclusions on imipramine are negative, criticize the positive studies. Cole and Brady state that samples in the negative studies were too small and Friedman *et al.* (1966) level the same criticism against the positive studies. An analysis of the number of patients in the studies reviewed by Brady gives a mean of 53 patients for the positive studies and 41 patients for the negative studies. The significance of the differences is hard to judge. In a review of both controlled and uncontrolled studies, Wechsler, Grosser, and Greenblatt (1965) found no significant correlation of result with sample size. Furthermore, Davis (1965) charges that the negative studies often used dosages that were too small; Klerman and Cole state that the effect of dosage is unknown; and Wechsler and his coworkers claim no correlation of result with dosage size. Davis asserts that the patient populations in the negative studies were too chronic while Brady states that they were too heterogeneous.

The possibility exists that imipramine may be effective in specific diagnostic groups and not effective in others. The reviewers are again in complete disagreement. Hordern (1965) says that imipramine is effective only with psychotics and not with neurotics; Friedman *et al.* say it is not effective with psychotic depressives at all and that the evidence on neurotics is unclear; Klerman and Cole assert that a differential effectiveness has not been established and the question is unclear; Overall *et al.* (1964) found that imipramine was superior to a phenothiazine in retarded depressions but not in anxious depressions.

Wechsler and his coworkers, examining controlled and uncontrolled studies, find a clearly superior response with depressions of recent onset. Klerman and Cole, looking only at controlled, double-blind studies, do not find a significant recent vs. chronic difference. Friedman *et al.* suggest that perhaps the improvement observed in so many studies is actually only an acceleration of spontaneous remissions during the first two or three weeks.

Summary: It is clear that the various double-blind studies comparing imipramine with a placebo have yielded contradictory results. Furthermore, there is disagreement among the authorities in evaluating the published studies. It is obvious, in any event, that the efficacy of imipramine has not been clearly established and that further studies are necessary to provide definite answers regarding its efficacy and indications. At the present time, a large-scale study of antidepressant drug treatment is being conducted by the Psychopharmacology Service Center of the United States Public Health Service to answer some of the questions raised in this chapter.

Amitriptyline, the other important tricyclic drug, has not been studied as extensively as imipramine. The reviewers are consistent in stating that four studies show amitryptyline as being superior to placebo and either none or one show no superiority (cf. Table 19–3) but the number of studies are too few to draw any definite conclusions.

Desipramine has been recently introduced with the claim of a more rapid action than imipramine. It has also been suggested that desipramine is the active principle in imipramine. Klerman and Cole cite two controlled studies which show no difference between these two drugs in terms of efficacy or speed of onset.

Table 19–3.

COMPARISON OF AMITRIPTYLINE (ELAVIL) WITH IMIPRAMINE
(TOFRANIL) AND PLACEBO

	Comparison with imipramine		Comparison with placebo	
Review	*Amitriptyline superior*	*Amitriptyline not superior*	*Amitriptyline superior*	*Amitriptyline not superior*
Cole (1964)	2	1	4	0
Hordern (1965)	2	3	2	0
Davis (1965)	3	2	4	1

MAO INHIBITORS

The reviewers who discuss the effectiveness of MAO inhibitors in comparison to placebo are Hordern (1965), Davis (1965), Cole (1964), and Wechsler, Grosser and Greenblatt (1965). Hordern and Cole both question the soundness of the studies of the MAO inhibitors.

The reviewers again differ as to how many studies have been published and what these studies show but there is more agreement here of both fact and opinion than with imipramine. The authors in general believe that at least one of the MAO inhibitors is effective although they differ about which one it is. Hordern says that iproniazid, now withdrawn from the market in the United States, was the best MAO inhibitor and that phenelzine is the best one now available. Davis agrees that phenelzine is the best but Cole asserts that tranylcypromine is best. Wechsler shows an equal range of im-

Table 19–4.

COMPARISON OF MAO INHIBITORS WITH PLACEBOS

	Hordern		Davis		Cole	
Drug	*Positive*	*Negative*	*Positive*	*Negative*	*Positive*	*Negative*
Iproniazid (withdrawn from use)	2	0	2	1	2	1
Tranylcypromine	1	0	2	0	2	0
Phenelzine	3	1	3	0	2	2
Isocarboxazid	1	2	3	2	3	2
Nialamide	0	1	1	1	1	3

provement on all the MAO inhibitors mentioned in his review with the exception of nialamide for which the improvement range is a little narrower.

The number of controlled, double-blind studies evaluating each drug, as stated by the reviewers who give such data, are shown in Table 19–4. It is clear from this data why Cole believes that tranylcypromine is the best MAO inhibitor, whereas Davis and Hordern choose phenelzine. (Again it is important to remember that all are reviewing the same literature through 1964.) Another important difference is that Davis and Cole both find two more studies favoring isocarboxazid than does Hordern. The number of studies is too small, however, for any definite conclusions about the efficacy of any of these drugs.

COMPARATIVE STUDIES

Davis (1965) has reviewed the comparative efficacy of the antidepressant drugs, the phenothiazines, and electroconvulsive therapy. A tabulation of the studies comparing imipramine with various MAO inhibitors showed a superiority of imipramine in four studies, no difference in six studies, and a superiority of the MAO inhibitors in none. In two studies, there was no difference in the relative efficacy of a phenothiazine and imipramine.

ECT was compared with imipramine in six studies. In three of these, ECT was judged to be clearly superior but in the other three, the effects of both treatments were judged to be equivalent.

OTHER DRUG TREATMENTS

There seems to be general agreement among the reviewers (Cole, Hordern, and Davis) that the amphetamine group of drugs is probably not effective in the treatment of moderate or severe depression. Hordern cites two double-blind studies in which the amphetamines were found to be no more effective than a placebo in relieving depression; in a third study, however, a combination of dextroamphetamine with amobarbitol was found to be as effective as imipramine, except in alleviation of agitation and in reduction of weight loss. Cole says that methylphenidate may be effective in the relief of nonpsychiatric patients with mild depressions.

Numerous isolated single studies support the effectiveness in depression of various miscellaneous drugs or combinations of known drugs. According to Cole, the evidence supporting the usefulness of Deaner is meager and the evidence regarding the efficacy of Deprol is equivocal.

Strömgren and Schou (1964) have reported favorable results using lithium salts in treating mania. They also believe lithium may have some positive effect in the depressive phase of manic-depressive psychosis. Schlagenhauf, Tupin, and White (1966) summarized the results reported in 18 studies from 1948–1963. Although the clinical consensus is that lithium is effective in manic excitement, the absence of controlled double-blind studies precludes any definite conclusions at this time.

METHODOLOGICAL PROBLEMS

The contradictory results reported in the previous sections suggest that some, if not all, of the studies of the pharmacotherapy of depression may be entangled in methodological problems.

RATER BIAS

The studies discussed in the previous sections have met the most basic criteria of pharmacological research design; they are both controlled and double-blind. But these criteria alone do not completely solve the problem of bias. Before any drug is subjected to controlled experimentation, its clinical value must first be estimated in a series of uncontrolled tests. These generally give a much more rosy picture of the effectiveness of the drug than do the eventual controlled studies (Cole, 1964; Wechsler, Grosser, and Greenblatt, 1965). Thus, before any controlled investigations are conducted, a clinical consensus on the efficacy of the antidepressant already exists. It is possible that this favorable attitude biases future controlled research; e.g., if an inactive placebo is used, the researcher can distinguish some drug subjects by the side-effects, and his ratings may be influenced toward a positive result. Or if an investigator gets a negative result, he may doubt its validity and, consequently, may look very closely for faults in research design. If he finds them, he may fail to publish the data at all.

To control side effects, atropine, which has similar autonomic effects to imipramine, has been used as an active placebo. When low or moderate doses of atropine were used, however, few imipramine-placebo differences were observed (Klerman and Cole). This suggests the possibility that the raters were unable to distinguish between the patients receiving imipramine and those receiving atropine, and consequently there was no bias in rating. Such a hypothesis suggests that imipramine is no more effective than atropine. Alternatively, it is possible that the side effects of atropine may work on the suggestibility of the patient to give a very high rate of placebo response.

PLACEBO RESPONSE

The rate of placebo response is radically different in different studies. It ranges from 0–77 per cent (Wechsler, Grosser, and Greenblatt, 1965; Friedman *et al.*, 1966). In the imipramine studies cited by Klerman and Cole (1965), the placebo response rate is 21 per cent in outpatients, 46 per cent in the newly hospitalized, and only 16 per cent in the chronic in-patients. In studies showing imipramine to be efficacious the rate of placebo response is 27 per cent. Where studies show imipramine to be ineffective it is 41 per cent. The rate of response to imipramine is respectively 70 per cent and 58 per cent, for the positive and negative studies. The difference between the two kinds of study does not depend solely on the placebo response rate.

The question of placebo response is connected with still another factor that may account for discrepancies in the data. The various experiments are not directly comparable because of differing time intervals between the initiation of the treatment and evaluation. The range in imipramine studies is 2 weeks to 2 1/2 months (Brady, 1963; Klerman and Cole, 1965). In the longer time periods, under conditions of high spontaneous remission, drug-placebo differences may be obscured.

Several other factors should be considered in evaluating the placebo response. (1) The improvement in the placebo group may reflect the natural history of the illness, i.e., the spontaneous remission. (2) Nondrug factors such as hospital milieu and psychotherapy may produce improvement in the placebo group. (3) The placebo effect itself may be therapeutic. It is possible that merely receiving medication may help to break the vise of hopelessness that grips the depressed patients. It is also possible that the patients report subjective improvement in order to please the rater even though the basic disorder has not improved. Studies that use no placebo in the control group should therefore be conducted.

NONRANDOM DISTRIBUTION OF VARIABLES

The rate of placebo response may be connected with another problem that affects not only each individual study but any comparisons of them. Each study must decide how to limit its patient sample. The descriptions "endogenous" and "reactive," "schizo-affective components," "neurotic," "agitated," etc., are widely used in the different studies and often undoubtedly in different ways. Thus, studies of depression can have either very broad sample groups, including schizophrenics, psychopaths, and mildly depressed individuals or very narrow sample groups. Since it is unknown what variables in the patient are related to the efficacy of the antidepressants, nonrandom distribution of patient characteristics into experimental and control groups may well occur (Snow and Rickels, 1964). Some variables not often considered crucial, e.g., socioeconomic status, may be of importance (Rickels, 1963; Rickels, Ward, and Schut, 1964). Also, a variable such as age, which may well be controlled for, may be important. Grosser and Freeman (1961), for example, have produced data indicating that patients under 40, or those with neurotic depressions, show a high placebo response rate. In a different setting, Friedman *et al.* (1966) have shown that inpatients of average age 60, with psychotic depressions, respond at an unusually high rate to placebo.

VARIABILITY OF MEASURES

A variety of measures have been used to evaluate the results of treatment, and the results seem to depend somewhat on the measure utilized. Klerman and Cole have made the following observations on the measures used in the imipramine studies. Eleven of 12 studies that used global ratings showed an imipramine-placebo difference, but only half the studies using total morbidity scores demonstrated such a difference. Seven studies showed differences on some factor scores representing aspects of psychopathology or on certain single measures of psychopathology. Two studies did not show either of these differences.

The reliability and validity of the measures are open to question and have generally not been systematically investigated. In several studies in which two different measures have been used the results have been contradictory (Snow and Rickels, 1963).

OTHER PROBLEMS

Many authors have claimed that a high or low dosage is responsible for a positive or negative result (e.g., Hordern, 1965; Davis, 1965). Others deny this (Klerman and Cole, 1965; Wechsler, Grosser, and Greenblatt, 1965) and the matter remains controversial.

There are a number of other factors, about which little is known, that may play a role in pharmacological studies. These factors have all been well outlined in the article by DiMascio and Klerman (1960). They include aspects of the researcher and research team other than bias, subject-researcher relations, the physical environment, and the social setting.

ADVERSE EFFECTS OF ANTIDEPRESSANT DRUGS

There seems to be a relatively strong consensus on the adverse effects of the tricyclic and MAO-inhibiting compounds (Ayd, 1964; Cole, 1964; Hordern, 1965; and Klerman and Cole, 1965).

Klerman and Cole point out a general problem in the assessment of side effects: It is necessary to have a control group and careful reporting of somatic complaints *prior* to the beginning of drug therapy. Otherwise, many of the symptoms noted as side effects may represent complaints that already exist or that would arise without the use of the drug.

TRICYCLIC DRUGS.

One of the more serious complications that can arise from the use of imipramine is jaundice. It has been reported in fewer than 0.5–1.0 per cent of patients taking the drug. The hepatitis resulting from the tricyclics is obstructive in type and does not primarily involve parenchymal tissue. It generally clears fairly quickly when drug administration is suspended.

Imipramine can also cause agranulocytosis. This type of hypersensitivity has appeared rarely: There have been 12 reports in the literature, including three fatalities. Also leukopenia, leukocytosis, and occasional low-grade eosinophilis have been observed. The danger of agranulocytosis seems to be greatest in elderly women. Ayd states that amitriptyline has proved safer than imipramine in producing less frequent hepatitis and agranulocytosis.

Imipramine and amitriptyline also produce various autonomic effects and cardiovascular complications. The most frequent autonomic effects are dry mouth, increased sweating, difficulties with visual accommodation, and constipation (Klerman and Cole). These are "annoying rather than serious," according to Cole.

Cardiovascular problems represent a greater danger. Postural hypotension and tachycardia are relatively frequent and have been observed in about 5 per cent of all patients treated. Such effects are usually mild and not seriously detrimental unless the patient is elderly and/or has previously existing cardiovascular disease. It is mostly with this type of patient that the serious cardiovascular incidents have been reported. Klerman and Cole say that these include coronary thrombosis, congestive heart failure, and pulmonary emboli. Other tricyclics—desipramine, protriptyline, and nortriptyline—have been said to produce fewer autonomic and cardiovascular side effects (Hordern). But they may yield other side effects and their effectiveness in ameliorating depression has been only sparsely studied so far.

Finally, there are the possibilities of brain and behavioral toxicity of the tricyclic compounds. A mild tremor has been reported in 10 per cent of the patients using imipramine. Dizziness and insomnia are common initially but are only transitory effects.

The possibility that imipramine may cause mania, hypomania, or schizophrenic excitements has been noted in occasional cases. Ayd, however, believes that true manic reaction is extremely rare and that the reported cases of such reaction are actually toxic psychokinetic stimulation. The two conditions have only a superficial resemblance and the toxic psychokinetic reaction, if caused by imipramine, clears up relatively quickly.

MAO INHIBITORS

The possible undesirable side effects of the MAO inhibitors have been discussed thoroughly by Ayd (1964). These effects are similar to those produced by the tricyclic drugs but are more numerous and more severe. Iproniazid, listed in Table 19–1 as being "withdrawn from use," is not now available in the United States because of the severity of certain side reactions.

The first major problem is cephalgia. Headache can be caused by all the antidepressants but in some cases the MAO inhibitors have caused severe cephalgia with hypertension. Accompanying symptoms may include apprehension, restlessness, muscle twitchings, dizziness, pallor, sweating, nausea, tachycardia or bradycardia, precordial pain, elevated blood pressure, and photophobia. Body temperature may change. The crisis may be acute for only a few hours but several days can pass before complete recovery. The most serious consequence of such an episode is intracranial hemorrhage, sometimes resulting in death.

There is no way of identifying the patients who will suffer such a hypertensive crisis. As with other adverse effects of the MAO inhibitors, there is wide individual variation in sensitivity to the drug. There is some indication that women and the elderly may be more prone to side reactions. These crises can occur at any time during the administration of the drug although they seem very often to be concomitant with the ingestion of other pharmacological agents. In particular, the concurrent consumption of hypertensive sympathomimetics or certain types of aged cheese (containing significant concentrations of pressor amines) may bring on hypertension with severe cephalgia or a cerebrovascular accident.

The hydrazine derivatives (isocarboxazid, nialamide, and phenelzine) may also cause hepatitis. There is some disagreement concerning the frequency of this reaction. Hordern, who minimizes the toxicity of the MAO inhibitors, states the frequency for iproniazid is only 1 in 10,000, significantly less than the 1 in 5,000 incidence of infectious hepatitis in the population at large. (It is extremely difficult to distinguish iproniazid-caused hepatitis from infectious hepatitis). Cole, who is concerned with the toxic effects of the MAO inhibitors, and who has less confidence in their efficacy than Hordern, states the frequency is 1 in 3,000. He questions whether the debatable effectiveness of the hydrazine derivatives merits their continued use in view of this incidence of hepatitis. The drug-associated hepatitis is similar to the viral hepatitis but has a much higher mortality rate. Cole's position may be correct if it is demonstrated that tranylcypromine is the most effective MAO inhibiting agent. Tranylcypromine is not a hydrazine MAO inhibitor, and thus far no hepatitis has been reported to result from treatment with the nonhydrazine derivatives. Among the hydrazine MAO inhibitors the most toxic is phenelzine, followed by isocarboxazid and, then, nialamide. This order may follow their order of hypothesized effectiveness (Hordern, 1965).

Two other dangers are widely agreed upon. One cannot use tricyclic and MAO inhibitors simultaneously or switch from one to the other without waiting at least a week. Reports of cases in which this precaution has not been taken describe "severe dizziness, tremor, restlessness, hallucinations, profuse sweating, vascular collapse, and extreme hyperpyrexia." (Klerman and Cole, 1965). Such consequences are less likely if the switch is from tricyclic to an MAO inhibitor than if it is the reverse.

The last danger is that a severely depressed patient may try to commit suicide with any of the drugs he may be taking. In those patients who have taken large doses of imipramine severe symptoms of various kinds have been present for two or three days, followed by complete recovery.

Chapter 20.
Electroconvulsive Therapy

Convulsions induced by substantial doses of camphor were used in the treatment of mental disorders as long ago as 1785. The treatment was revived in 1933 by Meduna who used camphor in the treatment of schizophrenic patients. Camphor was gradually replaced by more effective drugs such as Metrazol. In 1938, Cerletti and Bini refined the technique of producing convulsions when they introduced the technique of passing an electric current through two electrodes placed on the forehead. Consequently, a relatively safe, convenient, and painless method of convulsive therapy could be used in the treatment of mental disorders. Electroconvulsive therapy (ECT) was introduced into the United States by Kalinowski in 1939.

Although Metrazol is still used at several psychiatric centers for purposes of convulsive therapy, the most common method of producing therapeutic convulsions is at present electroshock.

PHYSIOLOGICAL EFFECTS

The physiological effects of ECT have been summarized by Holmberg (1963). Electroconvulsive therapy, when not modified by muscle relaxing agents, produces a grand mal seizure. Initially there is a tension or jerk produced by direct cortical stimulation. This is followed by a latent period and then by tonic and clonic convulsions. The electroencephalogram during the tonic phase is characterized by a generalized, intensive spike activity. During the clonic phase the EEG shows spike-wave activity that is not synchronous with the clonic movements. Immediately following the convulsion, the EEG shows a brief period of electrical silence followed by a gradual return of activity until the preconvulsive pattern is resumed.

Holmberg lists a variety of physiological changes that occur during the convulsion. Respiration is suspended as a result of spasm of the respiratory muscles and glottis. There is an elevation of the blood carbon dioxide tension and a substantial reduction of the oxygen tension. Although the cerebral circulation is markedly increased during the convulsion, the increased blood supply does not meet the demand of the tremendously increased brain metabolism. According to Holmberg, the discrepancy between the available cerebral circulation and the increased brain metabolism is the main reason for the spontaneous termination of the convulsion.

Anoxia is readily counteracted by the insufflation of oxygen prior to ECT. The heart rate is frequently rapid and irregular and there may be extreme fluctuations in blood pressure. The irregularity of the heart rate may be neutralized by premedication with atropine. Muscle relaxants may be used to reduce the increase in arterial pressure.

The immediate effects on the EEG following ECT are brief and reversible. The effects tend to be cumulative, however, over a series of treatments. They do not persist in general for more than a month following a course of treatment.

Some authors report a relationship between the degree of slowing of the EEG and clinical improvements. Others, however, deny the existence of such relationship.

Some investigators have reported an association between the severity of memory defects and the degree of EEG change. In other studies, however, no such correlation has been found. In general, the EEG changes are correlated more highly with memory defects than with the antidepressive effects.

ECT produces a variety of autonomic changes that are attributable to the excitation of the autonomic regulatory centers. One of the most prominent effects is psychomotor restlessness. A number of cholenergic effects such as transient arrhythmias may occur but these are easily controlled by the use of anticholenergic drugs. The increase in salivary and bronchial secretions may similarly be counteracted by preliminary atropinization.

BIOCHEMICAL EFFECTS

Holmberg discusses a number of biochemical and hormonal changes that have been reported in conjunction with ECT. Hyperglycemia of one to several hours duration is a constant phenomenon. There is also an increase in nitrogen compounds, potassium, calcium, phosphorous, and steroids in the blood. Several investigators have demonstrated an increase in the catecholamines and serotonin of the blood, but there is no evidence that this effect has anything to do with the therapeutic action of ECT.

Holmberg also lists certain specific biochemical changes within the brain. The serotonin level in the brain, and especially in the brain stem, is increased but there is no change in the brain amine oxidase activity. The increase in serotonin is attributed to the electrical stimulus and does not appear to be related to the intensity of the convulsion.

PSYCHOLOGICAL EFFECTS

Some impairment of memory occurs almost constantly with ECT. This impairment may range from a mild tendency to forget names or dates to a severe confusion. The amnesia may be both anterograde and retrograde. It is often disturbing to the patient and may continue for several weeks following the conclusion of treatment. The impairment of memory usually disappears within a month (Cronholm and Molander, 1964). There is no lasting impairment of memory even after as many as 250 treatments. Most authors believe that the efficacy of ECT in depression bears no relationship to the memory defects.

Holmberg suggests that very intensive treatment in elderly arteriosclerotic subjects may cause irreversible brain damage with resultant intellectual impairment. Others writers, however, do not believe that such a risk exists.

CLINICAL EFFICACY

Clinicians generally consider that the number of treatments necessary to clear a depression varies from 2–10. Frequently only four or five treatments are required and occasionally dramatic improvement is noted after only one treatment. There is some variability in the frequency of treatment, which may take place one to five times a week. Daily treatment may result in a cumulative confusion whereas treatments that are too widely spaced may increase the possibility of relapse.

Articles on the efficacy of ECT have reported improvement rates from 40 per cent to 100 per cent of patients in depressed states. Manic states are said to have a somewhat lower rate of response. The differences in results may be primarily due to differences of samples, but also may be influenced by variations in methods for assessing recovery. As has been observed in Chapter 3, depressed patients in the normal course of their illness show a very high percentage of spontaneous recovery. This varies from a median of 3–4 months among outpatients to a median of 6–18 months among inpatients. Despite the known tendency for spontaneous remission, the various psychiatric textbooks and the monographs on depression assert that ECT accelerates the improvement. On the other hand, manic-depressive patients who have received ECT seem to have a higher probability of recurrence and a shorter free interval period between attacks than patients who had a remission without receiving shock (Salzman, 1947).

Huston and Locher (1948) reported a recovery rate of 88 per cent in 74 manic-depressive patients who received ECT as compared with 79 per cent recovery rate for 63 patients who had been hospitalized before the introduction of ECT. The duration of illness was substantially less in the treated group (9 months vs. 15 months). Bond and Morris (1954) also compared patients hospitalized after the introduction of ECT with patients who were treated before the introduction of ECT. They found that the recovery rate for manic depressives was 72 per cent for the ECT group as compared with 59 per cent for the pre-ECT group. However, in those cases where 5-year follow-up studies could be completed, the differences were largely wiped out; the permanent recovery figures were 66 per cent for the patients of the current era and 64.5 per cent for the pre-ECT patients. One of the most conspicuous findings was the difference in the duration of hospitalization: 2.3 months for those admitted in the years after the introduction of ECT as compared with 4.5 months for patients admitted in the earlier period. The results with involutionals were much more dramatic. The five-year recovery rate of the treated cases was 56 per cent as compared with 27 per cent for the controls. The duration of hospitalization was 2 months and 12 months respectively.

There are a number of methodological difficulties in studies of this nature. One of the most common is that in follow-up it is easier to find records of patients who have relapsed than of those who have not. It is possible, also that the more careful follow-up available with the later cases may have spuriously inflated the ratio of recurrences. Furthermore, there is no evidence that the samples taken at different eras were similar, or that other therapeutic factors, such as milieu therapy, were equivalent.

The more recent controlled studies have compared improvement rates of patients assigned randomly to ECT and a control group. Riddell (1963), in a review of the effectiveness of ECT, was able to locate only three controlled studies of this nature. In one, ECT was significantly more effective than no treatment; in the second, ECT was significantly more effective than a placebo; in the third, ECT was significantly more effective than iproniazid although the ECT relapse rate may have been higher.

In his review of antidepressant drugs, Davis (1965) found six studies comparing ECT with imipramine. Three studies showed no significant differences in their effectiveness but three showed ECT to be superior. Lumping together Riddell's and Davis' reviews, we can conclude that ECT was superior to no treatment or placebo in two studies; it was more effective than antidepressant drugs in four studies; and it was equivalent to drug therapy in three studies.

Although there is not very extensive evidence, it is widely believed that ECT is effective in the treatment of psychotic depression. All the reviewers of the drug studies who mention ECT say that no drug has been shown to be superior to it. [However, Cole (1964) and Hordern (1965) do not believe that ECT is effective or advisable for neurotic depressions.] Hordern, Cole, Davis, Klerman, and Cole (1965) and Wechsler, Grosser, and Greenblatt (1965), assert that the available reports indicate that ECT is superior to, or at least equal to, any drug treatment for psychotic depressives. The meaning of the controlled studies would be clearer if the superiority of ECT to placebo or to no treatment was demonstrated in more carefully designed studies. For if, as in a number of studies, the ECT and imipramine effectiveness are equal, and conditions are such that imipramine is not effective, then what is proved is that ECT is equally ineffective.

Whether drugs or ECT should be used in practice has been the subject of many polemics. The two sides of the argument are summarized by Hordern (1965). Disagreement also exists on whether ECT produces improvement *more rapidly* than any drug (Cole, 1964) and is therefore preferable in the treatment of severe depressions, particularly those with a danger of suicide.

A number of investigators have attempted to determine whether there are any *types* of depression, or configurations of clinical factors, that are predictive of a favorable outcome with ECT. In general, the studies of this nature (Carney, Roth, and Garside, 1965; and Mendels, 1965) have found favorable prognostic signs among the clinical features generally associated with so-called endogenous depression.

COMPLICATIONS

The most frequent complications are fractures and dislocations produced by the muscular contractions during the convulsions. The most frequent fracture is a compression fracture of the dorsal vertebrae. These fractures are generally not of major clinical significance and generally do not require special treatment; in fact, many are observed only on routine x-ray examination. Back pain may persist for a few days or weeks.

Fractures can be eliminated by *softening procedures,* viz., the use of muscular relaxing agents. With well modified ECT the strain on any part of the locomoter system can be reduced or eliminated.

At the present time, the only really important risks are cardiovascular accidents. Cardiovascular accidents are most likely to occur if there is pre-existing pathology. Transient cardiac arhythmias may occur but their incidence may be reduced by premedication with acetycholine-blocking agents. Succinylcholine greatly reduces the strain on the heart.

In earlier studies, the mortality risk for a specific patient was approximately 3 in 1,000. With the more modern modifications of ECT, the fatality rate is reduced even more. Holmberg reports that of several thousand electroconvulsive treatments that he has administered with pentobarbital-succinlycholine relaxation over a 10-year period there have been no complications.

MECHANISM OF ACTION

Kalinowsky and Hoch (1961) describe a wide variety of theories of the mode of action of ECT. While the mechanism of action has still not been established, it has been possible to eliminate many factors previously considered to be of major importance in producing therapeutic effects. Among the factors that can be discarded as therapeutically important are anoxia, hypercapnia, muscular exertion, adrenal reactions, peripheral excretion of catecholamines, and other biochemical changes in the blood (Holmberg).

Changes in the central nervous system, as manifested by the slowing of the EEG and intellectual impairment, are frequently claimed to have been responsible for the therapeutic improvement with ECT; however, proof is lacking to substantiate these claims.

The effectiveness of ECT is dependent on the production of seizure activity in the brain. Subconvulsive treatment and nonconvulsive electro-stimulation of the diencephalon have been shown to be of no therapeutic value. Moreover it has been reported that reducing the convulsive activity by premedication with anticonvulsive drugs reduces the therapeutic effect of ECT. On the other hand, intensification of the convulsive activity by the use of muscular relaxants and oxygenation increases the therapeutic effects (Holmberg).

Chapter 21.
Psychotherapy

REVIEW OF LITERATURE

In his book, *Manic-Depressive Disease,* Campbell (1953) suggests the following steps in the psychologic therapy of manic depressives:

First Step–Proper Diagnosis: An explicit diagnosis should be made and positive treatment begun. The physician cannot reassure his patient if he is not convinced himself. In the absence of positive physical or laboratory findings and the presence of sufficient autonomic disturbance, there is "no diagnosis in medicine as dependable as that of manic-depressive psychosis."

Second Step–Explanation of Somatic Symptoms: The physician should give the patient a physiologic explanation of his somatic symptoms. This knowledge and reassurance is helpful in obtaining the patient's cooperation and in achieving his relaxation.

Third Step–Removal of Precipitating or Aggravating Environmental Factors: The physician must be aware of the detailed history and of any provoking circumstances in the patient's life. It may be necessary to interview those close to the patient to ascertain what disturbing situations in the environment may be blocking his efforts to rest and relax.

Fourth Step–Combat Conscientiousness: The physician should make the patient aware that his inordinate conscientiousness stems from inner feelings of guilt, from an over-strict conscience, and from keen feelings of insecurity, and should encourage him to expect less of himself, to dispossess himself of the drive for accomplishment, and to develop a more nonchalant outlook on life. These changes, which may be achieved by insight, logic, and reasoning, may not only help to relieve the present illness, but may prevent future depressive reactions.

Fifth Step–Psychotherapy: In addition to reeducation, reassurance, and explanation, Campbell recommends simply allowing the patient to talk. The physician can also explain that this illness is self-limiting and that the patient will get well.

Sixth Step–Advice to the Family and Friends: The family should be told that the "patient has a well-recognized disease which happens to manifest itself by depression, indecision, crying spells, etc." It should be explained to them that this illness requires rest and relaxation, and that the patient must avoid anything that increases his tension and anxiety.

Seventh Step—Rest and Relaxation: The objective of the preceding six steps is to prepare the patient to rest, to relax, and to allow his nervous system a respite. The patient must be trained to relax and to realize the importance of rest to his hypersensitive nervous system since work seems to be a compulsive phenomenon with the manic depressive.

Eighth Step—Occupational Therapy: Making or doing things with one's hands relieves anxiety, stimulates initiative and imagination, and produces a feeling of satisfaction. It is best if the patient discovers an avocation for himself rather than that the doctor assign one.

Ninth Step—Bibliotherapy: The patient should be encouraged to read to relax or to divert himself, rather than to improve his mind or personality; Campbell finds that there is not much benefit to be expected from the reading of books of an inspirational, religious nature.

In an article on the dynamics and psychotherapy of depression, Wilson (1955) points out that when the necessary state of personality equilibrium is disrupted, a "need-satisfaction sequence" is set up. Interruption of the need-satisfaction sequence produces anxiety. Turning on the self is a common substitute activity if the anxiety state cannot be satisfied by the actual object sought. The turning on the self produces a temporary or prolonged depression. Those people prone to an exaggerated depression show a special need as children for the approval of others. When young, they develop a technique by means of which they can obtain approval rather than developing a sense of self-worth or self-esteem. When the technique fails, the patient turns on himself, and becomes depressed.

Wilson recommends the following steps: (1) the therapist should show acceptance of the patient in spite of the patient's rejection of the therapist; (2) the patient should be shown how he continually seeks approval, how this has failed, and how he has turned on the self; (3) the therapist should show the patient how to be honest and direct; and (4) the therapist should support the patient in using more direct methods of self-expression.

Kraines, in his book *Mental Depressions and Their Treatment* (1957), stresses, as does Campbell, the physical basis of manic-depressive illness but considers psychotherapy essential to shorten the illness, to alleviate the patient's suffering, and to prevent complications. The therapy should be individualized according to the patient and to the phase of his illness and it may include medication, psychotherapy, direct guidance, and physical hygiene measures. Unlike Campbell, who feels that rest and relaxation are the major goals and who suggests curtailing of social contacts, Kraines believes that social activity should be encouraged. Both agree that in mild cases the patient does best when in his usual surroundings and both suggest institutional care and electric shock treatments when there is extreme agitation. Kraines and Campbell both stress "formulation to the patient," i.e. explaining to him the nature of his illness, emphasizing that he will be cured, and reassuring him that his illness has a physical basis. Both advise that relatives be informed that the patient is really ill despite the absence of objective medical tests.

The psychotherapy includes: (1) the *basic triad*,—understanding, hope, and plan; (2) utilization of the physician's personality; (Success depends not only on technical knowledge but on the ability to establish rapport.); (3) the four levels of psychotherapy—ventilation, symptom management, mental hygiene principles, and deep personality analysis; and (4) therapeutic guidance. (Direct advice can be of great value but must be used with discretion according to individual needs.)

Ayd, in his book *Recognizing the Depressed Patient* (1961), also stresses (as do Campbell and Kraines) that the physician start by telling the patient that his illness has a physical basis and that he will improve. He feels that encouragement is important and that the physician should dissuade the patient from trying what is likely to be difficult since failure only reinforces his sense of inadequacy and guilt. Ayd feels that "no advantage is gained by an intellectual understanding of the psychological aspects of the illness," although he notes that it is important that the precipitating factors be analyzed and eliminated if possible so that the patient can be prepared to cope with similar problems in the future. Ayd states that many physicians do not seem to take cognizance of the natural course and duration of a depression and come discouraged when the response is slow or the patient retrogresses. He suggests that the physician involve family and friends in assisting and cooperating in the treatment of the depressed patient. He believes that informed relatives can assist the melancholic to carry out the doctor's instructions, can help to make environmental changes, and can fortify his desire to recover.

Ayd says it is essential that the depressed person obtain rest and relaxation which can only be achieved by changing his attitudes and habits since the depressive, goaded on by self-imposed standards and incited by feelings of guilt, tends to deny his feelings of fatigue and nervousness.

Arieti (1962) states that "Depression is . . . a reaction to the loss of a normal ingredient of psychological life." The patient must reorganize his thinking "into different constellations which do not bring about sadness." Depression changes the thought processes, apparently to decrease the quantity of thoughts "in order to decrease the quantity of suffering."

Arieti distinguishes between a "claiming depression" and a "self-blaming depression." In a claiming depression the patient is dependent on a dominant other and becomes more demanding as he feels more deprived. The self-blaming depression is an attempt to retrieve loss of the relationship to the dominant other by expiation. The mechanism's pattern is guilt, atoning, attempted redemption.

In cases of moderate intensity, Arieti suggests that the therapist alter the environment, especially the relationship to the dominant other; relieve the patient's feeling of guilt, responsibility, unaccomplishment, and loss; and disallow depressive thoughts to expand into general mood of depression.

Gibson (1963) in an article on psychotherapy of manic-depressive states, singles out two technical difficulties in the psychotherapy of manic depressives. The therapist should recognize the patient's difficulty in establishing a relationship with the therapist in which meaningful communication can take place. The patient tends to recast the therapist's remarks and interpretations into his own predetermined way of perceiving relationships. This "constellation" can be expected to reappear again and again "as a resistance." It may help for the therapist to challenge the patient's view in order to introduce a new point of view.

The therapist must avoid the complementary role which the patient's personality patterns call for as the patient tries to gain the analyst's approval. (The patient may be aware of his manipulative tendencies but the defensive aspect of these tendencies is generally unconscious. It is part of the patient's standard method of dealing with people.) The therapist's active involvement may become necessary. He may need to be more directive. Interpretations may be made as emphatic statements. A hoped for result is that the patient see analysis as a new human experience.

Regan (1965), in an article entitled, "Brief psychotherapy of depression," is concerned with "tactics," a "circumscribed set of procedures aimed at a specific tactical goal." He advocates these tactical approaches in psychotherapy of depression:

1. Protection of patient. The therapist must anticipate the effects of his therapeutic efforts and the risk of patient's suicide.

2. Need for preparatory exploration. Since a conviction of hopelessness is a uniform feature of depression and leads to negativism about therapeutic efforts the therapist should arouse the patient into therapeutic activity by direct and aggressive questioning.

3. Interruption of the ruminative cycle. The psychotherapist prohibits the patient from engaging in activities in which he will fail and limits activities to a sphere in which he is sure the patent will succeed.

4. Use of physical therapy. For physical treatment to be lasting, the forces resulting in the depression must be eliminated simultaneously with the physical treatment.

5. Initiation of attitudinal change.

Bonime (1965) states that depression is a sick way of relating to other human beings. Characteristically, the depressive makes inordinate demands on others. Depressive living has a basic consistency pervading all its variations from neurotic sulking to psychotic mania, the elements of which are manipulativeness, aversion to influence, unwillingness to give gratification, hostility, and anxiety.

Bonime also states that the depressive's dreams show elements of anxiety and destructiveness, and reflect the way in which the patient reacts to people and the role he plays in producing the paralysis, anxiety, rage, and deprivations in his life. The therapist can help the patient to see possibilities of new choices and new consequences. The therapist must guard against subsidizing the depressive tactics of his patient. He must foster the patient's recognition of his role in bringing about his pain and the personal resources he (the patient) has for altering his practices.

SUPPORTIVE PSYCHOTHERAPY

Various methods used in the supportive treatment of depression have been described in detail by a number of authors (Appel, 1944); Campbell, 1953; Kraines, 1957; Ayd, 1961.) There seems to be a consensus regarding supportive therapy and the discussion below reflects the generally accepted procedures.

REASSURANCE

The authors agree on the importance of stressing that depression is a self-limited disorder to counteract the patient's belief that he will never get better. Kraines gives his patients lengthy explanations, both of the factors involved in depression and of the course of the illness, and concludes, "The thing for you to remember is that this exhaustion can and will be overcome. You will need patience and you will need to cooperate. It won't be easy; it will take time; *but you will recover.*" (p. 409) He states that a majority of the patients are comforted, sustained, and encouraged by a straightforward explanation of their illness and by positive reassurance of their recovery.

Ayd emphasizes to his patients that although it may take weeks or months for complete recovery, they will feel progressively better and will not remain at their current level of depression. Ayd reports that, after recovery, many patients remark that their confidence is the physician's promise of recovery and his constant assurances prevented suicide and made their existence more tolerable.

I have found that optimistic statements about the outcome may encourage the patient to become more active and may help to neutralize the all-pervasive pessimism. In mild or moderate depressions such positive predictions may have a noticeable ameliorating effect but severely depressed patients may view these optimistic statements with skepticism and may fail to be influenced by them.

The therapist may often be of help in reassuring the patient about other misconceptions and worries, e.g., that he will be unable to provide for his family, that he will be unable to meet the minimal demands of living, or that his physical health is deteriorating rapidly. Through appropriate encouragement the therapist can often increase the patient's self-confidence and can counteract his feeling of helplessness.

Reassurance should be administered judiciously and with an awareness of the way it is construed by the patient. A bluff, hearty manner by the therapist may be interpreted as insincerity or insensitiveness by the patient and may increase his sense of hopelessness.

A depressed medical student told his therapist that he felt isolated and alone and that these symptoms meant to him that he was suffering from chronic schizophrenia. The therapist launched into a lengthy discussion of the difference between depression and schizophrenia. The patient's reaction to this was: "He doesn't understand me." The patient wanted to ventilate his worries and he felt that the therapist had cut him off with a premature reassurance. As a result he felt even more isolated.

Another technique that is often helpful in counteracting the patient's low self esteem and hopeless feeling is a discussion of his positive achievements. If allowed to follow his inclinations, the patient is likely to dwell on past failures and traumatic experiences. The therapist, however, can foster a more realistic appraisal of the past and can raise the patient's self-evaluation by skillfully guiding him into describing his successes in detail.

VENTILATION AND CATHARSIS

It is worthwhile to draw the depressed patient into a discussion of the life situations and the relationships that are bothering him. Occasionally, the patient is helped by being able to express his problems and feelings to a permissive and understanding person. Some patients are inhibited in discussing their difficulties with their relatives or their closest friends, out of the fear that they will be criticized for complaining or because they anticipate humiliation from admitting they have emotional problems. They tend to equate emotional problems with weakness and character defects.

Some depressed patients experience considerable relief after ventilating their feelings and concerns to the therapist. The emotional release produced by crying occasionally produces a notable alleviation of the symptoms. Severely depressed patients, however, may react adversely to ventilation. After a discussion of their problems they may not only feel more overwhelmed and helpless but may, in addition, feel humiliated over having exposed themselves.

GUIDANCE AND ENVIRONMENTAL CHANGE

The need for some change in the patient's activities is often obvious and the therapist may draw on the therapeutic relationship to induce the patient to modify his routine. For instance, the therapist may act as a catalyst to redirect the patient from self-preoccupation to an interest in the outside world; he might suggest appropriate forms of recreational, manual, intellectual, or aesthetic activities.

Sometimes a change in the over-all pattern of living is helpful. For example, an ambitious businessman may be driving himself further into a depression by continuing his stressful activities and by denying himself any form of passive gratification. Since the patient might not reduce his absorption in business of his own volition the therapist may persuade him to take a vacation or to reduce his work load. When chronic marital tensions are contributing to a depression, marriage counselling or (in mild depressions) a period of separation from the spouse may be useful. Although these forms of reducing stress are often helpful in the *reactive* depressions, they must be used cautiously. Some depressed patients, particularly the severely depressed, may fare worse on vacation than if they continue with their regular occupations.

Severely depressed patients who are unable to continue with their usual occupation are often helped by being provided with a well-structured daily program. These patients experience a lack of organization, direction, and motivation. If left to their own inclinations they would stay in one place and brood. A daily program of scheduled hourly activities provides a tangible structure and tends to counteract the regressive, escapist wishes. The schedule, furthermore, helps these patients mobilize constructive motivations and organize their thinking around external goals. In short, this program serves both as an integrative force and also as a distraction from the depressive brooding.

In recommending activities to a depressed patient, the therapist should attempt to gauge both the patient's tolerance for the stress involved and the probabilities of success. The particular task should not be too difficult or too time consuming. We have found that the successful completion of a task by depressed patients *significantly increases optimism, level of aspiration, and performance on subsequent tasks* (Loeb *et al.*, 1966).

Hospitalization is a more extreme form of environmental change and is definitely indicated when there is a serious suicidal risk. The hospital, furthermore, not only removes the patient from domestic stress but can provide a therapeutic regimen that is not available at home. A structured program of occupational therapy, recreational therapy, and group and individual psychotherapy has been shown to reduce the duration of psychotic depressions (Friedman *et al.*, 1966).

COGNITIVE (INSIGHT) PSYCHOTHERAPY

Cognitive psychotherapy is based on the theory elaborated in Chapters 17 and 18. In brief, the theory postulates that the depressed or depression-prone individual has certain idiosyncratic cognitive patterns (schemas) which may become activated either by specific stresses impinging on specific vulnerabilities or by overwhelming, nonspecific stresses. When the cognitive patterns are activated, they tend to dominate the individual's thinking and to produce the affective and motivational phenomena associated with depression. Cognitive psychotherapy may be used symptomatically during depressions to help the patient gain objectivity toward his automatic reactions and counteract them. During nondepressed periods, the therapy is designed to modify the idiosyncratic cognitive patterns to reduce the patient's vulnerability to future depressions.

The techniques consist of: a *macroscopic* or longitudinal approach, aimed at mapping out the patient's sensitivities, exaggerated or inappropriate reactions, and the cause-effect relationships between external events and internal discomfort; a *microscopic* or cross-sectional approach, focused on recognizing and evaluating specific cognitions; and the identification and modification of the misconceptions, superstitions, and syllogisms that lead to maladaptive reactions.

Although cognitive psychotherapy may be used in conjunction with supportive therapy during the depressive episodes, its major application is in the postdepressed period. During this period, the patient may have transient periods of feeling blue but for the most part is functioning well enough to be able to examine objectively his life patterns, his automatic thoughts, and his basic misconceptions. This approach is designed to produce changes in the cognitive organization to reduce the patient's vulnerability to future depressions.

I have also found cognitive psychotherapy effective in certain types of depressed patients *during* the depression; these are generally cases that would be classified as *reactive* rather than *endogenous* depressions. The characteristics of these patients are: (*a*) They are not severely ill; (*b*) the precipitation of the depression is related to a significant environmental event such as a disruption of a close interpersonal relationship or a serious financial reversal; and (*c*) the illness does not follow the typical U-shaped curve described in Chapter 3, namely, a continuous downward progression, then a flattening out, and then a continuous improvement. The depressed patient who is amenable to cognitive psychotherapy generally shows wide fluctuations during the course of a day and also from day to day. These fluctuations, moreover, are related to specific environmental events; positive experiences diminish and negative experiences increase the degree of depression.

Delineating the Major Maladaptive Patterns

One of the first steps in the insight psychotherapy of the depressed patient is a survey of the life history data. In reviewing the patient's history of difficulties the therapist tries to identify the major patterns and sequences in the patient's life. It is generally possible to demonstrate to him that he responds *selectively* to certain types of experiences; i.e., he does not overreact to *every* type of difficult or unpleasant situation, but has a predilection to react excessively to *certain* events.

The therapist should attempt to reconstruct with the patient the stages in the development of his depression (Chapter 18). These include the formation of maladaptive attitudes as the result of early experiences, the sensitization to particular types of stresses, and the precipitation of the depression as the result either of a gross traumatic event or of more insidious influences. By reviewing his history in this way, the patient is able to see his psychological disturbance in terms of specific problems rather than in terms of symptoms. The increased objectivity and understanding removes the mystery and may then provide a measure of mastery of the problems.

A patient suffering from intermittent depression reported that he had been feeling blue all day. At first he had no idea what had initiated his depressed feeling. He recalled that when he awoke he felt quite good. As he reported this he remembered that he started to feel somewhat below par when his wife did not get up to prepare breakfast for him. In recounting this episode he became visibly upset. He then realized that he had felt rejected by his wife's not getting up—even though he knew that she was very tired from having been up most of the night with their baby.

Tracing back his patterns of reaction, the patient recognized that he generally responded adversely whenever he did not get much attention. In grade school, for instance, where he was the teacher's pet, he felt hurt whenever the teacher praised another student or did not pay him a compliment. That he got more praise than any other student in the class did not relieve his feelings on the few occasions when he did not get praise. He recalled that later he felt similarly rejected when any of his close friends did not show the usual amount of warmth or camaraderie. Both his parents were very warm and indulgent people and he was aware of always wanting their approval (which he usually got) as well as that of almost everybody else he met.

In reviewing the cause-and-effect sequences, the patient recognized that he had a pattern of reading rejection into any situation in which he did not get preferential treatment. He could see the inappropriateness of this reaction. He realized, furthermore, that he depended on getting constant approval to maintain his sense of worthwhileness. When the approval was not forthcoming he was prone to react with hurt feelings. In applying this formulation to his reaction to his wife's not getting up in the morning, he realized that he had misinterpreted her behavior. As he said, "I guess I got it all wrong. She wasn't rejecting me. She simply was too tired to get up. I took it though as a sign of her not liking me and I felt bad about it."

Among the more common situations that produce disproportionate or inappropriate reactions in the depression-prone patient are: failing to reach a particular goal, being excluded from a group, being rejected by another person, receiving criticism, and not receiving expected approval, encouragement, or guidance. Although such situations might be expected to produce transient unpleasant reactions in the average person, they may produce prolonged feelings of disappointment or hopelessness in the depression-prone person.

By being primed in advance to recognize his typical overreaction, the patient is fortified when the specific stress occurs and he is less likely to be overwhelmed by it. It is generally possible for the therapist to point out the precise characteristics of the exaggerated reaction, viz., that the patient is reacting according to a repetitive pattern rather than to the specific features of the reality situation. The patient feels overwhelmed or hopeless, for example, not because the situation is overwhelming or insoluble but because he construes it that way. By referring to the past history, the therapist can demonstrate how the maladaptive pattern got started and was repeated on various occasions.

One woman, for instance, felt sad and unwanted whenever a friend or acquaintance had a party and did not invite her. Intense and prolonged feelings of rejection were aroused although she was very popular and was, in truth, invited to more parties than she had time to attend. We were able to date the onset of this rejection pattern to early adolescence when she entered junior high school. At that time she was excluded from various cliques that the other girls formed. She vividly remembered sitting alone in the cafeteria and thinking that she was socially undesirable and inferior to the other girls. In therapy, she was able to recognize that the rejection pattern was mobilized inappropriately in her adult life. Her concept, "I have no friends and nobody wants me," was no longer valid. Until it was pointed out that she was simply re-living a past experience, as it were, she tended to believe that not being invited to a party indicated that she did not really have any friends.

Neutralizing "Automatic Thoughts"

The second approach in insight therapy consists of the patient's focusing on his specific depression-generating cognitions. In the mild or moderately ill depressed patient, these thoughts are often at the periphery of awareness and require special focusing in order for the patient to recognize them. In psychoanalytical terminology, they would probably be regarded as preconscious. In the more severely ill depressed patient, however, these thoughts are at the center of the patient's phenomenal field and tend to dominate the thought content.

This kind of depression-generating cognition seems to be a highly condensed representation of more elaborate ideas. The ideas are apparently compressed into a kind of shorthand and a rather complicated thought occurs within a split second. Albert Ellis (1962) refers to these thoughts as "self-statements" or "internalized verbalizations." He explains these thoughts as "things that the patient tells himself." I have labeled these types of cognitions as *automatic thoughts*.

As pointed out in Chapter 15, these self-statements or cognitions reflect the distortions that occur in the depressed state. As a result of these distortions, the patient experiences dysphoria. But when he can identify the distorted cognitions, and can acquire objectivity towards them and correct them, he can neutralize some of their pathogenic quality.

Pinpointing Depressive Cognitions

At the beginning of therapy the patient is generally aware only of the following sequence: event or stimulus → affect. He must be trained to fill in the link between the stimulus and the affect: stimulus → cognition → affect.

A patient, for example, reported that he felt blue every time he made a mistake, and he could not understand why he should feel this way. He fully accepted the notion that there was nothing wrong in making mistakes and that it was an inevitable part of living. He was instructed to focus on his thoughts the next time he felt an unpleasant affect in connection with making a mistake. At the next interview he reported the observation that whenever he made a mistake he would think "I'm a dope," or "I never do anything right," or "How can anybody be so dumb." After having one of these thoughts he would become depressed. By becoming aware of the self-criticisms, however, he was able to recognize how unreasonable they were. This recognition seemed to remove the sting from his blue reactions.

The automatic thoughts not only bear a relationship to unpleasant affect but also bear a relationship to many of the other phenomena of depression. Loss of motivation, for example, is based on such ideas as "I won't be able to do it," or "If I do this, I will only feel worse." Examples of the influence of the depressive thinking on motivation are found in Chapter 17.

As the patient becomes more adept at recognizing the precise wording of his automatic thoughts, he is less influenced by them. He can view them as though from a distance and can assess their validity. The processes of recognition and distancing are the initial steps in neutralizing the automatic thoughts.

Identifying Idiosyncratic Content

As the patient gains experience in recognizing his cognitions he becomes ready to identify the common themes among the cognitions that produce an unpleasant feeling. In order to help him to categorize his cognitions, I generally point out the major depressive themes, such as deprivation, self-reproach, or sense of inferiority. It is important to emphasize that of the inumerable ways in which he can interpret his life experiences he tends to perseverate in a few stereotyped interpretations or explanations; he may, for example, repeatedly interpret any interpersonal difficulty or dissension as indicating his own deficiency. It is also important to point out to him how these depressive cognitions actually represent distortions of reality.

It is often difficult for the patient to accept the idea that his interpretations are incorrect, or at least inaccurate. In fact, the more depressed the patient is, the more difficult it is for him to regard the depressive cognitions with any degree of objectivity.

Recognizing Formal Characteristics of Cognitions

To increase the patient's objectivity towards his cognitions and to help him evaluate them, it is often helpful to point out some of the characteristics of the cognitions. This not only helps him to identify them, but it also gives him a chance to question their authenticity.

It is often valuable to make a distinction for the patient between "two types of thinking." The first type is the *higher-level* type of thinking that involves judgment, weighing of the evidence, and consideration of alternative explanations (secondary process). The *lower-level* form of cognition, in contrast, tends to be relatively rapid and does not seem to involve any complicated logical processes (primary process).

One of the characteristics of the lower-level cognitions is that they tend to be *automatic*. They arise as if by reflex and are generally not the result of deliberation or careful reasoning. A patient observed that when she approached a task (preparing a meal, writing a letter, making a phone call) she immediately had the thought, "I can't do it." When she focused her attention on this thought, she recognized its arbitrariness and she was able to assume some detachment towards it. After the patient has been successful in specifying the idiosyncratic cognitions generated by certain specific situations, he is in a better position to prepare himself to deal with them when they arise.

Another important characteristic of the depressive cognitions is their *involuntary* quality. In the more severe cases, particularly, it is apparent that these cognitions continuously invade the phenomenal field and the patient has little power to ward them off or to focus his attention on something else. Even when he is determined to think rationally about a situation and to make an objective judgment he is apt to be diverted by the relentless intrusion of the depressive cognitions. This perseverating and compelling quality of the depressive cognitions may be so strong as to make any form of insight therapy fruitless at this stage.

In the less severely ill patient, the recognition of the involuntary aspect of the cognitions helps to drive home that they are not the result of any deliberation or reasoning. The patient is able to look upon them as a kind of obsession that intrudes onto his more rational thinking but that does not have to be given any particular truth value.

One of the crucial characteristics of these cognitions in terms of psychotherapy is that they seem *plausible* to the patient. Even normal people tend to accept the validity of their thoughts without subjecting them to any kind of careful scrutiny. The problem is compounded for the depressed patient because the idiosyncratic cognitions seem especially plausible or real. At times the more incongruous these cognitions may appear to the therapist the more plausible they may seem to the patient. The more reasonable the thought seems to be, the greater is the affective reaction. The converse also seems to be true; the more intense the affective state, the more credible the depressive cognitions are to the patient. When the intensity of the affect is reduced through antidepressant drugs, there is a diminution in the compelling quality of the cognitions. This seems to indicate an interaction between cognition and affect.

Distinguishing "Ideas" from "Facts"

After the patient becomes experienced in recognizing the idiosyncratic content and other characteristics of the cognitions, the therapeutic work consists of training him to evaluate their validity or accuracy. This procedure consists essentially of the application of the rules of evidence and logic to the cognitions and the consideration of alternative explanations or interpretations by the patient.

In examining the validity of a cognition, the patient first must learn to make a distinction between thinking and believing; i.e., simply because he *thinks* something does not, *ipso facto,* mean he should *believe* it. Despite the often apparent sophistication of the patient it is necessary to point out that thoughts are not equivalent to external reality, and, no matter how convincing they may seem, they should not be accepted unless validated by some objective procedure.

A patient, for instance, had the thought that his girlfriend no longer liked him. Instead of treating this notion as a hypothesis he accepted it as an actuality. He then used this notion to explain recent differences in his girlfriend's behavior and thus fortified his acceptance of the idea. The goal of therapy is to help the patient shift from this type of deductive analysis of experience to more inductive procedures. By checking his observations, by taking into account all the data, and by considering other hypotheses to explain the events, he is less prone to equate his automatic thoughts with reality.

Checking Observations

The validation of the patient's interpretations and judgments depends on checking the accuracy and completeness of the initial observations. On reflection, the patient frequently discovers that either his original impression of a situation was distorted or that he jumped to a conclusion too quickly and thus ignored or rejected salient details that were not compatible with that conclusion. A professor, for example, was downcast and complained that he was "slipping" because "nobody showed up" for a lecture. On re-examining the evidence, he realized that this was his initial impression, but that in actuality most of the seats in the lecture hall were filled. Having made an incorrect preliminary judgment, he had failed to correct it until he was helped to re-examine the evidence.

A woman told me she had "made a fool out of myself" in a job interview the day before. She felt humiliated and downcast up to the time of our appointment. I then inquired "What *actually happened* in the interview?" As she recounted the details of the interview, she realized that she had handled it rather well and that her negative judgment was based on only one short portion of the interview.

Responding to Depressive Cognitions

Once the patient has established that a particular cognition is invalid it is important for him (or the therapist) to neutralize its effects by stating precisely why it is inaccurate, inappropriate, or invalid. By verbalizing the reasons that the idea was erroneous, the patient is able to reduce the intensity and frequency of the idea as well as of the accompanying affect.

A depressed patient, for instance, found that no matter how fastidiously she cleaned a drawer or closet she thought that it was still dirty. This made her feel discouraged until she began to counter the thought with the following rebuttal: "I'm a good housekeeper—which I know and other people have told me. There's absolutely no sign of dirt. It's just as clean as it ever is when I'm not depressed. There may be a few specks of dust but that's not dirt." On another occasion, when she started to prepare a roast, she had the thought, "I won't be able to do it." She reasoned the problem through and verbalized to herself, "I've done this many times before. I may be a little slower than usual because I'm depressed but I know what to do and if I think it out step-by-step there's no reason why I can't do it." She felt heartened after this and finished preparing the meal.

It is often helpful for the patient to label the particular paralogical mechanisms involved in the depressive cognition, e.g., overgeneralization, arbitrary inference, selective abstraction, or magnification (Chapter 15). If he can say to himself, "I'm taking this out of context," or "I'm jumping to conclusions," or "I'm exaggerating," he may be able to reduce the power of the depressive cognition.

Weighing Alternative Explanations

Another method of neutralizing the inaccurate negative interpretations is the consideration of alternative explanations. For instance, a patient, who was exceptionally personable and popular, would characteristically interpret any reduction of enthusiasm toward her as a sign of rejection and also as evidence that she was unlikeable. After some training in dealing with her idiosyncratic cognitions, she reported the following incident. She was conversing on the telephone with an old friend when the friend said she had to hang up because she had a beauty parlor appointment. The patient's immediate thought was, "She doesn't like me," and she felt sad and disappointed. Applying the technique of alternative explanations, she countered with the following: "Marjorie has been my friend for many years. She has always shown that she likes me. I know she has a beauty parlor appointment today and that is obviously the reason why she had to hang up." Her initial interpretation was part of a stereotyped pattern and excluded the proffered explanation. When the patient reviewed the episode and considered the possible explanations she was able to accept her friend's explanation as more probable than her automatic interpretations.

VALIDATING BASIC PREMISES

Although the technique just described deals directly with the specific cognitions, the operation to be described in this section is directed towards the patient's underlying chronic misconceptions, prejudices, and superstitions about himself and his world. Allied to these are the assumptions basic to the way the individual sets goals, assesses and modifies his behavior, and explains adverse occurrences; these assumptions underlie the injunctions, debasements, criticisms, punitiveness, and blame that the patient directs to himself. The aim to modify these chronic attitudes and patterns (schemas) is based on the thesis that they partly determine the content of the individual's cognitions. It should follow that a basic modification or attenuation of these schemas would modify the way he organizes and interprets specific experiences, as well as how he sets his goals and goes about achieving them.

The content of the chronic attitudes may be readily inferred (Chapter 18) from the examination of the recurrent themes in the patient's cognitive responses to particular situations and in his free associations (themes of personal deficiency, debility, and hopelessness). Further information about his basic premises and assumptions may be obtained by asking him either what he bases a particular conclusion on, or his reasons for a specific judgment. An inquiry into his values, opinions, and beliefs will yield additional data. Some idea of the schemas used in approaching his problems or in attaining goals may be obtained by an examination of his self-instructions and self-reproaches. One of the useful features of this approach is that it attempts to correct the major premises or assumptions that form the basis for the deductive thinking. Since the predominance of deductive (as opposed to inductive) thinking is an important determinant of the cognitive distortions in depression, any correction of the invalid major premises will tend to reduce the erroneous conclusions.

Illustrative of the typical assumptions and premises underlying the cognitive distortions in depression are ideas such as the following: "It is very bad to make a mistake." "If anything goes wrong, it's my fault." "I'm basically unlucky and bring bad luck to myself and everybody else." "If I don't continue to make a lot of money, I will go bankrupt." "I really am quite stupid and my academic success is the result of clever faking." "Trouble with constipation is a sign of disintegration."

Let us say that a patient reports, "Everything I did today was wrong;" or "Everybody has been pushing me around;" or "I'm getting uglier every day." The therapist may review with the patient the evidence for these conclusions and may attempt to demonstrate that the ideas are exaggerations or frank misinterpretations. Often, however, the ideas are so strong that the patient cannot even contemplate the possibility that they could be inaccurate. In such cases, the force of the ideas may be weakened by dissecting the network of underlying assumptions.

A depressed woman of 40 had strong suicidal wishes. She justified these as follows: "What's the use of living. I've got to die some time anyhow. I'm just prolonging something that's deteriorating. It's a losing battle so I might as well get out now before I've deteriorated completely." Rebuttals to the effect she was still relatively young, attractive, and healthy and that she still had many potential years of happiness did not influence her thinking. She clung to the notion that she was decaying and that, if she lived, she would soon experience the horror of physical disintegration.

One day, in looking in the mirror, she observed that the image appeared to be that of her mother during her terminal illness. She turned her head in disgust and felt more depressed. Although she realized that the reflection was hers, not her mother's, she could not shake the belief that she had already deteriorated so much that she now looked like her dying mother.

Drawing on this information, I said to the patient, "Your whole idea of quitting life is based on one premise: You believe that you are following in your mother's footsteps. You got the notion when she was dying that when you reached her age (40 years) you would start to have strokes and would go to pieces. The truth of the matter is that all our tests have shown that your physical health is perfect. Your mother had severe diabetes since childhood and she became blind and had her strokes as a complication of the diabetes. However, you don't have diabetes and, in fact, you don't have any physical disease."

I explained to the patient how she had identified herself with her mother and how this formed the basis for the premise that she was starting to deteriorate. She had, without fully realizing it, adopted the formula: getting old (i.e. more than 40 years) equals becoming deteriorated and ugly. By pinpointing this formula, we were able to discuss its validity. As she was able to see the arbitrariness of this equation, her ideas that she was ugly and deteriorating started to fade as did her suicidal wishes.

Sometimes the patient can see the fallacy of his basic assumptions without any difficulty. However, the simple acknowledgement of their irrationality may not change them. They may continue to be manifest in repetitive automatic thoughts. It is often necessary to examine the invalid assumptions repeatedly and to encourage the patient to state the reasons they are invalid. Sometimes, I direct the patient to specify the argument in favor of the invalid assumption and then the argument against it. At other times I offer the argument supporting an invalid assumption and induce the patient to supply the rebuttal.

A scientist felt sad and empty whenever he failed to get recognition for his performance. We were able to establish that he had a set of interlocking premises: "It is of utmost importance that I become famous. The only gratification I can get out of life is by being acclaimed by everybody. If I do not achieve fame, then my life is worthless and meaningless." If these premises were correct, then it would be inevitable that he would feel ungratified and empty when he missed out on recognition. If they were invalid, then they could be modified and he would be less subject to feelings of desolation when he failed to get recognition.

To test the validity of these assumptions, I presented the following argument. "If these premises are true, we would expect the following to happen. One, that you never obtain gratification from anything except recognition. Two, that recognition has brought you gratification. Three, that nothing in life means anything or is worth anything to you except fame."

Upon hearing this argument, the patient was quick to provide a rebuttal. "I *have* gotten pleasure from lots of things that don't involve recognition. I enjoy my family and friends. I get a lot of satisfaction from reading and listening to classical records and going to concerts. Also I really do enjoy my work and would like what I'm doing even if I did not get any recognition at all. Besides, when I do get recognition, I don't get much feeling of satisfaction from it. Actually, I find that personal relationships are more satisfying than getting an article published."

After many discussions of this nature, the exaggerated emphasis on recognition was reduced, and the patient found that he was able to get more enjoyment out of his work because he was no longer continually worried about recognition. Furthermore, he was able to enjoy his nonprofessional activities more because activities not directed towards achieving fame no longer were regarded as a waste of time.

MODIFYING MOOD BY INDUCED FANTASIES

Some depressed patients report spontaneous fantasies (daydreams), which have a gloomy content such as deprivation, personal inadequacy, and thwarting. When he contemplates an event in the near or distant future, the patient has a pictorial image of a negative outcome.

A depressed woman sat down to prepare her list of items to be purchased at a grocery store. She then experienced the following fantasy, which she later reported to me: "I went into the supermarket with my marketing list. I went from counter to counter and I couldn't find what I wanted. I then noticed that people were looking at me peculiarly as though they thought I was crazy. I felt so humiliated I had to leave without buying anything." As a result she did not go to the market that day.

It is noteworthy that while she was having this fantasy, the patient experienced intense humiliation as though the fantasied event was occurring in reality. In an attempt to help her deal with the expectation of frustration and humiliation, I asked her to imagine the scene in the supermarket again. This time she felt less humiliation. After imaging the same scene three more times, she no longer felt any unpleasant affect in association with the fantasy. She remarked, "I can see that I was really exaggerating the problem in my daydream." Following this interview, the patient was able to do her marketing without any difficulty.

This example illustrates that a patient may react to his fantasies in much the same way that he reacts to his automatic thoughts. The patient may be trained to deal therapeutically with his fantasies in much the same way as he can deal with maladaptive ideas of a verbal nature.

By having the patient repeat the depressive fantasy during the therapy session, the therapist can help him gain greater objectivity towards the actual real life situation. This kind of *rehearsal* may then enable the patient to undertake a task that he had previously avoided.

Sometimes spontaneous modification of the content of the fantasy may be achieved by simple repetition of the fantasy. A patient was feeling pessimistic about his job and had a fantasy on the way to my office: "I went into my superior's office with a suggestion. He got very angry with me. I felt I had stepped beyond the proper bounds." The feeling that accompanied this fantasy was discouragement and humiliation. When I asked him to imagine the scene again, he experienced a repetition of the same unpleasant affects.

I then asked the patient to imagine the scene once more. This time the fantasy was as follows: "My boss was interested in what I had to say. He wanted more information. I felt that there was a mutual interchange between two professionals." The affect accompanying this fantasy was pleasant. Concomitantly, the patient's generally pessimistic mood about the anticipated events of the day lifted and he went to work feeling more optimistic and self-confident. The actual outcome of his interaction with his superior was similar to that in the pleasant fantasy.

I have found in other cases that it has been possible to alleviate pessimism by inducing the patient to have more realistic fantasies about anticipated events. Another technique of combatting the sense of inadequacy or deprivation is to suggest that the patient recall in pictorial form certain past successes or gratifications. Upon revivifying the past memories, the patients often experience a sense of gratification that persists for the rest of the day.

The technique of fantasy induction serves much the same purpose as examination of the maladaptive self-verbalizations. By examining his gloomy fantasies, the patient is able to loosen their grip on him, to reality test them, and to consider more favorable outcomes. Moreover, the induction of pleasant fantasies helps to neutralize his sadness and pessimism.

Appendix

DEPRESSION INVENTORY

A. (SADNESS)

0 I do not feel sad
1 I feel blue or sad
2a I am blue or sad all the time and I can't snap out of it
2b I am so sad or unhappy that it is quite painful
3 I am so sad or unhappy that I can't stand it

B. (PESSIMISM)

0 I am not particularly pessimistic or discouraged about the future
1a I feel discouraged about the future
2a I feel I have nothing to look forward to
2b I feel that I won't ever get over my troubles
3 I feel that the future is hopeless and that things cannot improve

C. (SENSE OF FAILURE)

0 I do not feel like a failure
1 I feel I have failed more than the average person
2a I feel I have accomplished very little that is worthwhile or that means anything
2b As I look back on my life all I can see is a lot of failures
3 I feel I am a complete failure as a person (parent, husband, wife)

D. (DISSATISFACTION)

0 I am not particularly dissatisfied
1a I feel bored most of the time
1b I don't enjoy things the way I used to
2 I don't get satisfaction out of anything any more
3 I am dissatisfied with everything

E. (GUILT)

0 I don't feel particularly guilty
1 I feel bad or unworthy a good part of the time
2a I feel quite guilty
2b I feel bad or unworthy practically all the time now
3 I feel as though I am very bad or worthless

333

F. (EXPECTATION OF PUNISHMENT)

    0 I don't feel I am being punished
    1 I have a feeling that something bad may happen to me
    2 I feel I am being punished or will be punished
    3a I feel I deserve to be punished
    3b I want to be punished

G. (SELF-DISLIKE)

    0 I don't feel disappointed in myself
    1a I am disappointed in myself
    1b I don't like myself
    2 I am disgusted with myself
    3 I hate myself

H. (SELF-ACCUSATIONS)

    0 I don't feel I am any worse than anybody else
    2 I am critical of myself for my weaknesses or mistakes
    2 I blame myself for my faults
    3 I blame myself for everything bad that happens

I. (SUICIDAL IDEAS)

    0 I don't have any thoughts of harming myself
    1 I have thoughts of harming myself but I would not carry them out
    2a I feel I would be better off dead
    2b I feel my family would be better off if I were dead
    3a I have definite plans about committing suicide
    3b I would kill myself if I could

J. (CRYING)

    0 I don't cry any more than usual
    1 I cry more now than I used to
    2 I cry all the time now. I can't stop it
    3 I used to be able to cry but now I can't cry at all even though I want to

K. (IRRITABILITY)

    0 I am no more irritated now than I ever am
    1 I get annoyed or irritated more easily than I used to
    2 I feel irritated all the time
    3 I don't get irritated at all at the things that used to irritate me

L. (SOCIAL WITHDRAWAL)

    0 I have not lost interest in other people
    1 I am less interested in other people now than I used to be
    2 I have lost most of my interest in other people and have little feeling for them
    3 I have lost all my interest in other people and don't care about them at all

M. (INDECISIVENESS)

    0 I make decisions about as well as ever
    1 I try to put off making decisions
    2 I have great difficulty in making decisions
    3 I can't make any decisions at all any more

N. (BODY IMAGE CHANGE)

0   I don't feel I look any worse than I used to
1   I am worried that I am looking old or unattractive
2   I feel that there are permanent changes in my appearance and they make me look unattractive
3   I feel that I am ugly or repulsive looking

O. (WORK RETARDATION)

0   I can work about as well as before
1a It takes extra effort to get started at doing something
1b I don't work as well as I used to
2   I have to push myself very hard to do anything
3   I can't do any work at all

P. (INSOMNIA)

0   I can sleep as well as usual
1   I wake up more tired in the morning than I used to
2   I wake up 1–2 hours earlier than usual and find it hard to get back to sleep
3   I wake up early every day and can't get more than 5 hours sleep

Q. (FATIGABILITY)

0   I don't get any more tired than usual
1   I get tired more easily than I used to
2   I get tired from doing anything
3   I get too tired to do anything

R. (ANOREXIA)

0   My appetite is no worse than usual
1   My appetite is not as good as it used to be
2   My appetite is much worse now
3   I have no appetite at all any more

S. (WEIGHT LOSS)

0   I haven't lost much weight, if any, lately
1   I have lost more than 5 pounds
2   I have lost more than 10 pounds
3   I have lost more than 15 pounds

T. (SOMATIC PREOCCUPATION)

0   I am no more concerned about my health than usual
1   I am concerned about aches and pains *or* upset stomach *or* constipation
2   I am so concerned with how I feel or what I feel that it's hard to think of much else
3   I am completely absorbed in what I feel

U. (LOSS OF LIBIDO)

0   I have not noticed any recent change in my interest in sex
1   I am less interested in sex than I used to be
2   I am much less interested in sex now
3   I have lost interest in sex completely

INSTRUCTIONS FOR ADMINISTRATION OF DEPRESSION INVENTORY

The following instructions have been developed in order to standardize the administration of the Depression Inventory. It is important that they be followed in order to provide uniformity and to minimize interviewer effects.

Routine of Administration

Say to the patient, "This is a questionnaire. On the questionnaire are groups of statements. I will read a group of statements. Then I want you to pick out the one statement in that group which best describes the way you feel today, that is, *right now!*"

At this point hand a copy of the questionnaire to the patient and say, "Here is a copy for you to follow as I read." Read the entire group of statements in the first category (do not read the numbers appearing before the statements); then say, "Now, which *one* of the statements best describes the way you feel right now?"

If the patient indicates his choice by responding with a number, read back the statement corresponding to the number given by the patient, in order to avoid confusion as to which statement is selected. If the patient says "the first statement," he may mean 0 or 1. After you are satisfied that the patient understands the numbering system, the numerical answer should be a sufficient indication of his choice.

Additional Notes

1. Make sure that each choice is indeed the patient's choice and not words you have put in his mouth. Get the patient to express, on his own, which statement is his choice.

2. If the patient indicates that there are two or more statements that fit the way he feels, then record the *higher* of the two values.

3. If the patient indicates that the way he feels is between, say, 2 and 3, being more than 2 but not quite 3, then record the value he is closer to, or 2.

4. Generally, the interviewer should continue to read aloud the statements comprising each category. Sometimes the patient will take the initiative and read the statements in a category silently, ahead of the interviewer, and start giving his preference. If the patient is alert and apparently knowledgeable, let him read the statements silently and then make his choice. Explain to such a patient that the reason you read the statements aloud is so that you can be sure he had read all the statements in the category before making his choice. Tell the patient that *if he will be sure to read all statements* in each group *before* making his choice, he may read silently. Use tact and diplomacy to encourage the patient to reflect sufficiently before making a choice.

5. The depression score should be entered on a record sheet. It is simply the sum of the weighted responses of items A through U. The weight is the numeral adjacent to each statement.

Appendix Table 1.
INTERCORRELATION OF DEPRESSION INVENTORY ITEMS ($n = 606$)

	(1)	(2)	(3)	(4)	(5)	(6)	(7)	(8)	(9)	(10)	(11)	(12)	(13)	(14)	(15)	(16)	(17)	(18)	(19)	(20)
1. Sadness																				
2. Pessimism	.52																			
3. Failure	.40	.41																		
4. Dissatisfaction	.49	.48	.41																	
5. Guilt	.36	.45	.48	.41																
6. Punishment	.27	.31	.31	.30	.39															
7. Self-dislike	.40	.38	.50	.41	.41	.32														
8. Self-accusations	.24	.28	.40	.31	.41	.28	.38													
9. Suicidal	.43	.46	.39	.35	.36	.33	.41	.31												
10. Crying	.26	.25	.27	.30	.23	.19	.28	.24	.29											
11. Irritability	.19	.17	.14	.22	.15	.05	.12	.12	.14	.18										
12. Withdrawal	.34	.35	.36	.45	.35	.28	.37	.27	.39	.30	.15									
13. Indecisive	.41	.42	.41	.39	.36	.23	.28	.36	.37	.34	.17	.40								
14. Self-image	.29	.28	.31	.30	.29	.19	.27	.27	.30	.22	.11	.25	.32							
15. Retarded	.32	.39	.26	.37	.28	.19	.27	.19	.25	.18	.05	.26	.34	.21						
16. Insomnia	.29	.31	.17	.28	.12	.19	.19	.12	.22	.14	.22	.22	.23	.22	.28					
17. Fatigue	.30	.36	.30	.36	.25	.22	.23	.20	.22	.20	.12	.29	.37	.24	.47	.25				
18. Anorexia	.37	.32	.14	.30	.22	.25	.21	.16	.26	.24	.10	.29	.28	.26	.23	.35	.20			
19. Weight loss	.18	.10	.07	.09	.05	.06	.03	.07	.05	.17	.10	.08	.13	.14	.08	.26	.07	.34		
20. Hypochondria	.26	.18	.19	.24	.20	.09	.15	.17	.10	.14	.13	.11	.17	.12	.23	.21	.24	.16	.14	
21. Libido loss	.33	.30	.23	.26	.17	.19	.15	.15	.22	.18	.07	.34	.22	.26	.30	.29	.29	.33	.25	.15

SCORING INSTRUCTIONS FOR "MASOCHISTIC DREAMS"

DEFINITION

The term "masochistic dream" designates a class of unpleasant dreams characterized by a specific thematic content. The image of the dreamer has negative characteristics and/or the outcome of the dream sequence is essentially a negative one. The dreamer is either represented as less fortunate or less attractive than he is in reality (such as defective, ugly, or sick) or he is subjected to an unpleasant experience (such as thwarting, rejection, or deprivation). The description of the dreamer, the action, the setting, or the outcome of the dream suggests that the dream is unpleasant.

SCORING

The dream is designated as "masochistic" if it contains any of the elements listed below. The scoring is dichotomous: Each dream is scored + if it contains one or more of these elements; 0 if it does not.

Negative Representation of the Self

The dreamer is portrayed in a negative way. He has unpleasant attributes that are not present in reality or are exaggerated in the dream. He is deficient or defective in some way. His appearance has changed so that he is less attractive.

Examples: "I was a bum."
"I was mentally defective."
"I had pus oozing out of all my pores."
"I was a cripple."
"I was blind."
"I was too weak to move."
"I had become old and ugly."
"I had a disgusting odor."
"I had tuberculosis."
"My hair fell out."
"I was very dirty."

The negative representation may be in terms of deficiencies in mental functioning or personality.

Examples: "Somebody gave me directions. My mind was all messed up and I didn't know what he was talking about."
"I had a repulsive personality and people shunned me."

When the dream is scored blindly, there may be no basis for deciding whether the negative characteristics are a correct portrayal or a distortion of reality. In such a case, the rule is to score the dream as "masochistic" since our experience has shown that the negative self-representations are almost always distortions or exaggerations of reality.

Physical Discomfort and Injury

Discomfort, suffering, or pathological changes are explicitly stated or are reasonable inferences from the dream content. Sometimes, this category overlaps the previous category.

Examples: "Leeches were crawling all over me."
"Blood was coming out of my nose."
"I was strapped down to a table."
"I was buried alive."
"I hurt myself."
"Our auto crashed. We were all taken to the hospital."
"A horse kicked me in the head."
"I was burned in a fire."

Thwarting

The dreamer does something or tries to do something but the outcome is unsatisfactory. His actions have an obvious goal and he is prevented from attaining it by an external factor. The thwarting must be something the dreamer does not deliberately bring on himself. It should be likely from the context or the wording that this kind of thwarting would produce distress if it happened in actuality (i.e., in the waking life).

Examples: "I rushed to get to my analytic session. When I got there, the door was locked."
"I made some toast. The popper did not work and the toast burned."
"I drove over to visit some old friends but ended up at the wrong house."
"I took careful aim and fired at the deer, but my gun didn't go off."
"I tried to save my daughter but my feet got stuck in the mud."
"I *looked* and *looked* and *looked*, but I couldn't find my notes."
"I got into a fight but my blows did not touch my opponent."

The following do *not* score because there is no indication that the goal is important to the dreamer or that thwarting occurs.

Examples: "I suggested lunch to the men but they weren't hungry. So we just sat around."

"I went into town to see a movie. I saw a parade and I followed it. I never did get to the movie."

"I was on my way to class. Then the scene shifted and I was skiing."

Deprivation

Disappointment: The patient wants or requests something but what he gets is less than he wanted or expected. Or he may receive something that he did not explicitly seek but which is obviously unsatisfactory. (This category sometimes overlaps the previous category.)

Examples: "I ordered rye and ginger. The bartender gave me warm beer and liquor, mixed."

"I bought some shoes but they were both for the left foot."

"I was in a restaurant but the waitress would not serve me."

"I put a dime in the coke machine. All that came out was fizz."

"My husband bought me furniture but it was in bad shape and the colors were horrible."

"My father gave me my allowance for the week. It was only a penny."

Loss: The dreamer has sustained the loss of something or someone.

Examples: All my friends had died."

"A robber stole my watch."

"I lost all my money."

Lack: The key factor is the lack of something important to the dreamer such as friendship, affection, food, or material possessions.

Examples: "I was single again. I had no friends, nobody to go to."

"I was all alone. I felt very lonely."

"I had nothing to eat."

"I was in a foreign country. I had nobody to turn to for help."

"I didn't have a cent to my name."

Physical Attack

Another person deliberately attacks (and presumably hurts) the dreamer. The attack is completed and not simply threatened. If the injury is not inflicted deliberately the dream element is scored under Category 2.

Examples: "A man fired a shot at me and it hit me in the arm."

"A gang of bullies beat me up."

"He beat me over the head."

The following do not score because the element of injury is absent.

Examples: "He kept hitting me but I didn't feel the blows."
"Somebody fired at me but missed."
"A man chased me."

Non-physical Attack

The patient is ridiculed, criticized, scolded, blamed, or mistreated.

Examples: "He called me a crybaby."
"My wife said she was disgusted with me."
"I made a fool of myself. Everybody laughed at me."
"They accused me of the crime."
"He cheated me."

Exclusions: Self-blame and self-criticism do not score +.
"It was all my fault."
"I felt I was a crybaby."

Simply being in an argument does not score. It is necessary that the dreamer is getting the worst of it. "He said I should shut up. I said he should shut up.": does not score. But, "He demolished everything I said.": does score.

Excluded, Superseded, or Abandoned

The dreamer is left out, rejected, or displaced by another person.

Examples: "I was the only one not invited to the party."
"My analyst said he didn't want to see me any more."
"My wife married another man."
"My mother gave my brother a ticket but not me."

Lost

The dreamer is lost.

Examples: "I was in a strange house and couldn't find my way out."
"I kept running through tunnels and I couldn't find the exit."
"I was in a city. I didn't know which way to go to get home."

Punishment

The dreamer receives punishment from a legal agency or an authority figure.

Examples: "I was in jail."
"My mother spanked me."
"I was expelled from school."
"I got a parking ticket."

Failure

The dreamer fails in a specific activity. There is no evidence in the dream that the lack of success is due to an external agent (as in Category 3).

Examples: "I flunked the exam."
"I came in last in the race."
"I aimed at the target and missed."
"I tried to solve the problem but I couldn't do it."
"I got up to make a speech and I couldn't think of anything to say."

EXCLUSIONS

No score is given for the following dream actions:

(1) When somebody else is the recipient of the unpleasant experience (even though the dreamer may be identified in some way with the other person).

Examples: "My father was hit by a car."
"A little girl, who looked like me, was lost."

(2) When there is doubt whether the experience is unpleasant.

(3) When the accompanying affect or other statement denies unpleasantness or when the damage is undone.

Examples: "I was shot through the stomach but I did not feel anything."
"I fell into a sewer. It did not bother me at all."
"My hair was messed up but I didn't care."
"Somebody stole my books but returned them to me."
"There was a plot against me but I foiled them."
"I lost my hat but I found it again."

"Threat Dreams"

These *do not score* as "masochistic dreams" unless one of the specific "masochistic" elements or themes listed in Section II is present. It is possible for a dream to score both as "threat" and "masochistic" if both kinds of themes are present. Threat dreams are frequently associated with anxiety states and have the following characteristics:

1. The *affect* is described as fright, fear, apprehension, or a synonym of these. In "masochistic dreams," on the other hand, the affect is stated to be sadness, loneliness, or frustration.

2. There is a danger or threat but no harm, injury, or loss occurs in the dream sequence. In the "masochistic" dream, in contrast, the negative experience occurs before the dream is terminated.

Examples: "A man was chasing me."
"I was falling into a pit."
"There was some dangerous force in the building."

The "masochistic" dreams corresponding to these themes would be:

"A man caught me and beat me."
"I fell into a pit and hit bottom."
"A dangerous force was crushing me."

Bibliography

ABRAHAM, K. (1911): "Notes on the Psychoanalytic Investigation and Treatment of Manic-Depressive Insanity and Allied Conditions," in *Selected Papers on Psychoanalysis*. New York, Basic Books, 1960, pp. 137–156.

ABRAHAM, K. (1916): "The First Pregenital Stage of the Libido," in *Selected Papers on Psychoanalysis*. New York, Basic Books, 1960, pp. 248–279.

ABRAHAM, K. (1924): "A Short Study of the Development of the Libido," in *Selected Papers on Psychoanalysis*. New York, Basic Books, 1960,. pp. 418–501.

ACKNER, B., and PAMPIGLIONE, G. (1959): An evaluation of the sedation threshold test. *J. Psychosom. Res. 3:*271–281.

ADLER, K. A. (1961): Depression in the light of individual psychology. *J. Individ. Psychol. 17:*56–67.

ALBEE, G. W. (1950): Patterns of aggression in psychopathology, *J. Consult. Psychol. 14:*465–468.

ALBEE, G. (1951): The prognostic importance of delusions in schizophrenia. *J. Abnorm. Soc. Psychol. 46:*208–212.

ALEXANDER, F., and WILSON, G. W. (1935): Quantitative dream studies: a methodological attempt at a quantitative evaluation of psychoanalytic material. *Psychoanal. Quart. 4:*371–407.

ALLPORT, F. H. (1955): *Theories of Perception and the Concept of Structure.* New York, Wiley.

AMERICAN PSYCHIATRIC ASSOCIATION (1952): *Diagnostic and Statistical Manual: Mental Disorders.* Washington, D.C.

AMERICAN PSYCHOLOGICAL ASSOCIATION (1954): Validity. Technical recommendations for psychological tests and diagnostic techniques. *Psychol. Bull. (suppl.) 51:*13–28.

ANASTASI A., and FOLEY, J. P. (1949): *Differential Psychology; Individual and Group Differences in Behavior.* New York, Macmillan.

ANDERSON, W. McC., and DAWSON, J. (1962): The clinical manifestations of depressive illness with abnormal acetyl methyl carbinol metabolism. *J. Ment. Sci. 108:*80–87.

APPEL, K. E. (1944): "Psychiatric Therapy," in *Personality and the Behavior Disorders,* ed. by HUNT, J. New York, Ronald Press, vol. II, pp. 1107–1163.

ARETAEUS (c. 150 A.D.): *The Extant Work of Aretaeus, the Cappadocian,* ed. and trans. by ADAMS, F. London, Sydenham Soc. Pub., 1856.

ARIETI, S. (1959): "Manic-Depressive Psychosis," in *American Handbook of Psychiatry,* ed. by ARIETI, S. New York, Basic Books, vol. I, pp. 419–454.

ARIETI, S. (1962): The psychotherapeutic approach to depression. *Amer. J. Psychother. 16:*397–406.

ARIETI, S. (1963): Studies of thought processes in contemporary psychiatry. *Amer. J. Psychiat. 120:*58–64.

ASCHER, E. (1952): A criticism of the concept of neurotic depression. *Amer. J. Psychiat.* *108:*901–908.

ASSAEL, M. and THEIN, M. (1964): Blood acetaldehyde levels in affective disorders. *Israel Ann. Psychiat.* 2:228–234.

ASTRUP, C., FOSSUM, A., and HOLMBOE, F. (1959): A follow-up study of 270 patients with acute affective psychoses. *Acta Psychiat. Scand. Suppl. 135.*

AYD, F. J., Jr. (1958): Drug-induced depression—fact or fallacy. *New York J. Med.* *58:*354–356.

AYD, F. J., Jr. (1961): *Recognizing the Depressed Patient.* New York, Grune & Stratton.

AYD, F. J. (1964): Chemical remedies for depression. *Med. Sci.* 15:37–44.

BALINT, M. (1952): New beginning and the paranoid and the depressive syndromes. *Int. J. Psychoanal.* 33:214–224.

BECK, A. T. (1961): A systematic investigation of depression. *Compr. Psychiat.* 2:162–170.

BECK, A. T., and HURVICH, M. S. (1959): Psychological correlates of depression. 1. Frequency of "masochistic" dream content in a private practice sample. *Psychosom. Med.* 21:50–55.

BECK, A. T., and STEIN, D. (1960): The self concept in depression. Unpublished study.

BECK, A. T., and VALIN, S. (1953): Psychotic depressive reactions in soldiers who accidentally killed their buddies. *Amer. J. Psychiat.* 110:347–353.

BECK, A. T., and WARD, C. H. (1961): Dreams of depressed patients: characteristic themes in manifest content. *Arch. Gen. Psychiat. (Chicago)* 5:462–467.

BECK, A. T., FESHBACH, S., and LEGG, D. (1962): The clinical utility of the digit symbol test. *J. Consult. Psychol.* 26:263–268.

BECK, A. T., SETHI, B., and TUTHILL, R. (1963): Childhood bereavement and adult depression. *Arch. Gen. Psychiat. (Chicago)* 9:295–302.

BECK, A. T., WARD, C. H., MENDELSON, M., MOCK, J., and ERBAUGH, J. (1961): An inventory for measuring depression. *Arch. Gen. Psychiat. (Chicago)* 4:561–571.

BECK, A. T., WARD, C. H., MENDELSON, M., MOCK, J. E., and ERBAUGH, J. K. (1962): Reliability of psychiatric diagnoses: 2. A study of consistency of clinical judgments and ratings. *Amer. J. Psychiat.* 119:351–357.

BECKER, J. (1960): Achievement-related characteristics of manic-depressives. *J. Abnorm. Soc. Psychol.* 60:334–339.

BECKER, J., SPIELBERGER, C. D., and PARKER, J. B. (1963): Value achievement and authoritarian attitudes in psychiatric patients. *J. Clin. Psychol.* 19:57–61.

BEERS, C. W. (1928): *A Mind that Found Itself; an Autobiography.* Garden City, N.Y., Doubleday.

BELLAK, L. (1952): *Manic-Depressive Psychosis and Allied Conditions.* New York, Grune and Stratton.

BERGER, H. (1908): Ueber periodische schwankungen in der schnelligkeit der aufeinanderfolge willkürlicher bewegungen. *Z. Psychol. Physiol. Sinnesorg* 1:321–331.

BIBRING, E. (1953): "The Mechanism of Depression," in *Affective Disorders,* ed. by GREENACRE, P. New York, Internat. Univ. Press, pp. 13–48.

BLEULER, E. (1911): *Dementia Praecox or the Group of Schizophrenia,* trans. by ZINKEN, J. New York, Internat. Univ. Press, 1950.

BLEULER, E. (1924). *Textbook of Psychiatry,* trans. by BRILL, A. A. New York, Macmillan.

BOARD, F., WADESON, R., and PERSKY, H. (1957): Depressive affect and endocrine function. *Arch. Neurol. Psychiat.* 78:612–620.

BOND, E. D., and MORRIS, H. H., JR. (1954): Results of treatment in psychoses—with a control series: III. Manic-depressive reactions. *Amer. J. Psychiat* 110:881–887

BONIME, W .(1965): A psychotherapeutic approach to depression. *Contemporary Psychoanalysis 2:*48–53.

BOYLE, H. (1930): Discussion on the diagnosis and treatment of the milder forms of the manic-depressive psychosis. *Proc. Roy. Soc. Med. 23:*890–892.

BRADLEY, J. J. (1963): Severe localized pain associated with the depressive syndrome. *Brit. J. Psychiat. 109:*741–745.

BRADY, J. P. (1963): Review of controlled studies of imipramine. Unpublished study.

BRIGHT, T. (1586): "Melancholy and the Conscience of Sinne," in *Three Hundred Years of Psychiatry 1535–1860,* ed. by HUNTER, R., and MACALPINE, I. London, Oxford, 1963, pp. 36–40.

BRODY, E. B., and MAN, E. B. (1950): Thyroid function measured by serum precipitable iodine determinations in schizophrenic patients. *Amer. J. Psychiat. 107:*357–359.

BROWN, F. (1961): Depression and childhood bereavement. *J. Ment. Sci. 107:*754–777.

BRUNER, J. S., GOODNOW, J. J., and AUSTIN, G. A. (1956): *A Study of Thinking.* New York, Wiley.

BUNNEY, W. E., and FAWCETT, J. A. (1965): Possibility of a biochemical test for suicidal potential: an analysis of endocrine findings prior to three suicides. *Arch. Gen. Psychiat. (Chicago) 13:*232–239.

BUNNEY, W. E., and HARTMANN, E. L. (1965): A study of a patient with 48-hour manic-depressive cycles: I. An analysis of behavioral factors. *Arch. Gen. Psychiat. (Chicago) 12:*611.

BUNNEY, W. E., HARTMANN, E. L., and MASON, J. W. (1965): Study of a patient with 48-hour manic-depressive cycles. II. Strong positive correlation between endocrine factors and manic-depressive patterns. *Arch. Gen. Psychiat. (Chicago) 12:*619.

BUNNEY, W. E., MASON, J. D., ROATCH, J. F., and HAMBURG, D. A. (1965): A psychoendocrine study of severe psychotic depressive crises. *Amer. J. Psychiat. 122:*72.

BURCHARD, E. M. L. (1936): Physique and psychosis: an analysis of the postulated relationship between bodily constitution and mental disease syndrome. *Compr. Psychol. Monogr. 13:*1.

BURTON, R. (1621): *The Anatomy of Melancholy,* ed. by DELL, F., and JORDAN-SMITH, P. New York, Tudor, 1927.

BUSFIELD, B. L., and WECHSLER, H. (1961): Studies of salivation in depression: a comparison of salivation rates in depressed, schizoaffective depressed, nondepressed hospitalized patients, and in normal controls. *Arch. Gen. Psychiat. (Chicago) 4:*10.

BUSFIELD, B. L., WECHSLER, H., and BARNUM, W. J. (1961): Studies of salivation in depression II. Physiological differentiation of reactive and endogenous depression. *Arch. Gen. Psychiat. (Chicago) 5:*472–477.

BUZZARD, E. F. (1930): Discussion of the diagnosis and treatment of the milder forms of the manic-depressive psychosis. *Proc. Roy. Soc. Med. 23:*881–883.

CADE, J. F. J. (1964): A significant elevation of plasma magnesium levels in schizophrenia and depressive states. *Med. J. Aust. 1:*195–196.

CAMERON, N. (1942): The place of mania among the depressions from a biological standpoint. *J. Psychol. 14:*181–195.

CAMERON, N. (1944): "The Functional Psychoses," in *Personality and the Behavior Disorders,* ed. by HUNT, J. McV. New York, Ronald Press, pp. 861–921.

CAMPBELL, J. D. (1953): *Manic-Depressive Disease.* Philadelphia, Lippincott.

CANDOLLE, A. P. de (1816): *Essai sur les propriétés medicales des plantes, comparées avec leurs formes extérieures et leur classification naturelle.* Paris, Crochard.

CARNEY, M. W. P., ROTH, M., and GARSIDE, R. F. (1965): The diagnosis of depressive syndromes and the prediction of E. C. T. response, *Brit. J. Psychiat. 3:*659–674.

CASSIDY, W. L., FLANAGAN, N. B., SPELLMAN, M. (1957): Clinical observations in manic-depressive disease: a quantitative study of 100 manic-depressive patients and 50 medically sick controls. *J. Amer. Med. Ass. 164:*1535–1546.

CASTELNUOVO-TEDESCO, P. (1961): *Depressions in Patients with Physical Disease.* Cranbury, N.J., Wallace Laboratories.

CHARCOT, J. M. (1890). Cited by White, R. W. in *The Abnormal Personality.* New York, Ronald Press, 1956, p. 25.

CHENEY, C. O. (1934): *Outlines for Psychiatric Examinations.* Albany, New York State Dept. of Mental Hygiene.

CLARK, J. A., and MALLET, B. A. (1963): Follow-up study of schizophrenia and depression in young adults. *Brit. J. Psychiat. 109:*491–499.

CLAYTON, P. J., PITTS, F. N., and WINOKUR, G. (1965): Affective disorder IV. Mania. *Compr. Psychiat. 6:*313.

CLEGG, J. L. (1935). The association of physique and mental condition. *J. Ment. Sci. 81:*297–316.

CLEGHORN, R. A., and CURTIS, G. C. (1959): Psychosomatic accompaniments of latent and manifest depressive affects. *Canad. Psychiat. Ass. J. Suppl. 4:*S13–S23.

CLYDE, D. J. (1961): *Clyde Mood Scale.* Washington, D.C., George Washington University.

COHEN, B., SENF, R., and HUSTON, P. (1956): Perceptual accuracy in schizophrenia, depression, and neurosis, and affects of amytal. *J. Abnorm. Soc. Psychol. 52:*363–367.

COHEN, M. B., BAKER, G., COHEN, R. A., FROMM-REICHMANN, F., and WEIGERT, E. V. (1954): An intensive study of twelve cases of manic-depressive psychosis. *Psychiatry 17:*103–137.

COLE, J. O. (1964): Therapeutic efficacy of antidepressant drugs. *J. Amer. Med. Ass. 190:*448–455.

COMREY, A. L. (1957): A factor analysis of items on the MMPI depression scale. *Educ. Psychol. Measurement 17:*578–585.

COPPEN, A. J., and SHAW, D. M. (1963): Mineral metabolism in melancholia. *Brit. Med. J. 2:*1439–1444.

CRAMMER, J. L. (1959): Water and sodium in two psychotics. *Lancet 1:*1122–1126.

CRICHTON-MILLER, H. (1930): Discussion of the diagnosis and treatment of the milder forms of the manic-depressive psychosis. *Proc. Roy. Soc. Med. 23:*883–886.

CRONBACH, L. J., and MEEHL, P. E. (1955): Construct validity in psychological tests. *Psychol. Bull. 52:*281–302.

CRONHOLM, B., and MOLANDER, L. (1964): Memory disturbances after electroconvulsive therapy: 5. Conditions one month after a series of treatments. *Acta Psychiat. Scand. 40:*212.

CURTIS, G. C., CLEGHORN, R. A., and SOURKES, T. L. (1960): The relationship between affect and the excretion of adrenaline, noradrenaline, and 17-hydroxycorticosteroids. *J. Psychosom. Res. 4:*176.

CUTLER, R. P., and KURLAND, H. D. (1961): Clinical quantification of depressive reactions. *Arch. Gen. Psychiat. (Chicago) 5:*280–285.

DAVIES, B. M., and GURLAND, J. B. (1961): Salivary secretion in depressive illness. *J. Psychosom. Res. 5:*269–271.

DAVIS, J. (1965): Efficacy of tranquilizing and antidepressant drugs. *Arch. Gen. Psychiat. (Chicago) 13:*552–572.

DELAY, J., PICHOT, P., LEMPERIERE, T., and MIROUZE, R. (1963): La nosologie des états dépressifs: rapports entre l'étiologie et la semiologie. 2. Résultats due Questionnaire de *Beck. Encéphale 52:*497–505.

DENISON, R., and YASKIN, J. C. (1944): Medical and surgical masquerades of the depressed state. *Penn. Med. J. 47:*703–707.

DIAZ-GUERRERO, R., GOTTLIEB, J. S., and KNOTT, J. R. (1946): The sleep of patients with manic-depressive psychosis, depressive type: an electroencephalographic study. *Psychosom. Med. 8:*399–404.

DIETHELM, O., and HEFFERMAN, T. (1965): Felix Platter and psychiatry. *J. Hist. Behav. Sci. 1:*10–23.

DIMASCIO, A., and KLERMAN, G. L. (1960): "Experimental Human Psychopharmacology: The Role of Non-drug Factors," in *The Dynamics of Psychiatric Drug Therapy,* ed. by SARWER-FONER, G. J. Springfield, Thomas, pp. 56–97.

DIXON, N. F., and LEAR, T. E. (1962): Perceptual regulation and mental disorder. *J. Ment. Sci. 108:*356–361.

DOVENMUEHLE, R. H., and VERWOERDT, A. (1962): Physical illness and depressive symptomatology. I. Incidence of depressive symptoms in hospitalized cardiac patients. *J. Amer. Geriat. Soc. 10:*932–947.

DREYFUS, G. (1907): Quoted in HOCH, A., and MACCURDY, J. T. (1922): The prognosis of involution melancholia. *Arch. Neurol. Psychiat. 7:*1–37.

DRIESS, H. (1942): Über der gestaltung und unterteilung in der involution auftretenden depressionen. *Z. Psych. Hyg. 14:*65–77.

DRIVER, M. V., and EILENBERG, M. D. (1960): Photoconvulsive threshold in depressive illness and the effect of E.C.T. *J. Ment. Sci. 106:*611–617.

DUNLOP, E. (1965): Use of antidepressants and stimultants. *Mod. Treatm. 2:*543–568.

EDITORIAL (1963): Thinking disorder in neurosis. *J. Amer. Med. Assoc. 186:*946.

ELLIS, A. (1962): *Reason and Emotion in Psychotherapy.* New York, Lyle Stuart.

ENGLISH, H. B., and ENGLISH, A. C. (1958): *A Comprehensive Dictionary of Psychological and Psychoanalytical Terms.* New York, Longmans.

FARBEROW, N. L., and SCHNEIDMAN, E. S. (1961): *The Cry for Help.* New York, McGraw-Hill.

FARBER, M. L. (1938): Critique and investigation of Kretschmer's theory. *J. Abnorm. Soc. Psychol. 33:*398.

FEINBERG, I. (1958): Current status of the Funkenstein Test. *Arch. Neurol. Psychiat. 80:*488.

FELDMAN, D., PASCAL, G. R., and SWENSON, C. H. (1954): Direction of aggression as a prognostic variable in mental illness. *J. Consult. Psychol. 18:*167.

FESHBACH, S. (1965): Personal communication.

FESTINGER, L. (1957): *A Theory of Cognitive Disonance.* Evanston, Harper & Row.

FISHER, S. (1964): Depressive affect and perception of up-down. *J. Psychiat. Res. 2:*25.

FLACH, F. (1964): Calcium metabolism in states of depression. *Brit. J. Psychiat. 110:*588

FLEMING, G. W. (1933): The revision of the classification of mental disorders. *J. Ment. Sci. 79:*753.

FOULDS, G. A. (1960): Psychotic depression and age. *J. Ment. Sci. 106:*1394.

FREMMING, K. (1951): *The Expectation of Mental Infirmity in a Sample of the Danish Population.* London, Cassell.

FREUD, S. (1917): "Mourning and Melancholia," in *Collected Papers,* vol. 4. London, Hogarth Press and the Institute of Psychoanalysis, 1950, pp. 152–172.

FREUD, S. (1938): *Basic Writings,* trans. by BRILL, A. A. New York, Modern Library.

FRIEDMAN, A. S. (1964): Minimal effects of severe depression on cognitive functioning. *J. Abnorm. Soc. Psychol. 69:*237–243.

FRIEDMAN, A. S. (1966): Personal communication.

FRIEDMAN, A. S., COWITZ, B., COHEN, H. W., and GRANICK, S. (1963): Syndromes and themes of psychotic depression: a factor analysis. *Arch. Gen. Psychiat. (Chicago) 9:*504–509.

FRIEDMAN, A. S., GRANICK, S., COHEN, H. W., and COWITZ, B. (1966): Imipramine (Tofranil) vs. placebo in hospitalized psychotic depressives. *J. Psychiat. Res. 4:*13–36.

FRIEDMAN, A. S., GRANICK, S., FREEMAN, L., and STEWART, M. (1965): Cross-validation of the low (EEG) sedation threshold of psychotic depressives. Paper presented at Annual Meeting of American Psychological Association. Chicago, September, 1965.

FUNKENSTEIN, D. H. (1954): "Discussion of Chapters 10–11: Psychophysiologic Studies of Depression: Some Experimental Work," in *Depression,* ed. by HOCH, P. H., and ZUBIN, J. New York, Grune & Stratton.

GERO, G. (1936): The construction of depression. *Int. J. Psychoanal. 17:423–461.*

GERSHON, S., and YUWEILER, A. (1960): Lithium ion: a specific psychopharmacological approach to the treatment of mania. *J. Neuropsychiat. 1:229–241.*

GIBBONS, J. L. (1960): Total body sodium and potassium in depressive illness. *Clin. Sci. 19:133–138.*

GIBBONS, J. L. (1963): Electrolytes and depressive illness. *Postgrad. Med. J. 39:19–25.*

GIBBONS, J. L. (1964): Cortisol secretion rate in depressive illness. *Arch. Gen. Psychiat. (Chicago) 10:572–575.*

GIBBONS, J. L., and McHUGH, P. R. (1962): Plasma cortisol in depressive illness. *J. Psychiat. Res. 1:162–171.*

GIBBONS, J. L., GIBSON, J. G., MAXWELL, A. E., and WILLCOX, D. R. C. (1960). An endocrine study of depressive illness. *J. Psychosom. Res. 5:32–41.*

GIBSON, R. W. (1957): *Comparison of the Family Background and Early Life Experience of the Manic-Depressive and Schizophrenic Patient.* Final Report on Office of Naval Research Contract (Nonr-751(00)). Washington, D.C., Washington School of Psychiatry.

GIBSON, R. W. (1963): Psychotherapy of manic-depressive states. *Psychiat. Res. Rep. Amer. Psychiat. Ass. 17:91–102.*

GILDEA, E. F., McLEAN, V. L., and MAN, E. B. (1943): Oral and intravenous dextrose tolerance curves of patients with manic-depressive psychosis. *Arch. Neurol. Psychiat. 49:852–859.*

GILLESPIE, R. D. (1929): Clinical differentiation of types of depression. *Guy Hosp. Rep. 79:306–344.*

GJESSING, R. (1938): Disturbances of somatic functions in catatonia with a periodic course, and their compensation. *J. Ment. Sci. 84:608–621.*

GOLDHIRSH, M. I. (1961): Manifest content of dreams of convicted sex offenders. *J. Abnorm. Soc. Psychol. 63:643–645.*

GOLDSTEIN, I. G. (1965): The relationship of muscle tension and autonomic activity to psychiatric disorders. *Psychosom. Med. 27:39–52.*

GOODMAN, L. S., and GILMAN, A. (1965): *The Pharmacological Basis of Therapeutics,* 3rd ed., New York, Macmillan.

GOTTLIEB, G., and PAULSON, G. (1961): Salivation in depressed patients. *Arch. Gen. Psychiat. (Chicago) 5:468–471.*

GOTTSCHALK, L., GLESER, G., and SPRINGER, K. (1963). Three hostility scales applicable to verbal samples. *Arch. Gen. Psychiat. (Chicago) 9:254–279.*

GRANICK, S. (1963): Comparative analysis of psychotic depressives with matched normals on some untimed verbal intelligence tests. *J. Consult. Psychol. 27:439–443.*

GREGORY, I. W. (1961): *Psychiatry: Biological and Social.* Philadelphia, Saunders.

GREGORY, I. W. (1966): Retrospective data concerning childhood loss of a parent: II. Category of parental loss by decade of birth, diagnosis and MMPI. *Arch. Gen. Psychiat. (Chicago) 15:362–367.*

GRESHAM, S. C., AGNEW, H. W., and WILLIAMS, R. L. (1965): The sleep of depressed patients: an EEG and eye movement study. *Arch. Gen. Psychiat. (Chicago) 13:503–507.*

GRINKER, R., MILLER, J., SABSHIN, M., NUNN, R., NUNNALLY, J. (1961): *The Phenomena of Depressions.* New York, Hoeber.

GROSSER, G. H., and FREEMAN, H. (1961): "Differential Recovery Patterns in the

Treatment of Acute Depression," in *Proceedings of the Third World Congress of Psychiatry.* University of Toronto Press and Montreal, McGill University Press, vol. 2, pp. 1396–1402.

HAMILTON, M. (1960a): A rating scale for depression. *J. Neurol. Neurosurg. Psychiat.* 23:56–61.

HAMILTON, M. (1960b): Quantitative assessment of the Mecholyl (Funkenstein) test. *Acta Neurol. Scand.* 35:156–162.

HAMILTON, M., and WHITE, J. (1959): Clinical syndromes in depressive states. *J. Ment. Sci.* 105:485–498.

HAMMERMAN, S. (1962). Ego defect and depression. Paper presented at Philadelphia Psychoanalytic Society. Philadelphia, November 7, 1962.

HARROWES, W. McC. (1933): The depressive reaction types. *J. Ment. Sci.* 79:235–246.

HARSCH, O. H., and ZIMMER, H. (1965): An experimental approximation of thought reform. *J. Consult. Psychology* 29:475–479.

HARVEY, O. J., HUNT, D. E., and SCHRODER, H. M. (1961): *Conceptual Systems and Personality Organization.* New York, Wiley.

HATHAWAY, W. R., and McKINLEY, J. C. (1942): A multiphasic personality schedule: III. The measurement of symptomatic depression. *J. Psychol.* 14:73–84.

HEMPHILL, R. E., HALL, K. R. L., and CROOKES, T. G. (1952): A preliminary report on fatigue and pain tolerance in depressive and psychoneurotic patients. *J. Ment. Sci.* 98:433–440.

HENDERSON, D., and GILLESPIE, R. D. (1963): *Textbook of Psychiatry,* 9th ed. London, Oxford Univ. Press.

HERON, M. J. (1965): A note on the concept endogenous-exogenous. *Brit. J. Med. Psychol.* 38:241.

HINSIE, L., and CAMPBELL, R. (1960): *Psychiatric Dictionary,* 3rd ed. London, Oxford Univ. Press.

HOCH, A. (1921): *Benign Stupors: A Study of a New Manic-Depressive Reaction Type.* New York, Macmillan.

HOCH, A., and MacCURDY, J. T. (1922): The prognosis of involution melancholia. *Arch. Neurol. Psychiat.* 7:1.

HOCH, P. H. (1953). Discussion of D. E. Cameron, "A Theory of Diagnosis," in *Current Problems in Psychiatric Diagnosis,* ed. by HOCH, P. H., and ZUBIN, J. New York, Grune & Stratton, pp. 46–50.

HOCH, P. H., and RACHLIN, H. L. (1941): An evaluation of manic-depressive psychosis in the light of follow-up studies, *Amer. J. Psychiat.* 97:831–843.

HOCH, P. H., and ZUBIN, J. (1953): *Current Problems in Psychiatric Diagnosis.* New York, Grune & Stratton.

HOLLINGSHEAD, A. B. (1957): *Two Factor Index of Social Position* (Mimeographed paper). New Haven, Conn., A. B. Hollingshead.

HOLMBERG, G. (1963): "Biological Aspects of Electro-convulsive Therapy," in *International Review of Neurobiology,* ed. by PFEIFFER, C., and SMYTHIES, J. New York, Academic Press, vol. 5, pp. 389–406.

HOPKINSON, G. (1963): Onset of affective illness. *Psychiat. Neurol. (Basel)* 146:133–140.

HOPKINSON, G. (1964): A genetic study of affective illness in patients over 50. *Brit. J. Psychiat.* 110:244–254.

HOPKINSON, G. (1965): The prodromal phase of the depressive psychosis. *Psychiat. Neurol. (Basel)* 149:1–6.

HORDERN, A. (1965): The antidepressant drugs. *New Eng. J. Med.* 272:1159–1169.

HORN, D. (1950): Intra-individual variability in the study of personality. *J. Clin. Psychol.* 6:43–47.

HORNEY, K. (1945): *Our Inner Conflicts.* New York, Norton.

HUNT, R. R., and APPEL, K. E. (1936): Prognosis in psychoses lying midway between schizophrenic and manic-depressive psychoses. *Am. J. Psychiat. 93:*313–339.

HUSTON, P. E., and LOCHER, L. M. (1948). Manic-depressive psychosis: course when treated with electric shock. *Arch. Neurol. Psychiat. 60:*37–48.

JACOBSON, E. (1953): "Contribution to the Metapsychology of Cyclothymic Depression," in *Affective Disorders,* ed. by GREENACRE, P. New York, Internat. Univer. Press, pp. 49–83.

JACOBSON, E. (1954): Transference problems in the psychoanalytic treatment of severely depressive patients. *J. Amer. Psychoanal. Ass. 2:*595–606.

JASPER, H. H. (1930): A measurement of depression-elation and its relation to a measure of extraversion-intraversion. *J. Abnorm. Soc. Psychol. 25:*307–318.

JELLIFFE, S. E. (1931): Some historical phases of the manic-depressive synthesis. *Ass. Res. Nerv. Ment. Proc. 11:*3–47.

KALINOWSKY, L. B., and HOCH, P. H. (1961): *Somatic Treatments in Psychiatry.* New York, Grune & Stratton.

KALLMANN, F. (1952): "Genetic Aspects of Psychoses," in Milbank Memorial Fund, *Biology of Mental Health and Disease.* New York, Hoeber, pp. 283–302.

KANTER, V. B. (1961): The British Hospital Progress Test: an attempt to measure depression and recovery from depression. Part I. Construction of the test. Paper presented at the Annual Meeting of the American Psychological Association. New York, August, 1961.

KASANIN, J. S. (1933): The acute schizoaffective psychoses. *Am. J. Psychiat. 13:*97–126.

KASANIN, J. S. (1944): *Language and Thought in Schizophrenia.* Berkeley, Univ. of Calif. Press.

KELLY, G. A. (1955): *The Psychology of Personal Constructs.* New York, Norton, vol. 1.

KENNEDY, F. (1944): The neuroses: related to the manic-depressive constitution. *Med. Clin. of N. Amer. 28:*452–466.

KENNEDY, F., and WIESEL, B. (1946): The clinical nature of "manic-depressive equivalents" and their treatment. *Trans. Amer. Neurol, Ass. 71:*96–101.

KILOH, L. G., and GARSIDE, R. F. (1963): The independence of neurotic depression and endogenous depression. *Brit. J. Psychiat. 109:*451–463.

KIRBY, G. H. (1908): Quoted in Titley, W. B. (1936). *Arch. Neurol. Psychiat. 36:*19–33.

KIRBY, G. H. (1913): The catatonic syndrome and its relation to manic-depressive insanity. *J. Nerv. Ment. Dis. 40:*694–704.

KLEIN, M. (1934): "A Contribution to the Psychogenesis of Manic-Depressive States," in *Contributions to Psycho-Analysis 1921–1945.* London, Hogarth Press and the Institute of Psychoanalysis, 1948, pp. 282–310.

KLEIN, R. (1950): Clinical and biochemical investigations in a manic-depressive with short cycles. *J. Ment. Sci. 96:*293–297.

KLEIN, R., and NUNN, R. F. (1945): Clinical and biochemical analysis of a case of manic-depressive psychosis showing regular weekly cycles. *J. Ment. Sci. 91:*79–88.

KLERMAN, G. L., and COLE, J. O. (1965): Clinical pharmacology of imipramine and related antidepressant compounds. *Pharmacol. Rev. 17:*101–141.

KLINE, N. (1964): Practical management of depression. *J. Amer. Med. Ass. 190:*732–740.

KOHN, M., and CLAUSEN, J. (1955): Social isolation and schizophrenia. *Am. Sociol. Rev. 20:*265–273.

KRAEPELIN, E. (1913). "Manic-Depressive Insanity and Paranoia," in *Textbook of Psychiatry*, trans. by BARCLAY, R. M. Edinburgh, Livingstone.

KRAINES, S. H. (1965): Manic-depressive syndrome: a diencephalic disease. Paper presented at Annual Meeting of the American Psychiatric Association. New York, May 6, 1965.

KRAINES, S. H. (1957): *Mental Depressions and Their Treatment.* New York, Macmillan.

KRAL, V. A. (1958): Masked depression in middle-aged men. *Canad. Med. Ass. J.* 79:1–5.

KREITMAN, N., SAINSBURY, P., MORRISSEY, J., TOWERS, J., and SCRIVENER, J. (1961): The reliability of psychiatric assessment: an analysis. *Brit. J. Psychiat.* 107:887–908.

KRETSCHMER, E. (1925): *Physique and Character,* trans. by SPROUT, W. J. H. New York, Harcourt.

KURLAND, H. D. (1964): Steroid excretion in depressive disorders. *Arch. Gen. Psychiat. (Chicago)* 10:554–560.

LANGE, J. (1926): Über Melancholie. *Z. Neurol. Psychiat.* 101:293–319.

LAXER, R. M. (1964): Self-concept changes of depressive patients in general hospital treatment. *J. Consult. Psychol.* 28:214–219.

LEHMANN, H. E. (1959): Psychiatric concepts of depression: nomenclature and classification. *Canad. Psychiat. Ass. J. Suppl.* 4:S1–S12.

LEWIS, A. (1934): Melancholia: a clinical survey of depressive states. *J. Ment. Sci.* 80:277–378.

LEWIS, A. (1938): States of depression: their clinical and aetiological differentiation. *Brit. Med. J.* 2:875–883.

LEWIS, N. D. C., and HUBBARD, L. D. (1931): The mechanisms and prognostic aspects of the manic-depressive schizophrenic combinations. *Res. Pub. Ass. Res. Nerv. Ment. Dis.* 11:539–608.

LEWIS, N. D. C., and PIOTROWSKI, Z. S. (1954): "Clinical Diagnosis of Manic-Depressive Psychosis," in *Depression,* ed. by HOCH, P. H., and ZUBIN, J. New York, Grune & Stratton, pp. 25–38.

LICHTENBERG, P. (1957): A definition and analysis of depression. *Arch. Neurol. Psychiat.* 77:516–527.

LOBBAN, M., TREDRE, B., ELITHORN, A., and BRIDGES, P. (1963): Diurnal rhythm of electrolyte excretion in depressive illness. *Nature (London)* 199:667–669.

LOEB, A., BECK, A. T., DIGGORY, J. C., TUTHILL, R. (1966): The effects of success and failure on mood, motivation, and performance as a function of predetermined level of depression. Unpublished study.

LOEB, A., FESHBACH, S., BECK, A. T., and WOLF, A. (1964): Some effects of reward upon the social perception and motivation of psychiatric patients varying in depression. *J. Abnorm. Soc. Psychol.* 68:609–616.

LOFTUS, T. A. (1960): *Meaning and Methods of Diagnosis in Clinical Psychiatry.* Philadelphia, Lea & Febiger.

LORR, M. (1954): Rating scales and check lists for the evaluation of psychopathology. *Psychol. Bull.* 51:119–127.

LORR, M. (1961): Classification of the behavior disorders. *Ann. Rev. Psychol.* 12:195–216.

LUBIN, B. (1965): Adjective checklists for measurement of depression. *Arch. Gen. Psychiat. (Chicago)* 12:57–62.

LUNDQUIST, G. (1945): Prognosis and course in manic-depressive psychoses. *Acta Psychiat. Neurol. Suppl. 35.*

MALAMUD, W., SANDS, S. L., and MALAMUD, I. (1941): The involutional psychoses: a socio-psychiatric study. *Psychosom. Med.* 3:410–426.

MALZBERG, B. (1929): A statistical study of the factor of age in manic-depressive psychoses. *Psychiat. Quart. 3:*590–604.

MAPOTHER, E. (1926). Discussion on manic-depressive psychosis. *Brit. Med. J. 2:*872–876.

MARTIN, I., and DAVIES, B. M. (1962): Sleep thresholds in depression. *J. Ment. Sci. 108:*466–473.

MARTIN, I., and DAVIES, B. M. (1965): The effect of Sodium Amytal on autonomic and muscle activity in patients with depressive illness. *Brit. J. Psychiat. 11:*168.

MEERLOO, J. A. M. (1962): *Suicide and Mass Suicide.* New York, Grune & Stratton.

MENDELS, J. (1965): Electroconvulsive therapy and depression. *Brit. J. Psychiat. 3:*675–681.

MENDELS, J., HAWKINS, D. R., and SCOTT, J. (1966): The psychophysiology of sleep in depression. Paper presented at Annual Meeting of the Association for the Psychophysiological Study of Sleep. Gainesville, Fla., March, 1966.

MENDELSON, M. (1960): *Psychoanalytic Concepts of Depression.* Springfield, Thomas.

MESSICK, M. (1960): Response style and content measures from personality inventories. *Educ. Psychol. Measurement. 22:*41–56.

METCALFE, M., and GOLDMAN, E. (1965): Validation of an inventory for measuring depression. *Brit. J. Psychiat. 111:*240–242.

MEYER, A. (1908): "The Problems of Mental Reaction Types," in *The Collected Papers of Adolf Meyer.* Baltimore, Md., Johns Hopkins Press, 1951, vol. 2, pp. 591–603.

MEZEY, A. G., and COHEN, S. I. (1961): The effect of depressive illness on time judgment and time experience. *J. Neurol. Neurosurg. Psychiat. 24:*269–270.

MICHAEL, R. P., and GIBBONS, J. L. (1963): "Interrelationships between the Endocrine System and Neuropsychiatry," in *International Review of Neurobiology,* ed. by PFEIFER, C., and SMYTHIES, J. New York, Academic Press.

MOSS, L. M., and HAMILTON, D. M. (1956): The Psychotherapy of the suicidal patient. *Amer. J. Psychiat. 112:*814–820.

MOTTO, J. A. (1965): Suicide attempts: a longitudinal view. *Arch. Gen. Psychiat. (Chicago) 13:*516–520.

MCCLELLAND, D. C. (1951): *Personality.* New York, Holt.

MACDONALD, J. M. (1964): Suicide and homicide by automobile. *Amer. J. Psychiat. 121:*366–370.

MCFARLAND, R. A., and GOLDSTEIN, H. (1939): The biochemistry of manic-depressive psychosis. *Amer. J. Psychiat. 92:*21–58.

MCNAIR, D. M., and LORR, M. (1964): An analysis of mood in neurotics. *J. Abnorm. Soc. Psychol. 69:*620–627.

NUSSBAUM, K., and MICHAUX, W. W. (1963): Response to humor in depression: a prediction and evaluation of patient change? *Psychiat. Quart. 37:*527–539.

NUSSBAUM, K., WITTIG, B. A., HANLON, T. E., and KURLAND, A. A. (1963): ·Intravenous nialamide in the treatment of depressed female patients. *Compr. Psychiat. 4:*105–116.

NYMGAARD, K. (1959): Studies on the sedation threshold: A. Reproducibility and effect of drugs. B. Sedation threshold in neurotic and psychotic depression. *Arch. Gen. Psychiat. (Chicago) 1:*530–536.

O'CONNOR, J., STEFIC, E., and GRESOCK, C. (1957): Some patterns of depression. *J. Clin. Psychol. 13:*122–125.

OSGOOD, C. E. (1957): "A Behavioristic Analysis of Perception and Language as Cognitive Phenomena," in Bruner, S. *et al.,* in *Contemporary Approaches to Cognition.* Cambridge, Harvard Univ. Press, pp. 75–119.

OSWALD, I., BERGER, R. J., JARAMILLO, R. A., KEDDIE, K. M. G., OLLEY, P. C., PLUNKETT, G. B. (1963): Melancholia and barbiturates: a controlled EEG, body and eye movement study of sleep. *Brit. J. Psychiat. 109:*66–78.

OVERALL, J. E. (1962): Dimensions of manifest depression. *J. Psychiat. Res. 1:*239–245.

OVERALL, J., and GORHAM, D. (1961): Basic dimensions of change in the symptomatology of chronic schizophrenics. *J. Abnorm. Soc. Psychol. 63:*597–602.

OVERALL, J. E., HOLLISTER, L. E., MEYER, F., KIMBELL, I., JR., and SHELTON, J. (1964): Imipramine and thioridazine in depressed and schizophrenic patients. *J. Amer. Med. Ass. 189:*605–608.

PALMER, H. D., and SHERMAN, S. H. (1938): The involutional melancholia process. *Arch. Neurol. Psychiat. 40:*762–788.

PALMER, H. D., HASTINGS, D. W., and SHERMAN, S. H. (1941): Therapy in involutional melancholia. *Amer. J. Psychiat. 97:*1086–1111.

PALMAI, G., and BLACKWELL, B. (1965): The diurnal pattern of salivary flow in normal and depressed patients. *Brit. J. Psychiat. 111:*334–338.

PARTRIDGE, M. (1949): Some reflections on the nature of affective disorders arising from the results of prefrontal leucotomy. *J. Ment. Sci. 95:*795–825.

PASAMANICK, B., DINTZ, S., and LEFTON, M. (1959): Psychiatric orientation and its relation to diagnosis and treatment in a mental hospital. *Amer. J. Psychiat. 116:*127–132.

PASKIND, H. A. (1929): Brief attacks of manic-depressive depression. *Arch. Neurol. Psychiat. 22:*123–134.

PASKIND, H. A. (1930a): Manic-depressive psychosis as seen in private practice: sex and age incidence of first attacks. *Arch. Neurol. Psychiat. 23:*152–158.

PASKIND, H. A. (1930b): Manic-depressive psychosis in private practice: length of attack and length of interval. *Arch. Neurol. Psychiat. 23:*789–794.

PAULSON, G. W., and GOTTLIEB, G. (1961): A longitudinal study of the electroencephalographic arousal response in depressed patients. *J. Nerv. Ment. Dis. 133:*524–528.

PAYNE, R. W., and HEWLETT, J. H. (1961): "Thought Disorder in Psychotic Patients," in *Experiments in Personality,* ed. by EYSENCK, H. H. London, Routledge, pp. 3–104.

PAYNE, R. W., and HIRST, H. L. (1957): Overinclusive thinking in a depressive and a control group. *J. Consult. Psychol. 21:*186–188.

PECK, R. E. (1959): The SHP Test: an aid in the detection and measurement of depress. *Arch. Gen. Psychiat. (Chicago) 1:*35–40.

PHILLIPS, L., and ZIEGLER, E. (1964): Role orientation, the action-thought dimension, and outcome in psychiatric disorder. *J. Abnorm. Soc. Psychol. 68:*381–389.

PIAGET, J. (1948): *The Moral Judgment of the Child,* trans. by GABAIN, M. Glencoe, Ill., Free Press.

PICHOT, P., and LEMPÉRIÈRE, T. (1964): Analyse factorielle d'un questionnaire d'auto-évaluation des symptomes dépressifs. *Rev. Psychol. Appl. 14:*15–29.

PICHOT, P. (1966): Personal communication.

PINEL, P. (1801): *A Treatise on Insanity,* trans. by DAVIS, D. D. New York, Hafner, 1962.

PITTS, F. N., JR., MEYER, J., BROOKS, M., and WINOKUR, G. (1965): Adult psychiatric illness assessed for childhood parental loss, and psychiatric illness in family members —a study of 748 patients and 250 controls. *Amer. J. Psychiat. Suppl. 121:*i–x.

POKORNY, A. D. (1964): Suicide rates in various psychiatric disorders. *J. Nerv. Ment. Dis. 139:*499–506.

POLLACK, H. M. (1931): Prevalence of manic-depressive psychosis in relation to sex, age, environment, nativity, and race. *Res. Publ. Ass. Res. Nerv. Ment. Dis. 11:*655–667.

POLYAKOVA, M. (1961): The effect of blood from manic-depressive psychotics on the higher nervous activity (behavior) of animals. *Zh. Nevropat. I Psikhiat. (Moscova) 61:*104–108.

POSTMAN, L. (1951): "Toward a General Theory of Cognition," in *Social Psychology at the Crossroads,* ed. by ROHRER, J. H., and SHERIF, M. New York, Harper.

PRYCE, I. G. (1958): Melancholia, glucose tolerance, and body weight. *J. Ment. Sci.* 104:421–427.

RACHLIN, H. L. (1935): A followup study of Hoch's benign stupor cases. *Amer. J. Psychiat.* 92:531.

RACHLIN, H. L. (1937): A statistical study of benign stupor in five New York state hospitals. *Psychiat. Quart.* 11:436–444.

RADO, S. (1928): The problem of melancholia. *Int. J. Psychoanal.* 9:420–438.

RAPAPORT, D. (1945): *Diagnostic Psychological Testing; the Theory, Statistical Evaluation, and Diagnostic Application of a Battery of Tests,* vol. 1. Chicago, Yearbook.

RAPAPORT, D. (1951): *Organization and Pathology of Thought.* New York, Columbia Univ. Press.

REES, L. (1944): Physical constitution, neurosis, and psychosis. *Proc. Roy. Soc. Med.* 37:635–638.

REES, L. (1960): "Constitutional Factors and Abnormal Behavior," in *Handbook of Abnormal Psychology,* ed. by EYSENCK, H. J. New York, Basic Books.

REGAN, P. F. (1965). Brief psychotherapy of depression. *Amer. J. Psychiat.* 122:28–32.

RENNIE, T. (1942): Prognosis in manic-depressive psychoses. *Amer. J. Psychiat.* 98:801–814.

RICHTER, P. R. (1965): *Biological Clocks in Medicine and Psychiatry.* Springfield, Ill., Thomas.

RICKELS, K. (1963): Psychopharmacological agents: a clinical psychiatrist's individualistic point of view: patient and doctor variables. *J. Nerv. Ment. Dis.* 136:540–549.

RICKELS, K., WARD, C. H., and SCHUT, L. (1964): Different populations, different drug responses: comparative study of two anti-depressants, each used in two different patient groups. *Amer. J. Med. Sci.* 247:328–335.

RIDDELL, S. A. (1963): The therapeutic efficacy of ECT. *Arch. Gen. Psychiat. (Chicago)* 8:546–556.

RIPLEY, H. S., SHORR, E., and PAPANICOLAOU, G. N. (1940): The effect of treatment of depression in the menopause with estrogenic hormone. *Amer. J. Psychiat.* 96:905–914.

ROBERTS, J. M. (1959): Prognostic factors in the electro-shock treatment of depressive states: II. The application of specific tests. *J. Ment. Sci.* 105:703–713.

ROBINS, E., GASSNER, S., KAYES, J., WILKINSON, R. H., and MURPHY, G. E. (1959): The communication of suicidal intent: a study of 134 consecutive cases of successful (completed) suicide. *Amer. J. Psychiat.* 115:724–733.

ROGERS, C. R. (1951): *Client-Centered Therapy.* Boston, Houghton-Mifflin.

ROSE, J. T. (1962): Autonomic function in depression: a modified metacholine test. *J. Ment. Sci.* 108:624–641.

ROSE, J. T. (1963): Reactive and endogenous depressions—responses to E.C.T. *Brit. J. Psychiat.* 109:213–217.

ROSENBLATT, B. P. (1956): The influence of affective states upon body image and upon the perceptual organization of space. Ph.D. Dissertation, Clark University, Worcester, Mass.

RUSSELL, G. F. M. (1960): Body weight and balance of water, sodium, and potassium in depressed patients given electroconvulsive therapy. *Clin. Sci.* 19:327–336.

SALZMAN, L. (1947): An evaluation of shock therapy. *Amer. J. Psychiat.* 103:669–679.

SANDIFER, M. G., JR., WILSON, I. C., and GREEN, L. (1966): The two-type thesis of depressive disorders. *Amer. J. Psychiat.* 123:93–97.

SANDLER, S. (1948): Depression masking organic diseases and organic diseases masking depression. *J. Med. Soc. New Jersey* 45:108–110.

SARBIN, T. R., TAFT, R., and BAILEY, D. E. (1960): *Clinical Inference and Cognitive Theory.* New York, Holt.

SAUL, L. J. (1947): *Emotional Maturity.* Philadelphia, Lippincott.

SAUL, L. J., and SHEPPARD, E. (1956): An attempt to quantify emotional forces using manifest dreams: a preliminary study. *J. Amer. Psychiat. Ass.* 4:486–502.

SCHAFER, R. (1948): *The Clinical Application of Psychological Tests.* New York, Internat. Univer. Press.

SCHILDKRAUT, J. (1965): The catecholamine hypothesis of affective disorders: a review of supporting evidence. *Amer. J. Psychiat.* 122:509–522.

SCHLAGENHAUF, G., TUPIN, J., and WHITE, R. B. (1966): The use of lithium carbonate in the treatment of manic psychoses. *Amer. J. Psychiat.* 123:201–207.

SCHOTTSTAEDT, W. W., GRACE, W. J., and WOLFF, H. G. (1956): Life situations, behaviour, attitudes, emotions, and renal excretions of fluid and electrolytes. IV. Situations associated with retention of water, sodium, and potassium. *J. Psychosom. Res.* 1:287–291.

SCHULTE, W. (1961): Nichttraurigseinkönnen im Kern melancholischen Erlebens. *Nervenartz* 32:314–320.

SCHWAB, J. J., BIALOW, M., MARTIN, P. C., and CLEMMONS, R. (1967): The use of the Beck Depression Inventory with medical inpatients. *Acta Psychiat. Scand.* (In press)

SCHWAB, J. J., BIALOW, M., and HOLZER, C. (1967): A comparison of two rating scales for depression. *J. Clin. Psychol.* 23:94–96.

SCHWAB, J. J., CLEMMONS, R. S., BIALOW, B., DUGGAN, V., and DAVIS, B. (1965): A study of the somatic symptomatology of depression in medical inpatients. *Psychosomatics* 6:273–277.

SCHWARTZ, D. A. (1961): Some suggestions for a unitary formulation of the manic-depressive reactions. *Psychiatry* 24:238–45.

SHAGASS, C., and JONES, A. L. (1958): A neurophysiological test for psychiatric diagnosis: results in 750 patients. *Amer. J. Psychiat.* 114:1002–1009.

SHAGASS, C., and SCHWARTZ, M. (1961): Cortical excitability in psychiatric disorder—preliminary results. *Third World Congr. of Psychiatry Proc.* 1:441–446.

SHAGASS, C., and SCHWARTZ, M. (1962): Cerebral cortical reactivity in psychotic depressions. *Arch. Gen. Psychiat. (Chicago)* 6:235–242.

SHAGASS, C., NAIMAN, J., and MIHALIK, J. (1956): An objective test which differentiates between neurotic and psychotic depression. *Arch. Neurol. Psychiat.* 75:461–471.

SHAPIRO, M. B., CAMPBELL, D., HARRIS, and DEWSBERRY, J. P. (1958): Effects of E.C.T. upon psychomotor speed and the "distraction effect" in depressed psychiatric patients. *J. Ment. Sci.* 104:681–695.

SHEPPARD, E., and SAUL, L. J. (1958): An approach to a systematic study of ego function. *Psychoanal. Quart.* 27:237–245.

SHIELDS, J. (1962): *Monozygotic Twins Brought Up Apart and Brought Up Together.* London, Oxford Univer. Press.

SHIELDS, J., and SLATER, E. (1960): "Heredity and Psychological Abnormality," in *Handbook of Abnormal Psychology,* ed. by EYSENCK, H. J. London, Pittman.

SHIP, I. I., and BURKET, L. W. (1965): "Oral and Dental Problems," in *Clinical Features of the Older Patient,* ed. by FREEMAN, J. T. Springfield, Ill., Thomas.

SIMONSON, M. (1964): Phenothiazine depressive reaction. *J. Neuropsychiat.* 5:259–265.

SLATER, E. (1953): Psychiatric and neurotic illnesses in twins. *Medical Research Council Special Report Series,* No. 278. London, Her Majesty's Stationery Office.

SLOANE, R. B., LEWIS, D. J., and SLATER, P. (1957): Diagnostic value of blood pressure responses in psychiatric patients. *Arch. Neurol. Psychiat.* 77:540–542.

SNOW, L. H., and RICKELS, K. (1964): The controlled evaluation of imipramine and amitriptyline in hospitalized depressed psychiatric patients. *Psychopharmacologia (Berlin)* 5:409–416.

SØRENSON, A., and STRÖMGREN, E. (1961): Frequency of depressive states within geographically delimited population groups. *Acta Psychiat. Scand. Suppl.* 162:62–68.

SPIELBERGER, C. D., PARKER, J. B., and BECKER, J. (1963): Conformity and achievement in remitted manic-depressive patients. *J. Nerv. Ment. Dis. 137:*162–172.

STATE OF NEW YORK DEPARTMENT OF MENTAL HYGIENE (1963): *1960 Annual Report.* Albany.

STEEN, R. (1933): Prognosis in manic-depressive psychoses: with report of factors studied in 493 patients. *Psychiat. Quart. 7:*419–429.

STENGEL, E. (1959): Classification of mental disorders. *Bull. WHO 21:*601–663.

STENGEL, E. (1962): Recent research into suicide and attempted suicide. *Amer. J. Psychiat. 118:*725–727.

STENSTEDT, A. (1952): A study in manic-depressive psychosis: clinical, social, and genetic investigations. *Acta Psychiat. Scand. Suppl. 79.*

STENSTEDT, A. (1959): Involutional melancholia: an etiologic, clinical and social study of endogenous depression in later life, with special reference to genetic factors. *Acta Psychiat. Scand. Suppl. 127.*

STRAUSS, E. B. (1930): Discussion on the diagnosis and treatment of the milder forms of the manic-depressive psychosis. *Proc. Roy. Soc. Med. 23:*894–895.

STRECKER, E. A., APPEL, K. E., EYMAN, E. V., FARR, C. B., LA MAR, N. C., PALMER, H. D., and SMITH, L. H. (1931): The prognosis in manic-depressive psychosis. *Res. Publ. Ass. Res. Nerv. Ment. Dis. 11:*471–538.

STRÖMGREN, E., and SCHOU, M. (1964): Lithium treatment of manic states. *Postgrad. Med. 35:*83–86.

STRONGIN, E. I., and HINSIE, L. E. (1938): Parotid gland secretions in manic-depressive patients. *Amer. J. Psychiat. 94:*1459.

TELLENBACH, H. (1961): *Melancholie.* West Berlin, Springer.

TEMOCHE, A., PUGH, T. F., and MACMAHON, B. (1964): Suicide rates among current and former mental institution patients. *J. Nerv. Ment. Dis. 136:*124–130.

THALBITZER, S. (1905): Cited by Lundquist, G. Prognosis and course in manic-depressive psychoses. *Acta Psychiat. Scand. Suppl. 35:*8, 1945.

THORNDIKE, R. L. (1942): Two screening tests of verbal intelligence. *J. Appl. Psychol. 26:*128.

TIENARI, P. (1963): Psychiatric illness in identical twins. *Acta Psychiat. Scand. Suppl. 171.*

TITLEY, W. B. (1936): Prepsychotic personality of patients with involutional melancholia. *Arch. Neurol. Psychiat. 36:*19–33.

TUCKER, J. E., and SPIELBERG, M. J. (1958): Bender-Gestalt Test correlates of emotional depression. *J. Consult. Psychol. 22:*56.

UNITED STATES BUREAU OF THE CENSUS (1963): *Statistical Abstract of the United States.* 84th Edition. Washington, D.C. U.S. Government Printing Office.

UNITED STATES WAR DEPARTMENT (1945): Tech. Bull. Med. 203. *Nomenclature and Method of Recording Diagnoses.* October 19, 1945.

VAILLANT, G. E. (1963a): Natural history of remitting schizophrenias. *Amer. J. Psychiat. 120:*367–375.

VAILLANT, G. E. (1963b): Manic-depressive heredity and remission in schizophrenia. *Brit. J. Psychiat. 109:*746–749.

VAILLANT, G. E. (1964a): An historical review of the remitting schizophrenias. *J. Nerv. Ment. Dis. 138:*48–56.

VAILLANT, G. E. (1964b): Prospective prediction of schizophrenic remission. *Arch. Gen. Psychiat. (Chicago) 11:*509–518.

VON HAGEN, K. O. (1957): Chronic intolerable pain; discussion of its mechanism and report of 8 cases treated with electroshock. *J. Amer. Med. Ass. 165:*773–777.

WADSWORTH, W. V., WELLS, B. W. P., and SCOTT, R. F. (1962): A comparative study of the fatigability of a group of chronic schizophrenics and a group of hospitalized non-psychotic depressives. *J. Ment. Sci. 108:*304–308.

WAPNER, S., WERNER, H., and KRUS, D. M. (1957): The effect of success and failure on space localization. *J. Personality 25:*752–756.

WARD, C. H., BECK, A. T., MENDELSON, M., MOCK, J. E., and ERBAUGH, J. K. (1962): The psychiatric nomenclature: reasons for diagnostic disagreement. *Arch. Gen. Psychiat. (Chicago) 7:*198–205.

WATTS, C. A. (1957): The mild endogenous depression. *Brit. Med. J. 1:*4–8.

WECHSLER, H., GROSSER, G., and BUSFIELD, B. (1963): The depression rating scale: a quantitative approach to the assessment of depressive symptomatology. *Arch. Gen. Psychiat. (Chicago) 9:*334–343.

WECHSLER, H., GROSSER, G., and GREENBLATT, M. (1965): Research evaluating antidepressant medications on hospitalized mental patients: a survey of published reports during a five year period. *J. Nerv. Ment. Dis. 141:*231–239.

WESSMAN, A. E., and RICKS, D. F. (1966): *Mood and Personality.* New York, Holt.

WEXBERG, E. (1928): Zur Klinik und Pathogenese der leichten Depressionzustände. *Z. Neurol. Psychiat. 112:*549–574.

WHATMORE, G. B., and ELLIS, R. M., JR. (1959): Some neurophysiologic aspects of depressed states: an electromyographic study. *Arch. Gen. Psychiat. (Chicago) 1:*70–80.

WHATMORE, G., and ELLIS, R. M. (1962): Further neurophysiologic aspects of depressed states: an electromyographic study. *Arch. Gen. Psychiat. (Chicago) 6:*243–253.

WHEAT, W. D. (1960): Motivational aspects of suicide in patients during and after psychiatric treatment. *Southern Med. J. 53:*273–278.

WHITTIER, J. R., KORENZI, C., GOLDSCHMIDT, L., and HAYDU, G. (1964): The serum cholesteral "sign" test in depression. *Psychosomatics 5:*27–33.

WILSON, D. C. (1951): Families of manic-depressives. *Dis. Nerv. Syst. 12:*362–369.

WILSON, D. C. (1955): Dynamics and psychotherapy of depression. *J. Amer. Med. Ass. 158:*151–153.

WILSON, W. P., and WILSON, N. J. (1961): Observations on the duration of photically elicited arousal responses in depressive illness. *J. Nerv. Ment. Dis. 133:*438–440.

WINOKUR, G., and PITTS, F. N. (1965): Affective disorder. IV. A family history study of prevalances, sex differences, and possible genetic factors. *J. Psychiat. Res. 3:*113–123.

WITTMAN, P., SHELDON, W., and KATZ, C. J. (1948): A study of the relationship between constitutional variations and fundamental psychotic behavior reactions. *J. Nerv. Ment. Dis. 108:*470–476.

YASKIN, J. C. (1931): Nervous symptoms as earliest manifestations of carcinoma of the pancreas. *J. Amer. Med. Ass. 96:*1664–1668.

YASKIN, J. C., WEISENBERG, T. H., and PLEASANTS, H. (1931): Neuropsychiatric counterfeits of organic visceral disease. *J. Amer. Med. Ass. 97:*1751–1756.

ZETZEL, E. R. (1966): The predisposition to depression. *Canad. Psychiat. Ass. J. Suppl. 11:*236–249.

ZILBOORG, G. (1933): "Manic-Depressive Psychoses," in *Psychoanalysis Today: Its Scope and Function,* ed. by LORAND, S. New York, Covici, Friede, pp. 229–245.

ZILBOORG, G. (1941): *A History of Medical Psychology.* New York, Norton, p. 67.

ZUBIN, J., SUTTON, S., SALZINGER, K., SALZINGER, S., BURDOCK, E., PERETZ, D. (1961): "A Biometric Approach to Prognosis in Schizophrenia," in *Comparative Epidemiology of the Mental Disorders,* ed. by HOCH, P. H., and ZUBIN, J. New York, Grune & Stratton, pp. 143–203.

ZUCKERMAN, M., and LUBIN, B. (1965): *Manual for the Multiple Affect Adjective Check List.* San Diego, Calif., Education and Industrial Testing Service.

ZUNG, W. W. K. (1965): A self-rating depression scale. *Arch. Gen. Psychiat. (Chicago) 12:*63–70.

ZUNG, W. W. K., WILSON, W. P., and DODSON, W. E. (1964): Effect of depressive disorders on sleep EEG responses. *Arch. Gen. Psychiat. (Chicago) 10:*439–445.

Name Index

Page numbers in *italics* refer to an author whose name does not appear on this page. Instead, his name is represented by *et al.* in the bibliographic citation on this page.

Subject Index

Acetylcholine-blocking agents, cardiac arrhythmia reduced by, 310
Acetylmethylcarbinal, 137
Acute onset, of episode, 48, 49, 59
Acute remitting schizophrenia, 113, 118
Acute schizo-affective psychosis, 112–113
Addison's disease, 74
Adrenalin, 135, 140
Affect
  in benign stupor, 110
  and cognition, 287–289
  in depression, 237–238, 254, 255, 256, 261–263
  in schizophrenia, 119, 120, 140
  and value judgments, 276–278
Aggression
  in depression, 248–249
  patterns of, and prognosis in schizophrenia, 120–121
  repressed, 80
Agitated depression, 7, 42–43, 64, 101, 104, 105, 266, 267, 274
Alcoholism, 31, 57, 67, 169
Amitriptyline (Elavil), 294, 296, 297, 302
Amnesia, 307
Amobarbital, 145, 152, 298
Amphetamine (Benzedrine), 294
Anal eroticism, 245
Anemias, 74
Anger, relative absence of, in depression, 288, 290
Anorexia, 10, 335, 337
Antidepressant drugs, 62, 122, 203, 293, 294–297, 298, 301, 308
  adverse effects of, 302–304
Anxiety reaction, 11, 14, 15, 68, 72, 191, 193, 268
  differentiated according to cognitive content, 270–271
  distinguished from depression, 200–201
Apathy, 20, 74, 293
Appearance, 39–41, 193
Appetite
  loss of, 33–34, 40, 69, 85, 91, 204
  variable, of manic patients, 91, 95
Arbitrary inference, defined, 234
Arteriosclerosis, cerebral, 7, 73
Arthritis, rheumatoid, 74
Asthma, 74
Atropine, 306
  as placebo, 299
Attachment, increased, to people and activities, 91, 92

Auto-eroticism, 245
Automatic thoughts, neutralizing of, 321–326
Autonomic function, in depression, 142–145
Autonomous depression, 63
Autonomous melancholia, 148
Avoidance wishes, 29, 30, 263, 264

Background variables, correlations of, with DI scores and depth of depression, 205
Basal metabolic rate, in affective disorders, 135
Beck Depression Inventory. *See* Depression Inventory.
Behavioral tests, of depression, 177
Bender-Gestalt scores, 155
Benign stupor, 42, 109, 110–112, 115, 266
Bereavement, childhood, and adult depression, 218–227
Biochemical studies, of depression, 132–139, 244–**245**
"Biological clocks," 98
Biological studies, of depression, 125–153, 243–244
Biphasic single episode, 46 and *n*.
Blame, assignment of, in manic patient, 91, 93
Blood glucose, 133, 135
Blood pressure
  and adrenalin, 135
  responses to Mecholyl, 142–143
Body build, 68, 127
  leptosomatic, 71, 127, 128
  pyknic, 68, 71, 126 and *n*., 127, 128
Body image, distortion of, 21, 22, 335
British Classification, 60

Calcium
  in blood of manic depressive, 133
  metabolism in endogenous depression, 138
California Fascism Scale, 163
Camphor, 305
Cardiovascular disease, 74, 302, 310
Caries, dental, 145
Catalepsy, 110
Catatonia, 42, 108, 109, 110, 111
  periodic, 136
Catecholamine hypothesis, of affective disorders, 244, 245
Catharsis, in supportive psychotherapy, 316, 317
Cerebral arteriosclerosis, 7, 73
Childhood bereavement, and adult depression, 218–227
Chloride
  in blood of manic depressive, 134
  excretion in endogenous depression, 137